Medical and Surgical Complications of Sickle Cell Anemia

Ahmed Al-Salem

Medical and Surgical Complications of Sickle Cell Anemia

Springer

Ahmed Al-Salem
Department of Surgery
Dar A lAlafia Medical Company
Qatif
Saudi Arabia

ISBN 978-3-319-24760-1 ISBN 978-3-319-24762-5 (eBook)
DOI 10.1007/978-3-319-24762-5

Library of Congress Control Number: 2015957249

Springer Cham Heidelberg New York Dordrecht London

Printed on acid-free paper

Springer International Publishing AG Switzerland is part of Springer Science+Business Media
(www.springer.com)

Preface

Sickle cell anemia is one of the common hemoglobinopathies in the world and it results from a single change of amino acid, valine instead of glutamic acid at the 6th position of the 146 amino acids of the beta chain of the hemoglobin. A single change of one amino acid can lead to so much morbidity and mortality. Sickle cell anemia can affect every part of the body leading to so much morbidity and mortality. Awareness of sickle cell anemia and its complications is important for early diagnosis and management, taking into consideration the recent advances in the management of sickle cell anemia including the use of hydroxyurea, bone marrow transplantation, and the promising gene therapy. This book is written as an outline of sickle cell anemia and its medical and surgical complications. It is written in a simple way and easy to read. It covers most aspects of sickle cell anemia with emphasis on the medical and surgical complications of sickle cell anemia and the most important points relevant to the patient's presentation, diagnosis, and management. This book is well illustrated and includes clinical, operative, radiological, histopathological, and hand-drawn illustrations. I hope this book will be useful to consultant pediatricians, consultant internists, consultant hematologists, specialists, fellows, and residents. The book should be useful also to general practitioners, general surgeons, accident and emergency doctors, trainees, medical students, and nurses.

Qatif, Saudi Arabia

Ahmed H. Al-Salem

Acknowledgment

I would like to express special thanks of gratitude to my family who supported me and made this project possible. I would also like to thank all my colleagues who reviewed chapters of this book.

Contents

History of Sickle Cell Anemia 1

- Sickle cell anemia is an inherited disease that existed in Africa for at least 5000 years but there have been no records of its existence till it was discovered in 1904.
- It is interesting to note that the deer is the only living creature other than humans known to suffer from sickle cell disease.
- In 1840, the British zoologist Gulliver observed under the microscope sickle-shaped red blood cells in the blood of a variety of exotic deer belonging to the London Zoological Garden.
- In North America, the white-tailed deer is occasionally encountered dying in sickle cell vaso-occlusive crisis in the forests of Michigan.
- The first description of sickle red blood cells in humans was published in 1899 when Dr. Hayem, a French colonial physician, reported his microscopic discovery from Africa. He erroneously explained that the crescent shape of these red blood cells represented a normal variation of erythrocyte morphology.
- In 1905, two French colonial physicians, Dr. Sargent and Dr. Sargent, examined the blood of 243 natives of Algiers and published a report describing "half-moon corpuscles" in 5 % of their African patients. Since all these patients suffered from malaria, the authors incorrectly attributed the presence of the sickle erythrocytes to malaria itself.
- The first report of the sickle red blood cells in North America was published in 1904 by Dr. Dresbach where in a histology class at Ohio State University, one mulatto student sketched ellyptoid erythrocytes which he observed under his own microscope.
- The first clinical description of sickle cell anemia was recorded by James Bryan Herrick in 1910.
- James Bryan Herrick was an American cardiologist and professor of medicine at the Chicago Presbyterian Hospital. He was also a major figure in the history of medical science and worked and taught at several hospitals in Chicago. He was born on August 11, 1861, in Oak Park, Illinois, and died in 1954.

A. Al-Salem, *Medical and Surgical Complications of Sickle Cell Anemia*,
DOI 10.1007/978-3-319-24762-5_1

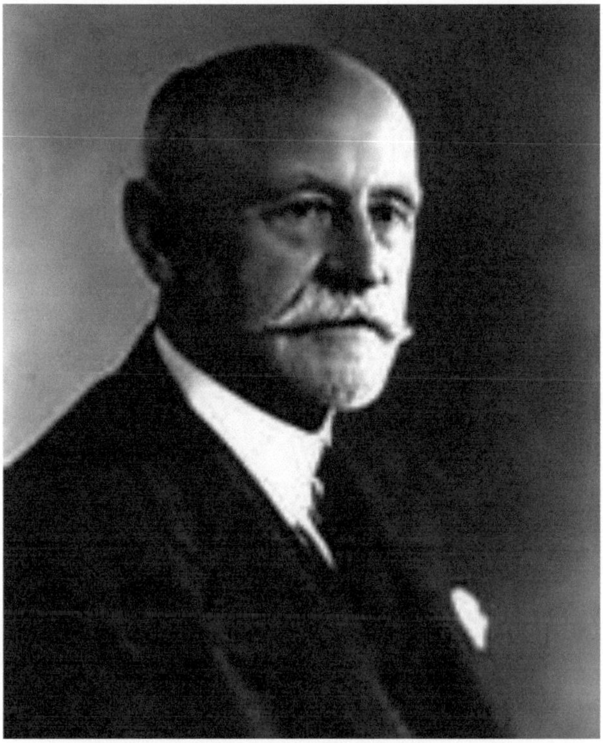

Professor James Bryan Herrick (1861–1954)

- In December 1904, a patient named Walter Clement Noel, a 20-year-old first-year dental student from the island of Grenada, was admitted to the Chicago Presbyterian Hospital suffering from painful episodes and symptoms of anemia. Prior to this, Walter Clement Noel suffered from an ulcer on the ankle which was painful and healed with conservative treatment.
  - Mr. Walter Clement Noel belonged to an affluent African family which owned the Duquesne estate, a large plantation on the island of Grenada.
  - His father had died at the age of 36 years, reportedly of kidney failure, and his sister also died prematurely at the age of 24 years, presumably of pulmonary tuberculosis.
  - Mrs. Noel decided to send her 20-year-old son to study in the United States where he was the only African student accepted to the Chicago College of Dental Surgery.

- He sailed to the United States in 1904 for the purpose of studying dentistry.
- When Mr. Walter Clement Noel disembarked from the ocean liner *SS Cearense* in New York on September 5, 1904, he already was suffering from chronic ankle ulcers. This was treated by a physician who applied iodine to the skin ulcers, which healed within a week.
- He then traveled by train to Chicago and enrolled at the Chicago College of Dental Surgery.
- By Christmas time, he became ill with pneumonia or what today would be referred to as acute chest syndrome and presented himself to the Presbyterian Hospital of Chicago. He was also anemic and was examined by Dr. Ernest Irons, an intern who performed a complete blood count including microscopic examination of the red blood cells.
- Mr. Walter Clement Noel appeared pale and his red blood cell count as documented on December 31, 1904, was only 2,880,000 cells per cubic milliliter.
- By January 22, 1905, he had recovered completely from acute chest syndrome, a complication of sickle cell disease which even today is associated with significant mortality.
- During his 3 years of study at the Chicago College of Dental Surgery, Mr. Walter Clement Noel would be treated on several other occasions by Dr. Ernest Irons and Dr. James Herrick for various clinical complications of his sickle cell anemia.
- Walter Clement Noel was readmitted several times over the next 3 years for "muscular rheumatism" and "bilious attacks."
- He managed to survive all of his sickle cell crises, completed his studies, graduated from dental school and returned to the capital of Grenada (St. George's) to practice dentistry in 1907.
- Upon return to his native land of Grenada, Mr. Walter Clement Noel established a successful dental practice and remained in more or less satisfactory health for almost 10 years.
- He must have suffered several life-threatening crises during his stay in St. George, Grenada. On the day of his death, he went to Grenville on the other side of the island in order to watch a horse race and returned the same day to the capital. He felt very tired, became ill with pneumonia, and died in 1916 at the age of 32 years from what looks like an acute chest syndrome (pneumonia). He was buried in the Catholic cemetery at Sauteurs in the north of Grenada next to his sister and father and their tombs are still intact today in Grenada.

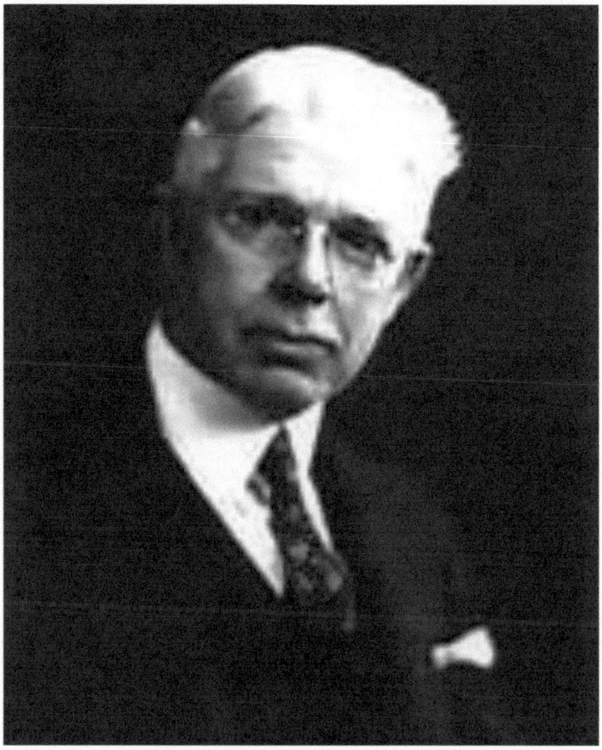

Dr. Ernest Edward Irons (1877–1959)

- Professor Herrick had an intern named Ernest Edward Irons (1877–1959). Ernest Irons was looking at Noel's blood film when he noticed the irregularity in the shape of the blood cells. He called them "peculiar, elongated, and sickle-shaped" red blood cells (Fig. 1.1).
- On December 31, 1904, Irons drew a rough sketch of these erythrocytes, the first pictures of sickled cells (Fig. 1.1).
- In 1910, Dr. James Herrick presented the case of Mr. Walter Clement Noel to the Association of American Physicians in Washington DC and in the same year published a report in the Archives of Internal Medicine.
- In 1910, Herrick published the findings with illustration and it was the first time the connection between the irregularities of the shape of red blood cells with sickle cell anemia was discovered and identified.
- This was published in the November 1910 issue of "Archives of Internal Medicine," when James B. Herrick of Chicago reported on "Peculiar Elongated and Sickle-Shaped Red Blood Corpuscles in a Case of Severe Anemia."

> This case is reported because of the unusual blood findings, no duplicate of which I have ever seen describe. (James B. Herrick, M.D.)

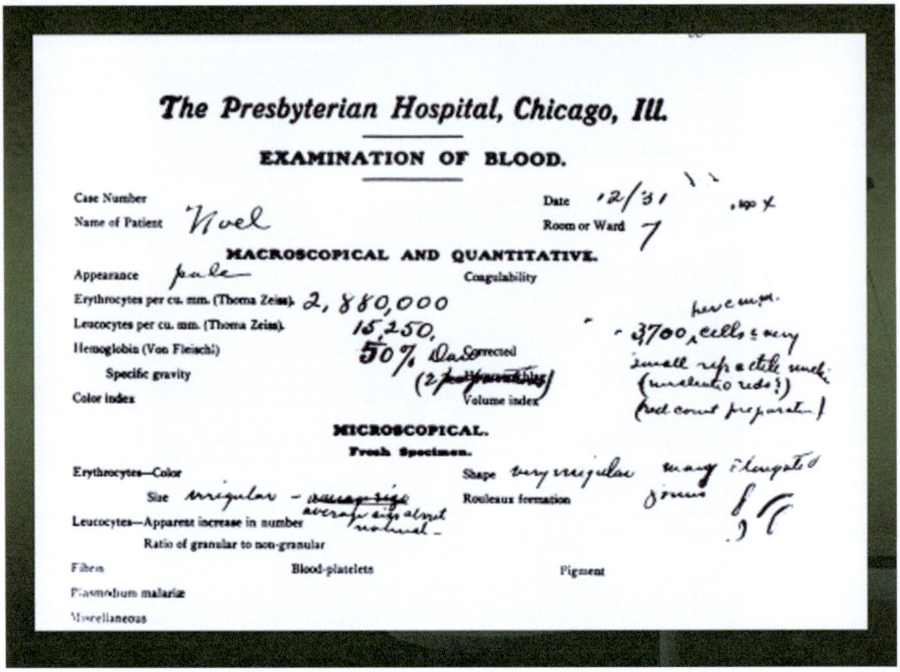

The Presbyterian Hospital, Chicago, Ill.

EXAMINATION OF BLOOD.

Case Number

Date 12/31, 190 4

Name of Patient Noel

Room or Ward 7

MACROSCOPICAL AND QUANTITATIVE.

Appearance pale

Coagulability

Erythrocytes per cu. mm. (Thoma Zeiss) 2,880,000

Leucocytes per cu. mm. (Thoma Zeiss) 15,250

Hemoglobin (Von Fleischl) 50%

Specific gravity

Color index

Volume index

MICROSCOPICAL.

Fresh Specimen.

Erythrocytes—Color

Size irregular

Shape very irregular many elongated

Rouleaux formation

Leucocytes—Apparent increase in number

Ratio of granular to non-granular

Fibrin

Blood-platelets

Pigment

Plasmodium malariæ

Miscellaneous

Fig. 1.1 Diagrammatic drawing of the blood film of Mr. Walter Clement Noel as was seen by Dr. Ernest Edward Irons. Note the detailed description of the blood film showing a pale patient with a total red blood cells number of 2,880,000 per cubic mm. The red blood cells appear very irregular and many elongated

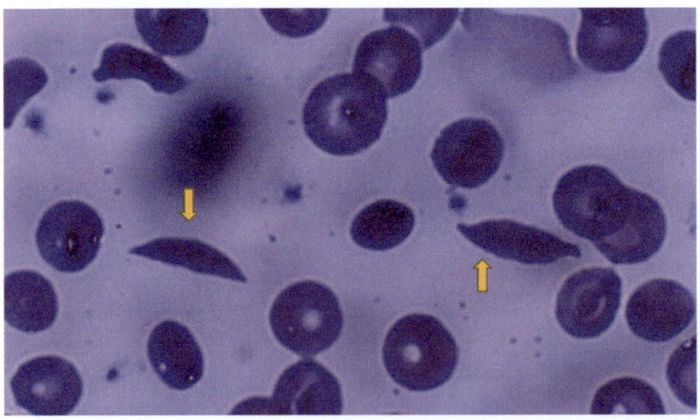

Fig. 1.2 A blood film showing sickle shaped red blood cells. Note also the normal looking red blood cells

- 1910 is regarded as the year of the discovery of sickle cell anemia.
- In the beginning and for some time, this condition was called Herrick's syndrome (Herrick's anemia) because of his contributions to the discovery of sickle cell anemia (Fig. 1.2).

- It is interesting to note that Dr. James Herrick was also the first physician to describe the pathology of heart attack or myocardial infarction and again received no lasting recognition for it. He later became Dean of Rush Medical School and died in 1954.
- Dr. Ernest Irons, the house officer who saw the sickle cells and sought no credit or recognition out of respect for his mentor, Dr. James Herrick, also had an illustrious career, becoming President of the American Medical Association in 1949.
- Some elements of sickle cell anemia, however, had been recognized earlier than this but were not well documented. In 1846, a paper in the "Southern Journal of Medical Pharmacology" described the absence of a spleen in the autopsy of a runaway slave. The African medical literature also reported this condition in the 1870s, when it was known locally as "ogbanjes" ("children who come and go") because of the very high infant mortality rate caused by this condition. A history of the condition tracked reports back to 1670 in one Ghanaian family. Also, the practice of using tar soap to cover blemishes caused by sickle cell sores was prevalent in the black community.
- In 1922, Verne Rheem Mason (Wapello, Iowa, August 8, 1889 – Miami, Florida, November 16, 1965) an eminent internist named the disease as "sickle cell anemia" based on the description of Ernest Irons. She received a B.S. from the University of California, Berkeley, in 1911, and an M.D. from Johns Hopkins University in 1915. As a medical resident at Johns Hopkins in 1922, Mason gave the disease the name of sickle cell anemia.

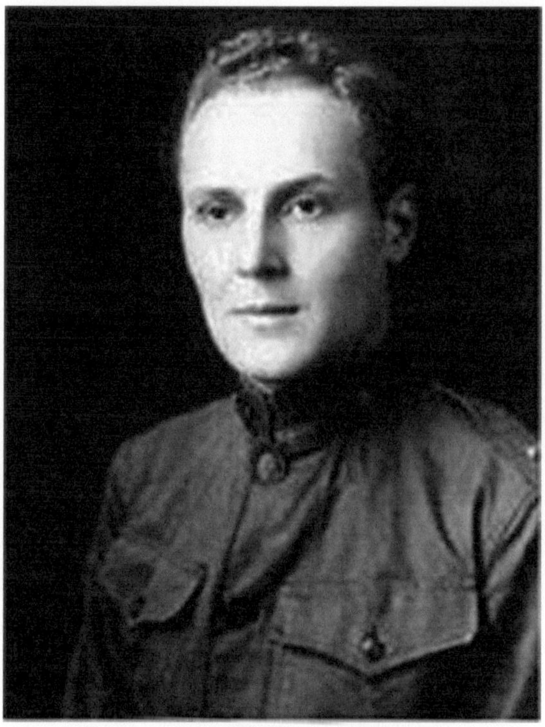

Dr. Verne Rheem Mason (1889–1965)

- In 1927, Hahn and Gillespie discovered that red blood cells from persons with the disease could be made to sickle by removing oxygen. There were also people at that time, often relatives of the patients, whose red blood cells were sickling when deprived of oxygen but who had no symptoms. These became known as "sickle trait." Hahn and Gillespie were the first to associate the red cell sickling to low oxygen and acidic conditions.
- The first splenectomy for the treatment of sickle cell anemia was reported by Hahn and Gillespie in 1927.
- In the late 1940s and early 1950s, the nature of the disease began to become clearer.
- In 1949, sickle cell disease was shown to be an inherited condition and that people with sickle trait were heterozygous (carriers or AS) for the gene, whereas people with the disease were homozygous, i.e., had a double dose of the gene (SS).
- This was proven and published simultaneously by two physicians, a military doctor in Mozambique named Col. E. A. Beet and Dr. James V. Neel (James Van Gundia Neel: March 22, 1915 – February 1, 2000), Chairman and founder of the Department of Human Genetics at the University of Michigan.

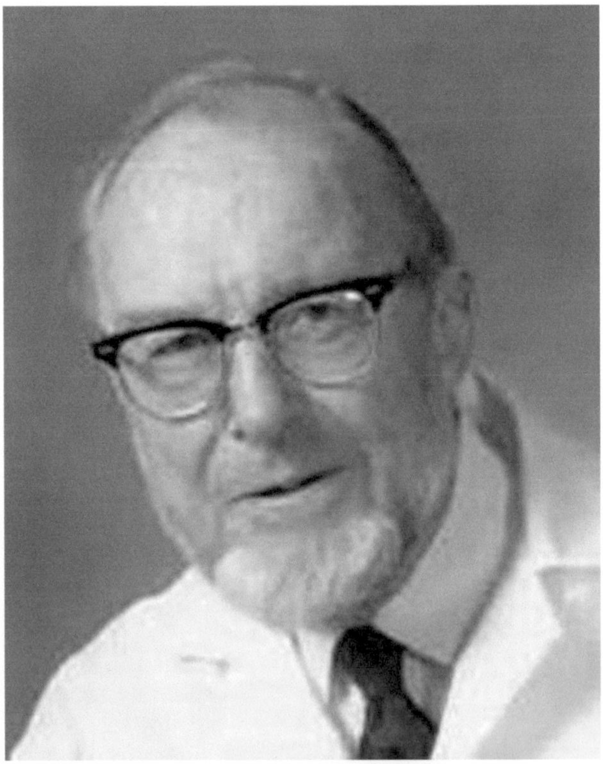

Dr. James Van Gundia Neel

- Many people however feel that Dr. Neel gets the credit for the discovery because of an earlier paper he published in 1947 showing that sickle cell anemia is hereditary.
- In 1940, Sherman (a student at Johns Hopkins Medical School) noted a birefringence of deoxygenated red cells, suggesting that low oxygen altered the structure of the hemoglobin in the molecule.
- Janet Watson, a pediatric hematologist in New York, suggested in 1948 that the paucity of sickle cells in the peripheral blood of newborns was due to the presence of fetal hemoglobin in the red cells, which consequently did not have the abnormal sickle hemoglobin seen in adults.
- In 1945, Dr. William Castle, a prominent hematologist, was traveling by train with Dr. Linus Carl Pauling (February 28, 1901 – August 19, 1994). He told the latter that the sickle cells showed a birefringence under the microscope in polarized light, suggesting that they may contain a hemoglobin different from the normal hemoglobin A. Back at the California Institute of Technology, Dr. Pauling asked Dr. Harvey Akio Itano (November 3, 1920 – May 8, 2010) to look into this interesting problem. It took 4 years for Dr. Itano to isolate the abnormal hemoglobin S and demonstrate its low electrophoretic mobility compared with normal hemoglobin A.

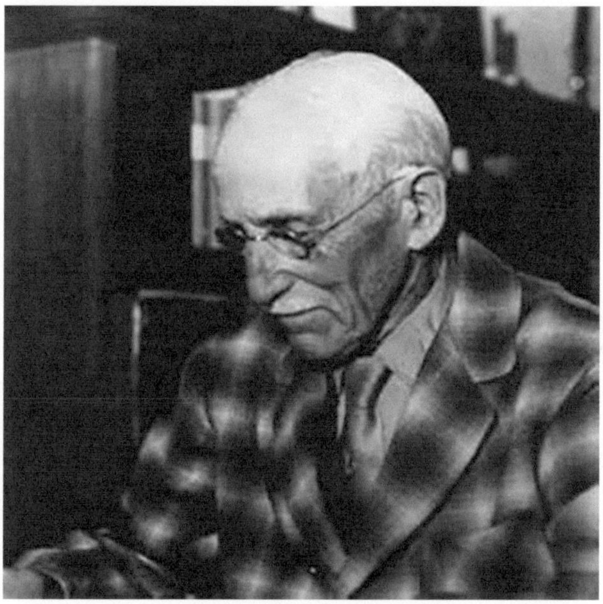

Dr. William Castle

- In 1949, the famous Nobel Prize-winning chemist Dr. Linus Carl Pauling (February 28, 1901 – August 19, 1994) and his colleague Dr. Harvey Itano were the first to show that the cause of the disease was an abnormality in the hemoglobin molecule. They demonstrate that sickle cell anemia occurs as a result of an abnormality in the hemoglobin molecule. They discovered that the red, oxygen-carrying protein called "hemoglobin" had a different chemical structure in persons with sickle cell anemia. They coined the term "molecular disease."

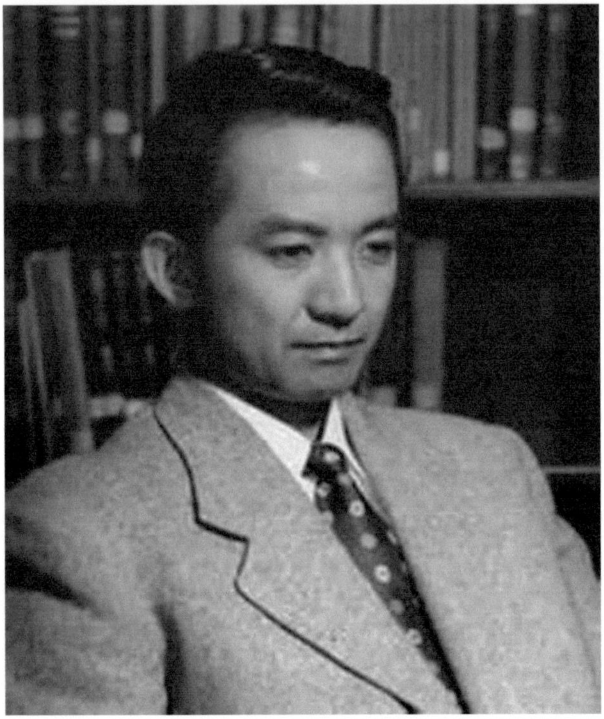

Dr. Harvey Akio Itano

- Thus sickle cell anemia became the first molecular disease ever described and Dr. Linus Pauling received the first of his two Nobel Prizes.
- This was the first time a genetic disease was linked to a mutation of a specific protein, a milestone in the history of molecular biology. They published their findings in 1951 in the paper titled "Sickle Cell Anemia, a Molecular Disease."
- Dr. Linus Pauling many years later become the recipient of the Nobel Peace Prize for his effort to end the testing of the atomic bomb.
- The details of the abnormality were worked out by Dr. Vernon Ingram in 1956.
- In 1956, Dr. Ingram discovered that a single amino acid substitution is responsible for the molecular abnormality that leads to sickle cell anemia. Dr. Ingram was able to isolate the abnormal beta globin chain, digest it with trypsin, and

demonstrate by two-dimensional electrophoresis that of the total of 146 amino acids of the beta globin chain, only one amino acid differed from normal. At position 6, counting from the amino terminal, there was the amino acid valine in the place of glutamic acid.

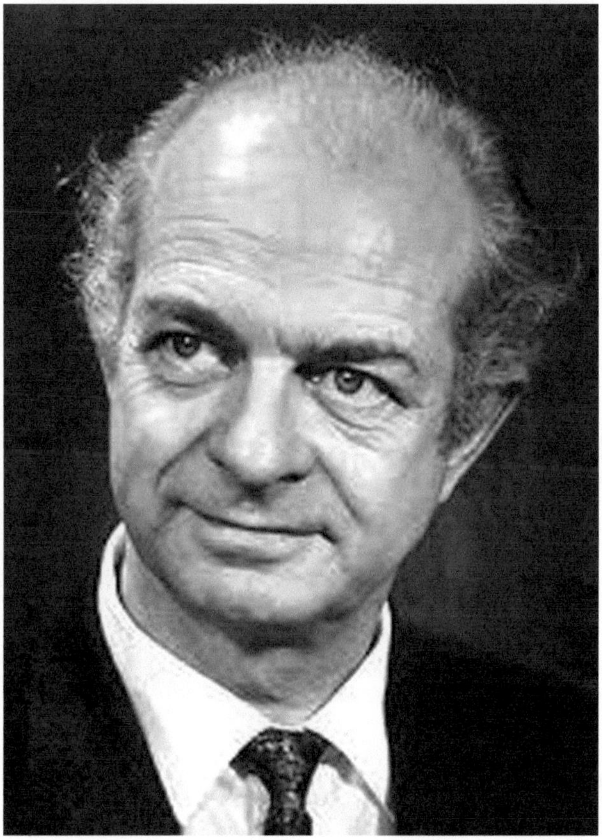

Dr. Linus Pauling (1901–1994)

- In 1956, Vernon Ingram, then at the MRC in England, and J.A. Hunt sequenced sickle hemoglobin and showed that a glutamic acid at position 6 was replaced by a valine in sickle cell disease. Dr. Vernon Martin Ingram (May 19, 1924 – August 17, 2006) was a German American professor of biology at the Massachusetts Institute of Technology. Using the known information about amino acids and the codons that coded for them, he was able to predict the mutation in sickle cell disease. This made sickle cell disease the first genetic disorder whose molecular basis was known.

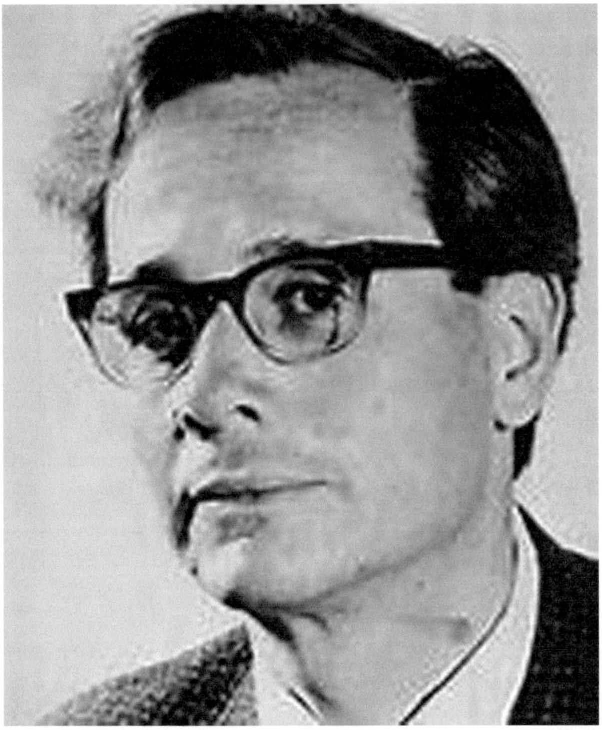

Dr. Vernon Ingram

- The origin of the mutation that led to the sickle cell gene was initially thought to be in the Arabian Peninsula, spreading to Asia and Africa. It is now known, from evaluation of chromosome structures, that there have been at least four independent mutational events, three in Africa and a fourth in either Saudi Arabia or central India. These independent events occurred between 3,000 and 6,000 generations ago, approximately 70–150,000 years.
- In the 1970s, more details of how this abnormal structure affects the red blood cells were revealed and better tests for the detection of the disease were developed.
- Nowadays we know quite clearly that the sickle mutation occurred in the beta globin gene inside chromosome 11 at the first exon where the triplet codon guanine-adenine-guanine has mutated to guanine-thymine-guanine. The result is replacement of glutamic acid at the sixth position of the 146 amino acids of the beta chain of hemoglobin by valine. This will lead to alteration in the structure of hemoglobin and sickling of red blood cells (Figs. 1.3, 1.4, and 1.5).

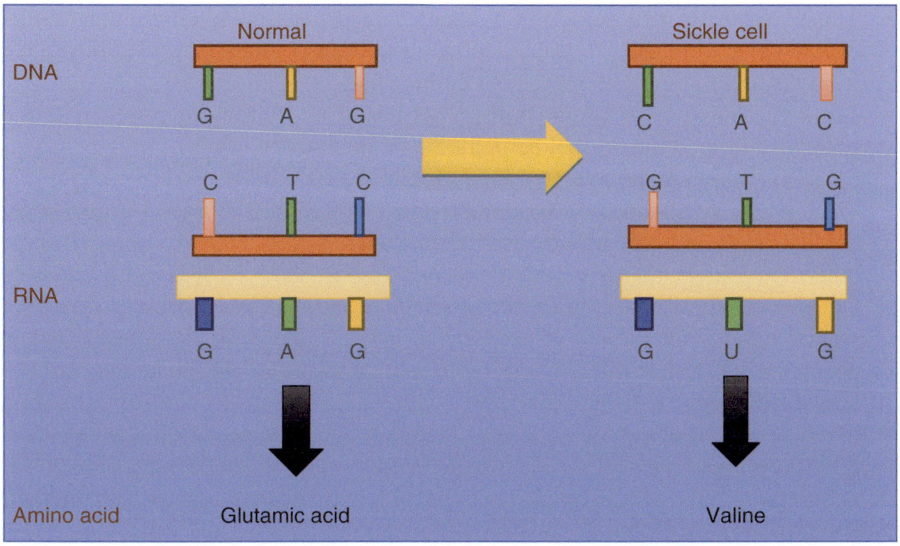

Fig. 1.3 Diagrammatic representation showing the change in the amino acid coding between normal and sickle cell anemia. The triplet codon guanine-adenine-guanine has mutated to guanine-thymine-guanine which leads to the production of valine instead of glutamic acid at the sixth position of the beta chain of hemoglobin

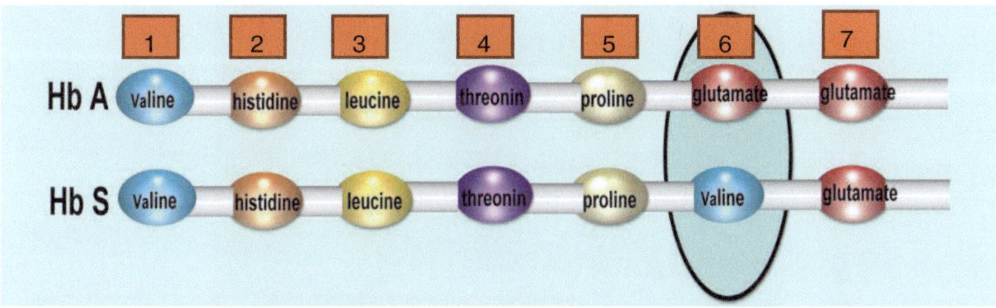

Fig. 1.4 Diagrammatic representation of the change in the amino acid sequence of the beta chain of hemoglobin where valine replaces glutamic acid at the sixth position among the 146 amino acids that makes up the beta chain of hemoglobin

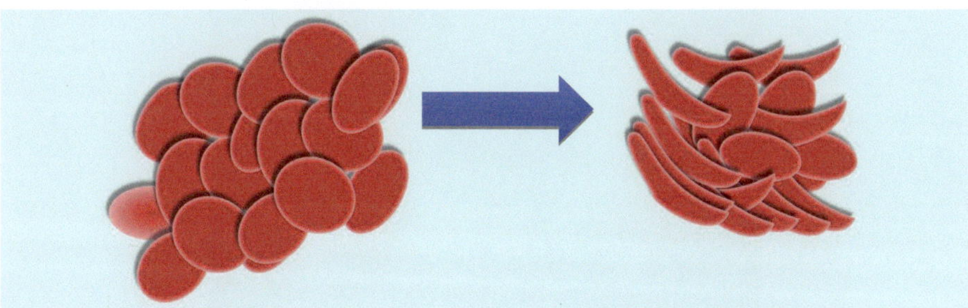

Fig. 1.5 Diagrammatic representation of the normal and sickled red blood cells as a result of the single amino acid change among the 146 amino acids of the beta chain of hemoglobin

- Transcription to messenger RNA resulted in a guanine-uracil-guanine triplet codon which ultimately translated to valine instead of glutamic acid at position 6 from the amino terminal of the beta globin chain.
- The hemoglobin molecule contains at its center an iron atom located within a porphyrin ring. In the normal hemoglobin A, this iron-porphyrin complex is surrounded by two alpha and two beta globin chains. The beta globin chain is a linear protein composed of 146 amino acids, coiled into its own 3-dimensional configuration, with the amino terminal at one end and the carboxy terminal at the other.
- Dr. Makio Murayama, a biological chemist at the National Institute of Health, reported that since the amino acid valine is hydrophobic, it will place itself in proximity to another valine normally located at position 1 of the amino acid terminal. This approximation of valine 1 and valine 6 leads to the formation of a ring-like structure, a process called cyclization of the valine ring. This ring structure serves as a chemical site for attachment to a complementary structure on the alpha chain of the next hemoglobin molecule, with the mutated valine 6 interacting with the beta globin of the adjacent hemoglobin S.
- This in turn leads to linear cord-like stacking of the hemoglobin S molecules and eventual sickling of the entire defective red blood cell.

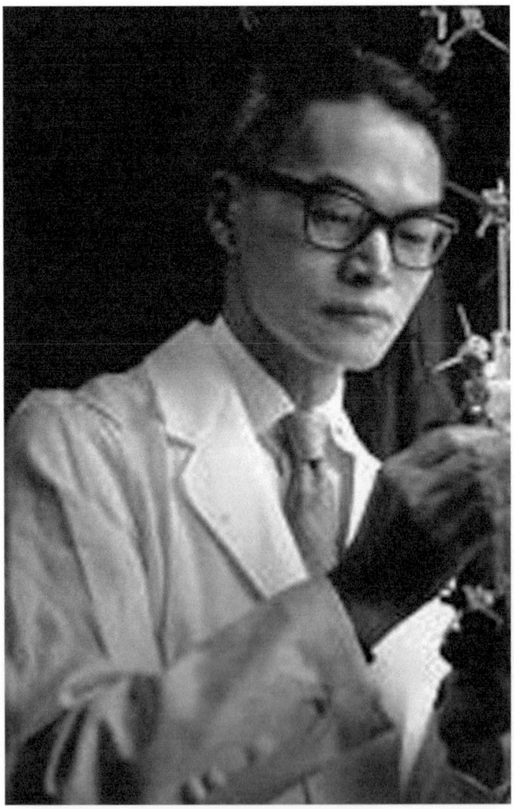

Dr. Makio Murayama

- In the years following, better ways of treating sickle cell patients and potential treatments appeared. The life span and the quality of life of patients were improved. Genetic counseling became an important tool for informing people about the risks of having a child with sickle cell disease.
- Physicians and scientists continue to work for better understanding of the disease and new ways to treat it.
- Currently, the term *sickle cell disease* (SCD) describes a group of inherited red blood cell disorders. Patients with SCD have abnormal hemoglobin, called *hemoglobin S* or sickle hemoglobin, in their red blood cells. When a person has two hemoglobin S genes, Hemoglobin SS, the disease is called *sickle cell anemia*. This is the most common and often most severe type of SCD.
- Other forms of sickle cell disease include:
  - Hemoglobin SS
  - Hemoglobin SC
  - Hemoglobin $S\beta^0$ thalassemia
  - Hemoglobin $S\beta^+$ thalassemia
  - Hemoglobin SD
  - Hemoglobin SE
- In 1973, the average lifespan of a person with sickle cell anemia in the United States was only 14 years. Currently, the life expectancy of a person with sickle cell anemia in the United States is about 40–60 years. This is attributed to advances in the diagnosis and care of patients with sickle cell anemia.
- Sickle cell anemia is a lifelong disease. The severity of the disease, however, varies widely from person to person. Fortunately, there are effective treatments that can reduce their symptoms, prevent and treat complication, and prolong their life.
- Early diagnosis and regular medical care to prevent complications also contribute to improved well-being of these patients.
- A significant figure in the history of sickle cell anemia is Dr. Charles F. Whitten who contributed so much to the sickle cell disease awareness. During the early 1970s, he realized that services for patients with sickle cell disease and their families were sorely lacking. Out of his pioneering efforts to advocate for the needs of patients with sickle cell disease, the Sickle Cell Disease Association of America (SCDAA) was born.
- Dr. Charles F. Whitten was born in Wilmington, Delaware, on February 2, 1922. A major area of Dr. Whitten's research has been sickle cell anemia. In 1971, with the help of other concerned citizens, he formed the Sickle Cell Detection and Information Center, the most comprehensive community program in the country. In the same year, he facilitated the creation of the National Association for Sickle Cell Disease. He died Aug 13, 2008.

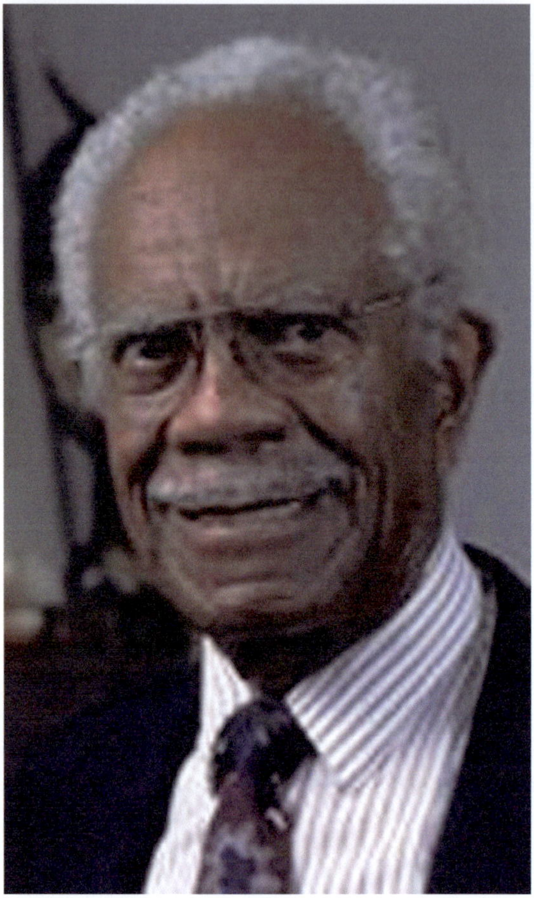

Dr. Charles F. Whitten (1922–2008)

- The treatment of patients with sickle cell anemia continued to be symptomatic, treating their pain and preventing or treating the complications.
- Till now there is no cure for sickle cell anemia and the goal of a total cure has not been reached but great progress has been made.
- Currently, about 90 % of patients with sickle cell anemia survive to age 20, and about 50 % survive beyond the fifth decade. The estimated mean survival for patients with sickle cell anemia is 53 years old for men and 58 years old for women.
- This is attributed to several factors including early diagnosis, better understanding of sickle cell anemia, and related complications as well as new therapeutic and preventive measures.

- Blood transfusions are often used in the management of patients with sickle cell anemia.
- This is to treat acute events such as acute anemia, acute splenic sequestration crisis, acute chest syndrome, stroke, and priapism.
- Blood transfusions are also used to prevent complications such as reducing the risk of first stroke or silent stroke when transcranial Doppler (TCD) ultrasonography shows abnormal increased cerebral blood flow velocities and also to reduce the risk of recurrent stroke and additional silent strokes, acute chest syndrome, and recurrent splenic sequestration crisis.
- Hydroxyurea:
  - Hydroxyurea was the first approved drug for the treatment of sickle cell anemia in 1995.
  - Hydroxyurea became the first drug proven to prevent complications of sickle cell disease in the Multicenter Study of Hydroxyurea in Sickle Cell Anemia which was completed in 1995.
  - Hydroxyurea was shown to be beneficial for patients with sickle cell anemia:
    - It decreases the number and severity of vaso-occlusive attacks.
    - It reduces the number of hospitalizations.
    - It reduces the frequency of acute chest syndrome.
    - It also reduces the need for blood transfusions.
    - Hydroxyurea reduces the overall hospital visits.
    - It reduces the overall hospital admissions.
  - Blood and bone marrow stem cell transplant is the only known cure for sickle cell anemia. This was established in 1984.
  - In 1984, bone marrow transplantation in a child with sickle cell anemia produced the first reported cure of the disease. The transplantation was done to treat acute leukemia. The child's sickle cell disease was cured as a side event. The procedure nonetheless set the precedence for later transplantation efforts directed specifically at sickle cell disease.

Benefits of Hydroxyurea Treatment for Patients with Sickle Cell Anemia

- It decreases the number and severity of vaso-occlusive attacks.
- It reduces the number of hospitalizations.
- It reduces the frequency of acute chest syndrome.
- It also reduces the need for blood transfusions.
- Hydroxyurea reduces the overall hospital visits.

- There are however several factors that makes bone marrow transplant not readily available option. These include:
  - Bone marrow transplant is not available in every country.
  - It is a very expensive treatment.
  - Patients with sickle cell anemia are less likely to find a matching donor. This is because of the genetic complications associated with sickle cell anemia.

  - Regular blood transfusion which is common in patients with sickle cell anemia leads to the production of antibodies which could potentially affect the success of a future transplant.
  - Bone marrow transplantation is a risky procedure with a high morbidity and mortality, including the chance that about one child in ten will die from the procedure itself. The risks of bone marrow transplantation are higher in older children and adults.
- Gene therapy:
  - Recently, there is progress in research for possible cure for sickle cell anemia using gene transfer to permanently increase fetal hemoglobin levels.
  - This depends on a technique to insert the gene for gamma-globin into blood-forming cells using a harmless viral carrier. It is hoped that those cells would permanently generate red blood cells containing fetal hemoglobin, which alleviate the disease.
  - These results are encouraging and hopefully it will be possible to correct sickle cell anemia with genetic therapy to produce fetal hemoglobin.
- Counseling and testing for sickle cell prior to marriage is important to dilute the gene in the communities and decrease the number of affected siblings.

Further Readings

Heeney MM, Ware RE. Hydroxyurea for children with sickle cell disease. Pediatr Clin North Am. 2008;55(2):483–501.

Herrick JB. Peculiar elongated and sickle shaped red blood corpuscles in a case of severe anemia. Arch Intern Med. 1910;6:517.

Ingram VM. Gene mutations in human haemoglobins: the chemical difference between normal and sickle cell haemoglobin. Nature. 1957;180:326.

Pauling L, Itano H, Singer SJ, Wells IC. Sickle cell anemia: a molecular disease. Science. 1949;110:543.

Strouse JJ, Lanzkron S, Beach MC, et al. Hydroxyurea for sickle cell disease: a systematic review for efficacy and toxicity in children. Pediatrics. 2008;122(6):1332–42.

Vichinsky EP, Haberkern CM, Neumayr L, et al. A comparison of conservative and aggressive transfusion regimens in the perioperative management of sickle cell disease. The preoperative transfusion in sickle cell disease study group. N Engl J Med. 1995;333(4):206–13.

Walters MC, Patience M, Leisenring W, et al. Bone marrow transplantation for sickle cell disease. N Engl J Med. 1996;335(6):369–76.

Yawn BP, Buchanan GR, Afenyi-Annan AN, Ballas SK, Hassell KL, James AH, et al. Management of sickle cell disease: summary of the 2014 evidence-based report by expert panel members. JAMA. 2014;312(10):1033–48.

Genetics and Pathophysiology of Sickle Cell Anemia

2

2.1 Introduction

- The normal hemoglobin is made up of two parts, heme and protein. The protein is made up of four polypeptide chains (Fig. 2.1):
  - 2 alpha chains (141 amino acids long)
  - 2 beta chains (146 amino acids long)
- There is a gene responsible for the alpha globin peptide chain and another gene for the beta globin peptide chain.
- The HBB gene which is responsible for the beta globin chains is located on the short arm of chromosome 11.
- There are many known mutations in the HBB gene. These lead to a variety of inherited diseases.
- A mutation in the HBB gene produces abnormal versions of beta-globin such as hemoglobin C (HbC), hemoglobin E (HbE), and hemoglobin S (HbS). Sickle cell anemia is caused by a mutation in the HBB gene.
- Sickle cell anemia is due to an autosomal recessive allele which is found on the short arm of chromosome 11.
- The major sickle genotypes described so far include the following:
  - HbSS disease or sickle cell anemia (homozygous for the S globin): This is the most common form with usually severe or moderately severe symptoms.
  - HbS/b-0 thalassemia (double heterozygous for HbS and b-0 thalassemia): This is clinically indistinguishable from sickle cell anemia.
  - HbS/b+thalassemia: This is characterized by mild to moderate severity with variability in different ethnicities.
  - HbSC disease (double heterozygous for HbS and HbC): This is characterized by moderate clinical severity.
  - HbS/hereditary persistence of fetal Hb (S/HPHP): This is characterized by very mild or asymptomatic phenotype.

A. Al-Salem, *Medical and Surgical Complications of Sickle Cell Anemia*,
DOI 10.1007/978-3-319-24762-5_2

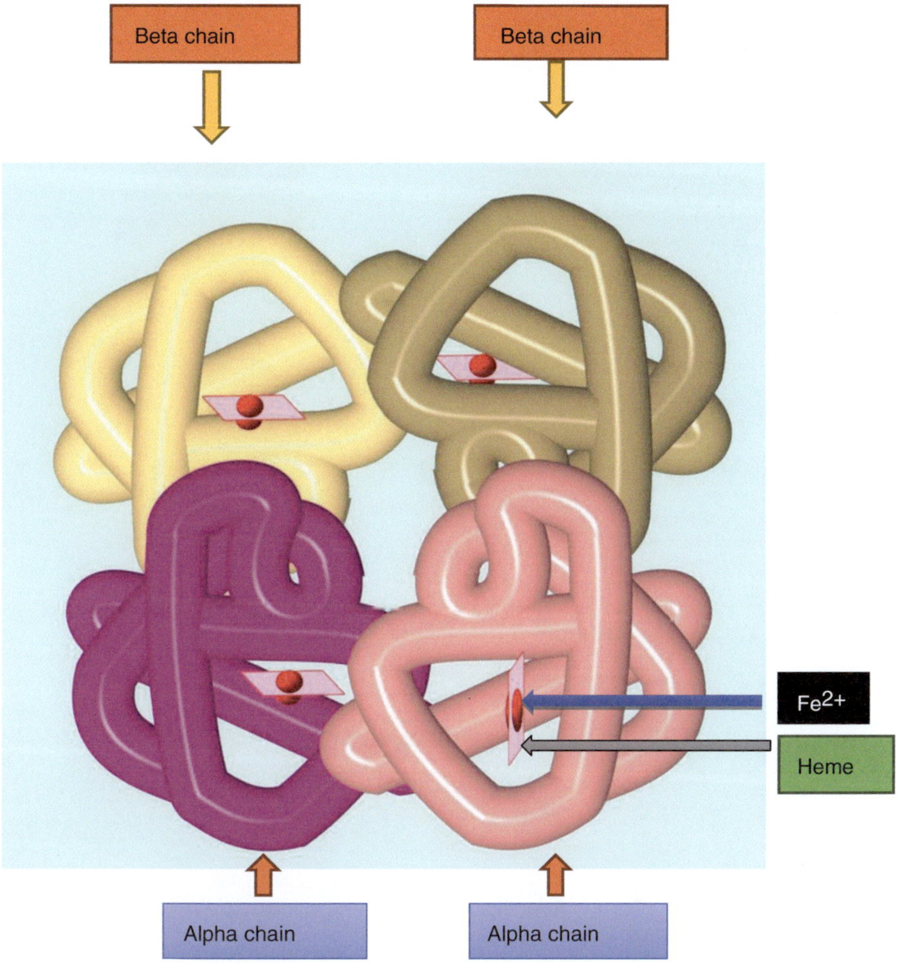

Fig. 2.1 Diagrammatic representation of the normal hemoglobin which is made up of heme and globin (2 alpha chains and 2 beta chains)

  - HbS/HbE syndrome: This is very rare with a phenotype usually similar to HbS/b + thalassemia.
  - Rare combinations of HbS with other abnormal hemoglobins such as HbD Los Angeles, G-Philadelphia, HbO Arab, and others.
- In sickle cell anemia, the genetic code is altered leading to the substitution of a single amino acid where the amino acid glutamic acid is replaced by valine in the sixth position of the 146 amino acids of the beta chain of hemoglobin (Figs. 2.2, 2.3, 2.4, and 2.5).
- The mutation causing sickle cell anemia is a single nucleotide substitution (A to T) in the codon for amino acid 6. The change converts a glutamic acid codon (GAG) to a valine codon (GTG). As a result of this change, a modified hemoglobin is produced. This is referred to as HbS (Figs. 2.6, 2.7, and 2.8).

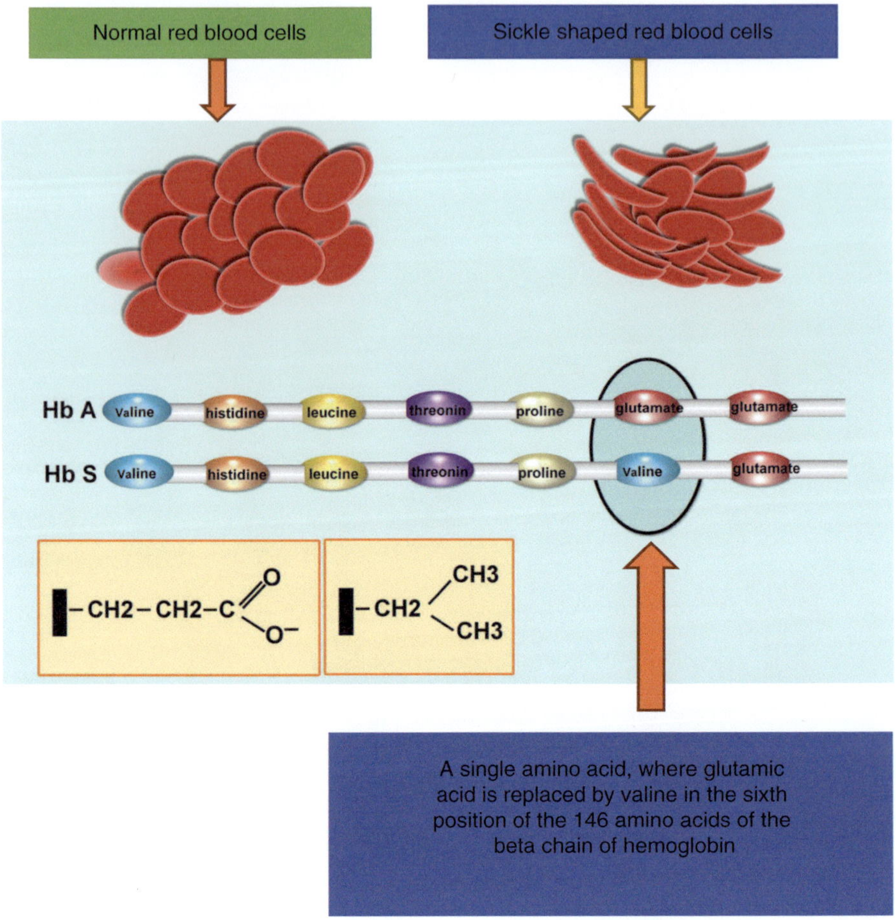

Fig. 2.2 Diagrammatic representation showing the change of a single amino acid, where glutamic acid is replaced by valine in the sixth position of the 146 amino acids of the beta chain of hemoglobin. This leads to the formation of hemoglobin S and a change of the normal red blood cells to sickle-shaped red blood cells

SEQUENCE FOR NORMAL HEMOGLOBIN

ATG	GTG	CAC	CTG	ACT	CCT	GAG	GAG	AAG	TCT	GCC
START	Val	His	Leu	Thr	Pro	Glu	Lys	Ser	Ala	Val

SEQUENCE FOR SICKLE CELL HEMOGLOBIN

Fig. 2.3 Diagrammatic representation showing the amino acids sequence in the normal hemoglobin and sickle cell hemoglobin. The change is at the sixth position among the 146 amino acids of the beta chain of hemoglobin where glutamic acid is replaced by valine

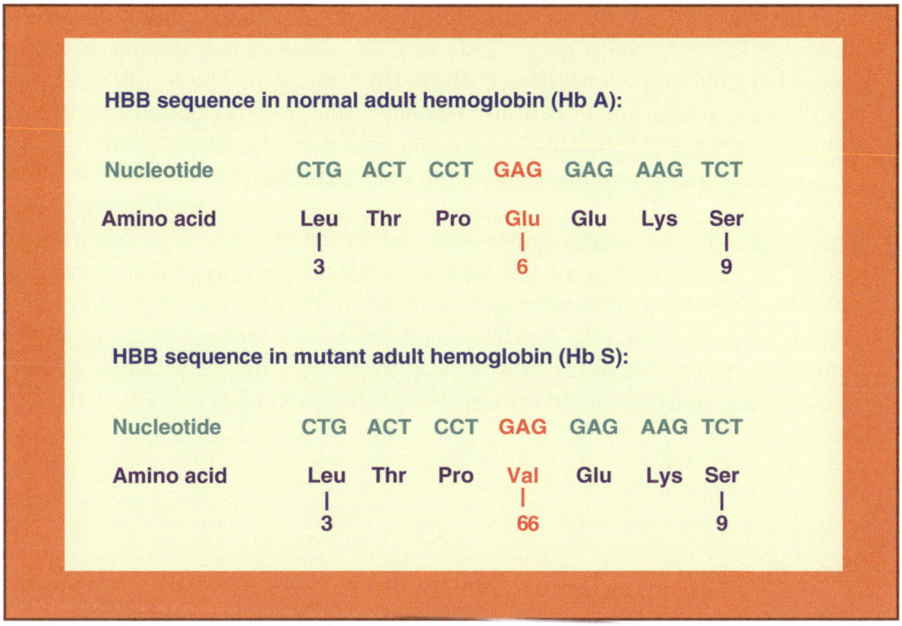

Fig. 2.4 Diagrammatic representation showing the nucleotide and amino acids sequence in the normal hemoglobin and sickle cell hemoglobin. The change is at the sixth position among the 146 amino acids of the beta chain of hemoglobin where glutamic acid nucleotide (*GAG*) is replaced by valine nucleotide (GTG). This will lead to the replacement of valine instead of glutamic acid

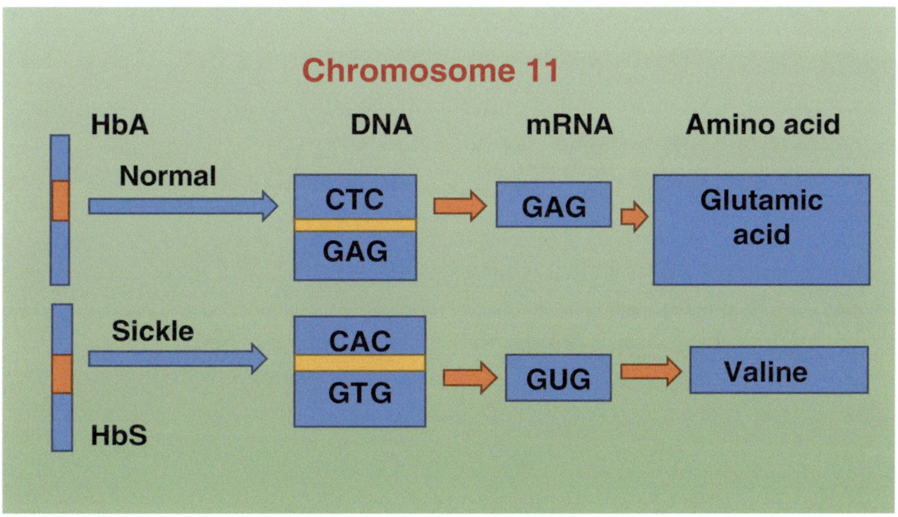

Fig. 2.5 Diagrammatic representation showing chromosome 11 and the changes in the nucleotide and amino acids sequence in the normal hemoglobin and sickle cell hemoglobin. The change will lead to the replacement of valine instead of glutamic acid

- HbS arises from a mutation substituting thymine for adenine in the sixth codon of the beta-chain gene, GAG to GTG. This causes coding of valine instead of glutamate in position 6 of the Hb beta chain. The resulting Hb has the physical properties of forming polymers under deoxy conditions. It also exhibits changes in solubility and molecular stability. These properties are responsible for the profound clinical expressions of the sickling syndromes.
- This single change of one amino acid, valine for glutamic acid substitution, results in hemoglobin tetramers that aggregate into arrays upon deoxygenation in the tissues. This aggregation leads to deformation of the red blood cell, changing them into sickle-shaped cells and making them relatively inflexible and unable to traverse the capillary beds. Repeated cycles of oxygenation and deoxygenation lead to irreversible sickling (Figs. 2.9, 2.10, 2.11 and 2.12).

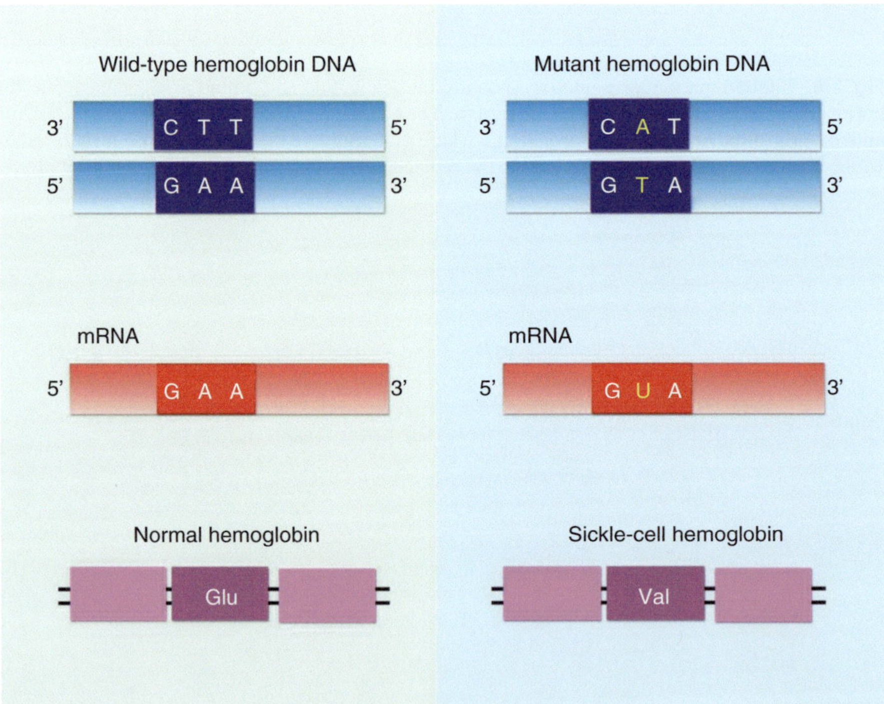

Fig. 2.6 Diagrammatic representation showing a single nucleotide substitution (A to T) in the codon for amino acid 6. Glutamic acid is coded by either GAA or GAG. Valine is coded by GUA, GUC, and GUU or GUG. In the mRNA, the change converts a glutamic acid codon (GAG or GAA) to a valine codon (GUA, GUC, GUU, or GUG)

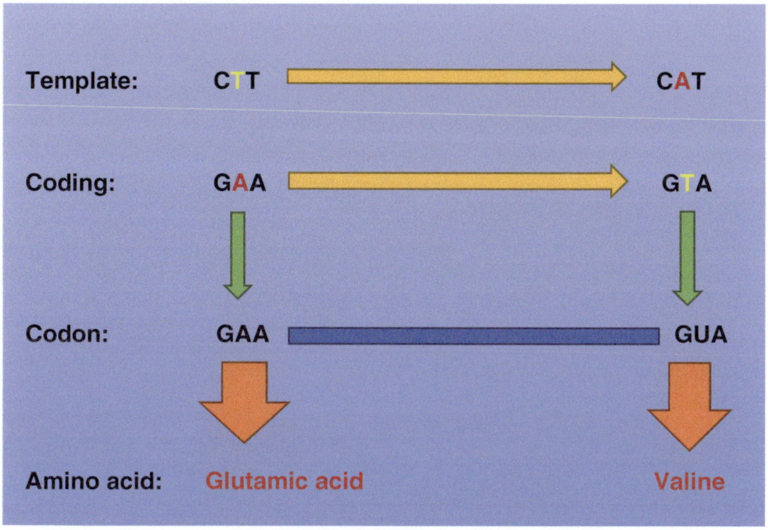

Fig. 2.7 Diagrammatic representation showing a single-nucleotide substitution (A to T) in the codon for amino acid 6 in patients with sickle cell anemia. The end result is a change of the codon for glutamic acid (*GAA*) to the codon for valine (GUA). This leads to the production of the amino acid valine instead of glutamic acid in the sixth position of the beta chain of hemoglobin

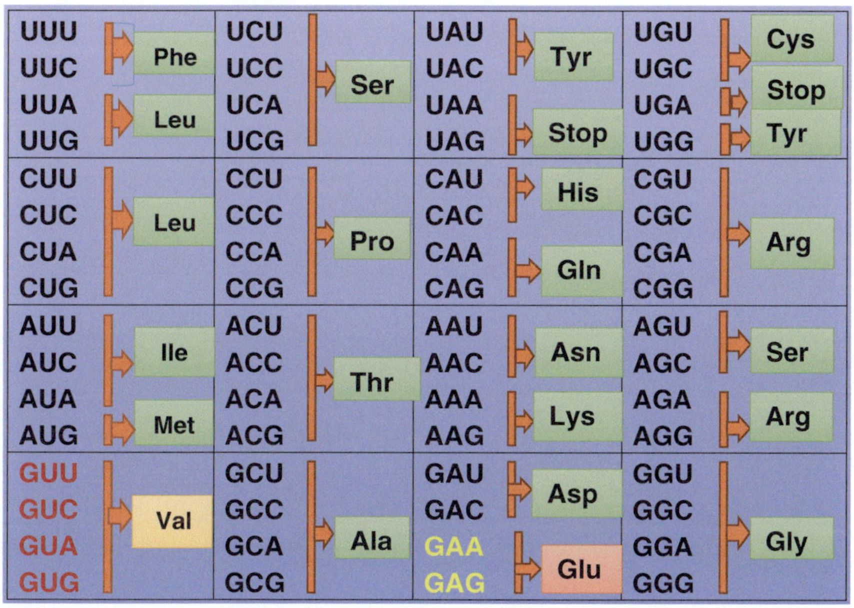

Fig. 2.8 Diagrammatic representation showing the codons for each amino acid. Glutamic acid is coded by either GAA or GAG. Valine is coded by GUA, GUC, and GUU or GUG. In patients with sickle cell anemia, there is a single change of one amino acid where glutamic acid at the sixth position among the 146 amino acid of the hemoglobin beta change is replaced by valine. This leads to a change and alteration of the hemoglobin and the hemoglobin tend to stick to each other, forming long insoluble fibers of hemoglobin within the red blood cell. The red blood cells become more fragile, adhering to each other and rupturing easily

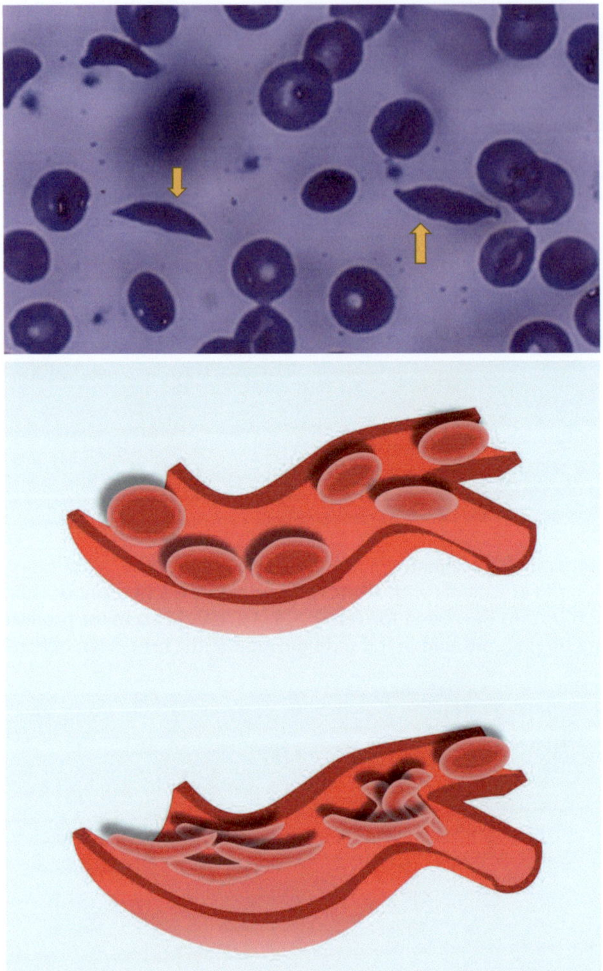

Figs. 2.9 and 2.10 A blood film showing sickled red blood cells and a diagrammatic representation of normal and sickled red blood cells causing occlusion of blood vessels

- As a result of this:
  - The hemoglobin molecule is altered so that it becomes more hydrophobic.
  - When the altered hemoglobin chains fold into their three-dimensional shape, they tend to stick to each other, forming long insoluble fibers of hemoglobin within the red blood cell.
  - The red blood cells are deformed by this altered hemoglobin. They become more fragile, rupturing easily and adhering to each other leading to closure of the small blood vessels.
- Sickle cell anemia is an autosomal recessive disorder. Affected individuals must carry two copies (homozygous genotype = SS) of the HbS gene. Individuals who are heterozygous (genotype = AS) have what is referred to as sickle cell trait.

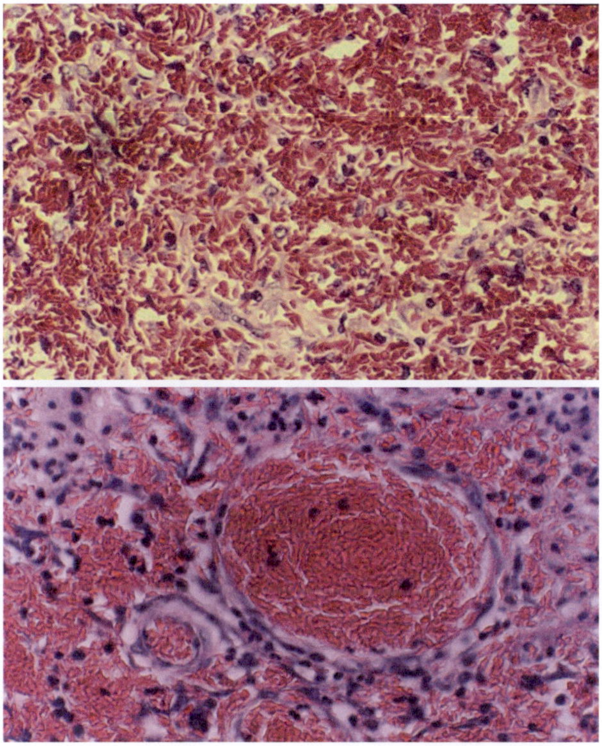

Figs. 2.11 and 2.12 A microscopic picture showing sickling of red blood cells and hemosiderosis. In the lower picture, note also the sickled cells within the blood vessel

2.2 Risk of Inheritance

- People inherit a pair of genes that regulate the production of hemoglobin.
- One gene comes from each parent.
- Sickle cell anemia:
  - This results from inheritance of two sickle genes, one from each parent.
- Sickle cell trait:
  - This occurs if a person inherits one normal hemoglobin gene and one sickle cell gene.
- People who have sickle cell trait are healthy, but they are "carriers" who can pass the disease on to their children.
- They are also prone to develop sickle cell anemia like symptoms but under certain conditions.
- The risk of a child inheriting sickle cell anemia or sickle cell trait is as follows:
- If both parents have sickle cell trait (each has one normal hemoglobin gene and one sickle cell gene) (Fig. 2.13):

- The child has a 50 % chance of inheriting sickle cell trait (one normal gene, one sickle cell gene).
- The child has a 25 % chance of inheriting sickle cell anemia (two sickle cell genes).
- The child has a 25 % chance of not inheriting either the trait or the disease (two normal genes).

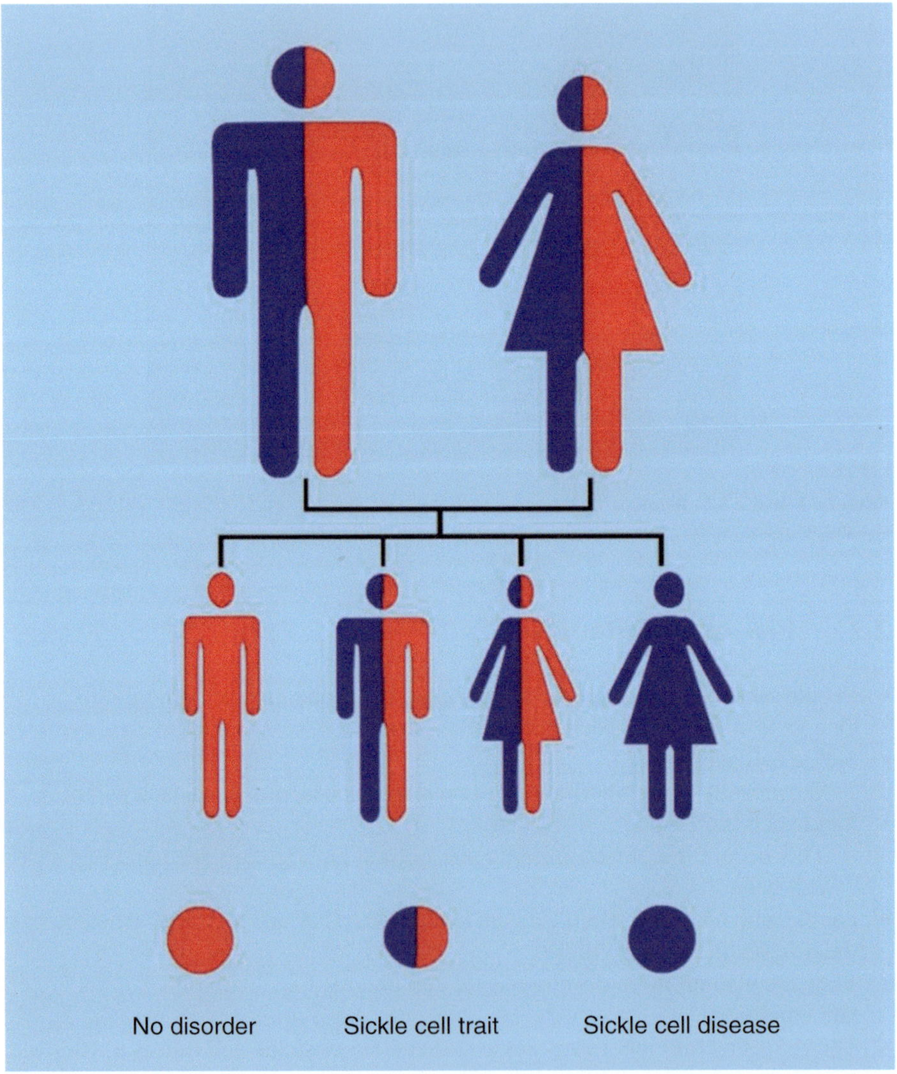

Fig. 2.13 Diagrammatic representation of inheritance if both parents have sickle cell trait

- If one parent has sickle cell trait (one normal gene and one sickle cell gene) and the other parent has two normal hemoglobin genes (Fig. 2.14):
  - The child has a 50 % chance of inheriting sickle cell trait (one normal gene and one sickle cell gene).
  - The child has a 50 % of inheriting neither the trait nor the disease (two normal genes).

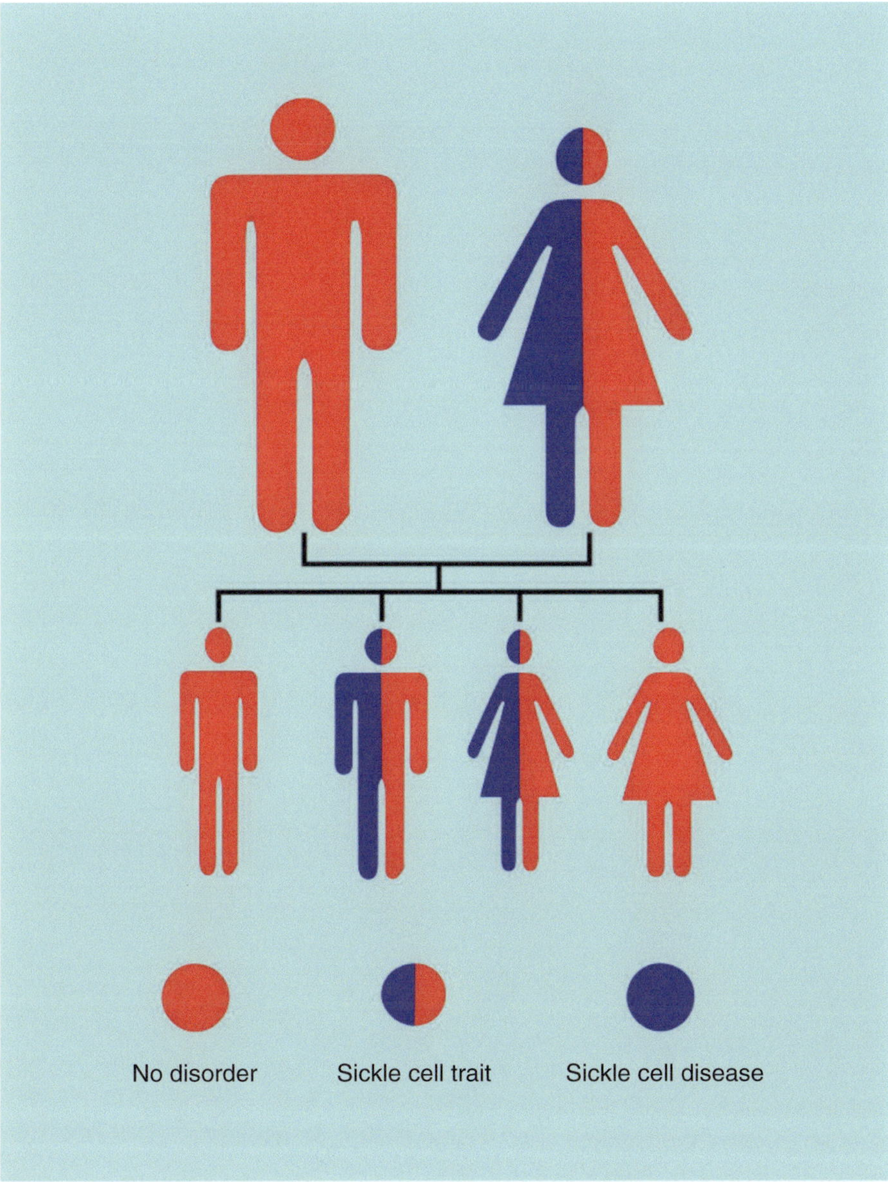

Fig. 2.14 Diagrammatic representation of inheritance if one parent has sickle cell trait

  - The child is not at risk of inheriting sickle cell anemia.
- If one parent has sickle cell anemia (two sickle cell genes) and the other parent has sickle cell trait (one normal gene, one sickle cell gene) (Fig. 2.15):
  - The child has a 50 % chance of inheriting sickle cell trait.
  - The child has a 50 % chance of inheriting sickle cell anemia.

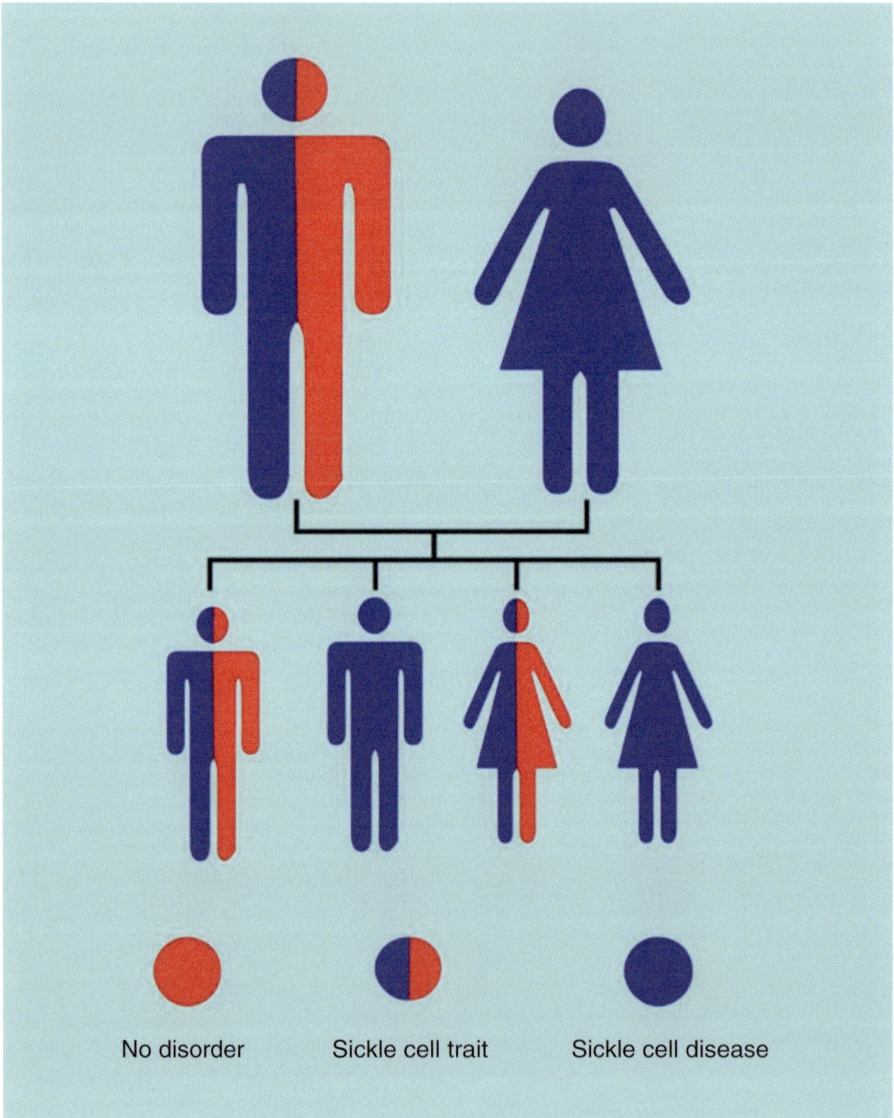

Fig. 2.15 Diagrammatic representation of inheritance if one parent has sickle cell trait and the other has sickle cell anemia

- If one parent has sickle cell anemia and the other parent has two normal hemoglobin genes, the child has a 100 % chance of inheriting sickle cell trait but not the disease (Fig. 2.16).

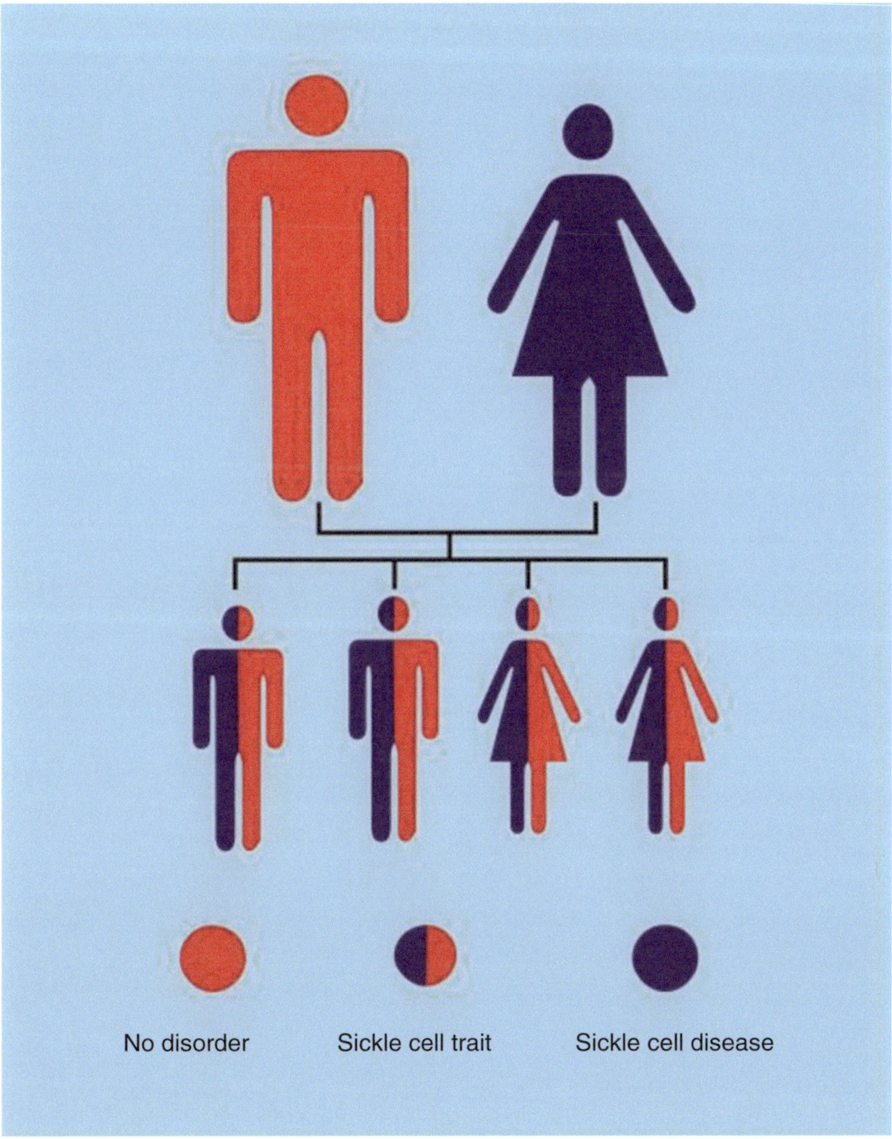

Fig. 2.16 Diagrammatic representation of inheritance if one parent has sickle cell anemia and the other is normal

- If both parents have sickle cell anemia, the child has a 100 % chance of inheriting the disease (Fig. 2.17).
- The child will inherit one sickle cell gene from each parent.
  - All children will be affected by sickle cell anemia.
  - None of the children will be normal.
  - None of the children will have sickle cell trait.

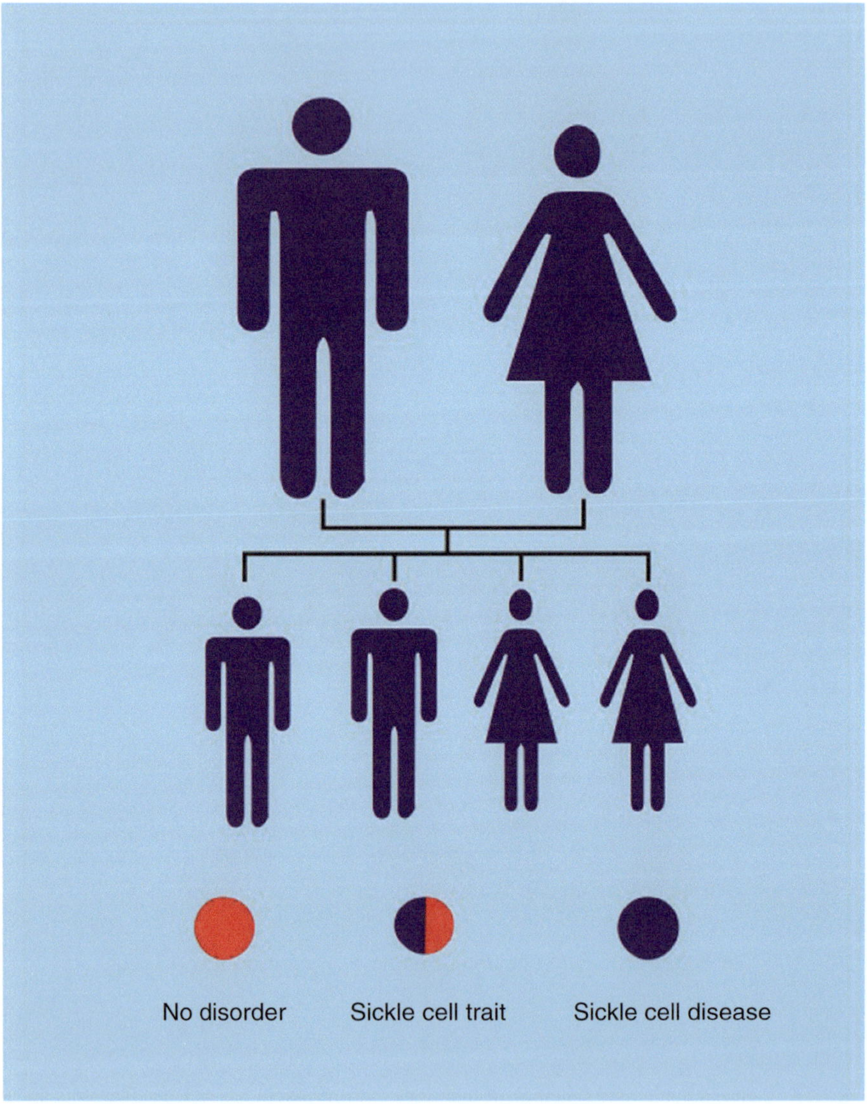

Fig. 2.17 Diagrammatic representation of inheritance if both parents have sickle cell anemia

2.3 Sickle Cell Trait

- People who inherit both copies of the HbS gene develop sickle cell anemia.
- Those who inherit just a single gene are referred to as having the sickle trait.
- Patients with sickle cell trait (the carrier state or the heterozygous form) are characterized by the presence of around 40 % HbS on electrophoresis.
- These people are usually asymptomatic and sickle cell trait provides a survival advantage over people with normal hemoglobin in regions where malaria is endemic. People with sickle cell trait are protected against malaria. This is especially when *Plasmodium falciparum* is the causative organism.
- Patients with sickle cell anemia on the other hand are not protected from malaria. In fact, malaria is more serious in these patients.
- The precise mechanism for this phenomenon in people with sickle cell trait is not known but several factors are believed to be responsible.
  - Infected red blood cells tend to have lower oxygen tension, because it is significantly reduced by the parasite. This causes sickling of that particular red blood cell and phagocytosis to get rid of the cell and hence the parasite within.
  - Since the sickling of parasite-infected cells is higher, these selectively get removed by the reticuloendothelial system, thus sparing the normal erythrocytes.
  - Excessive vacuole formation occurs in those parasites infecting sickle cells.
  - Sickle trait red blood cells produce higher levels of the superoxide anion and hydrogen peroxide than do normal red blood cells; both are toxic to malarial parasites.
- The sickle cell trait was found to be 50 % protective against mild clinical malaria, 75 % protective against admission to the hospital for malaria, and almost 90 % protective against severe or complicated malaria.
- There are however several complications known to occur in patients with sickle cell trait.
- Patients with sickle cell trait can develop vaso-occlusive attacks under low oxygen tension such as high altitude and travelling in an unpressurized aircraft.
- Renal medullary carcinoma, a cancer affecting the kidney, is a very rare complication seen in patients with sickle cell trait.
- Hematuria.
- Renal papillary necrosis.
- Hyposthenuria (inability to concentrate urine or excretion of urine of low specific gravity).
- Splenic infarcts at high altitude.
- Urinary tract infection.
- Rarely, sudden deaths during physical exertion.

Presentations of Patients with Sickle Cell Trait

- They are usually asymptomatic.
- Patients with sickle cell trait can however develop complications under low oxygen tension such as high altitude and travelling in an unpressurized aircraft. These complications include:
  - Vaso-occlusive attacks.
  - Renal medullary carcinoma, a cancer affecting the kidney, is a very rare complication seen in patients with sickle cell trait.
  - Hematuria.
  - Renal papillary necrosis.
  - Hyposthenuria (inability to concentrate urine or excretion of urine of low specific gravity).
  - Splenic infarcts at high altitude.
  - Urinary tract infection.
  - Rarely, sudden deaths during physical exertion.

2.4 Pathophysiology of Sickle Cell Anemia

- Sickle cell hemoglobin (HbS) arises from a mutation substituting thymine for adenine in the sixth codon of the beta-chain gene, GAG to GTG (Fig. 2.18).
- This causes coding of the amino acid valine instead of glutamate in the 6th position of the Hb beta chain (Fig. 2.19).
- The resulting Hb has the physical properties of forming polymers under deoxy conditions. It also exhibits changes in solubility and molecular stability. These properties are responsible for the profound clinical features of sickle cell anemia.
- Under deoxy conditions, HbS undergoes several changes including:
  - Marked decrease in solubility.
  - Increased viscosity.
  - Polymer formation.
  - It forms a gel-like substance containing Hb crystals called tactoids. The gel-like form of Hb is in equilibrium with its liquid-soluble form. A number of factors influence this equilibrium, including:
    - Oxygen tension
    - Concentration of Hb S
    - The presence of other hemoglobins
  - Oxygen tension is an important factor in the polymer formation which occurs only in the deoxy state. If oxygen is present, the liquid state prevails.

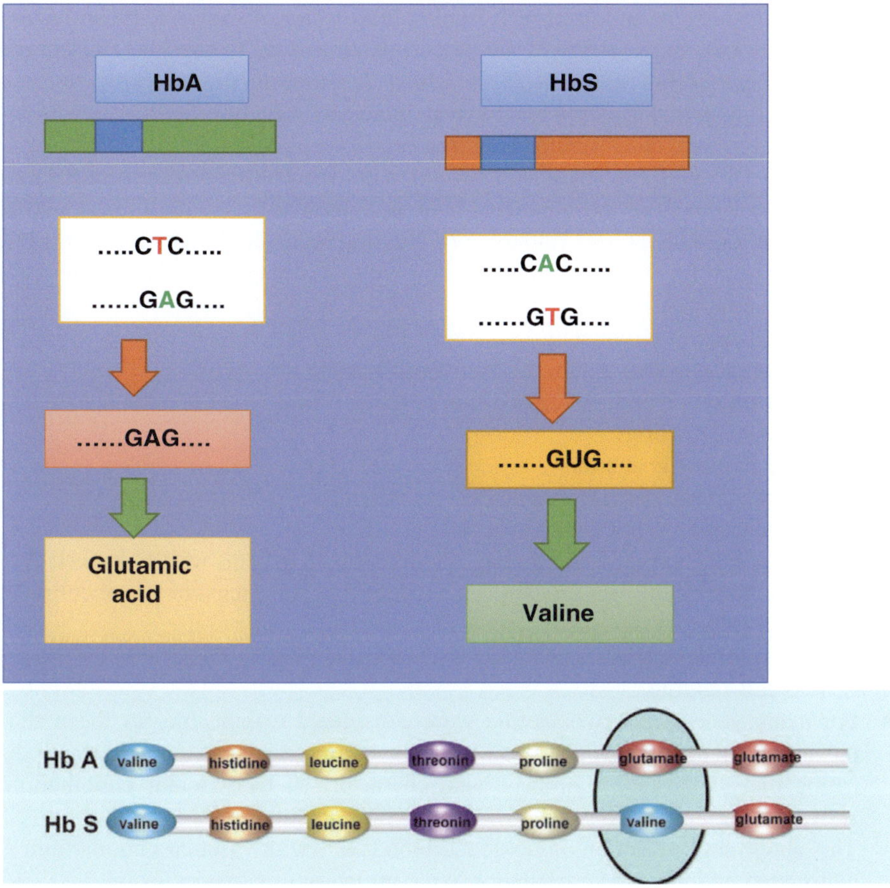

Figs. 2.18 and 2.19 Diagrammatic representation showing the mutation substituting thymine for adenine in the sixth codon of the beta-chain gene, GAG to GTG nucleotide and amino acid sequence in the normal hemoglobin and sickle cell hemoglobin. This causes coding of the amino acid valine instead of glutamate in the 6th position of the Hb beta chain

  - Concentration of Hb S is another factor in the formation of the gel-like form of HbS which occurs at concentrations greater than 20.8 g/dL (the normal cellular Hb concentration is 30 g/dL).
  - The presence of other hemoglobins is a factor in that normal adult hemoglobin (HbA) and fetal hemoglobin (HbF) have an inhibitory effect on the formation of the gel form of Hb. This is one factor why patients with high HbF have a milder disease when compared with those with low HbF.
- Affected patients with sickle cell anemia present with a wide range of clinical problems that result from vascular obstruction and ischemia.
- Although sickle cell anemia can be diagnosed at birth, clinical manifestations usually do not occur before age 6 months.

- This is attributed to an initial high level of HbF which is known to be protective and ameliorate the severity of sickle cell anemia. Add to this the subsequent development of functional asplenia which develops in the majority of these patients. Functional asplenia results in an increased susceptibility to overwhelming infection with encapsulated bacteria.
- Newborn screening for sickle hemoglobinopathies is considered an essential part of the management of these patients in areas known to have a high frequency of sickle cell anemia. This is valuable not only in diagnosing affected patients but also important for their subsequent follow-up and management when they present to the emergency room.
- Sickle cell anemia is characterized by:
  - Persistent episodes of chronic hemolytic anemia
  - The occurrence of acute episodes of sickling crises
  - Repeated infections
  - Acute hemolytic anemia
  - Recurrent vaso-occlusive episodes
  - Complications related to these episodes
- Red blood cells normally live for 90–120 days, but in patients with sickle cell anemia, they live for only 10–20 days. This will lead to persistent chronic anemia.
- The main pathophysiological defects of sickle cell anemia are:
  - HbS polymerization
  - Red cell sickling
- For many years these two factors were considered responsible for the pathophysiological changes of sickle cell anemia, but there is growing evidence indicating that sickle cell anemia is also characterized by vascular endothelium activation and increased blood cell-endothelium interactions.
- This abnormal interaction of sickle red blood cells with vascular endothelium is considered an important contributor to the initiation of vaso-occlusion.
- This abnormal adhesion of sickle red cells to the vascular endothelium is induced by:
  - Repeated sickling
  - Expression of adhesion molecules
  - Dense red cell formation
  - Upregulation of endothelial adhesion molecules
- Ischemia and reperfusion in the microcirculation is also an important factor which may lead to endothelial oxidant generation, endothelial activation, and upregulation of adhesion molecules.
- Inflammatory activation of endothelium and increased leukocyte recruitment in combination with adhesion of sickle red cells may further contribute to stasis.
- Sickle red cell adhesion in postcapillary venules can cause increased microvascular transit times and initiate vaso-occlusion.
- Add to this, involvement of an array of adhesion molecules expressed on sickle red cells including:
  - CD36
  - α-4-β-1 integrin

  - ICAM-4
  - Basal cell adhesion molecule (B-CAM)
  - Activated endothelium:
    - P-selectin
    - Vascular cell adhesion molecule-1 (VCAM-1)
    - Alpha-V-beta-3 integrin
- Plasma factors and adhesive proteins:
  - Thrombospondin (TSP)
  - von Willebrand factor (vWf)
  - Laminin
- Sickle cells express very late antigen-4 (VLA-4) on the surface. VLA-4 interacts with the endothelial cell adhesive molecule, vascular cell adhesive molecule-1 (VCAM-1). VCAM-1 is upregulated by hypoxia and inhibited by nitric oxide.
- The induction of VCAM-1 and P-selectin on activated endothelium is known to enhance sickle RBC interactions.
- In addition, a-V-ß-3 integrin is upregulated in activated endothelium in patients with sickle cell anemia.
- A-V-ß-3 integrin binds to several adhesive proteins (TSP, vWf, red-cell ICAM-4, and, possibly, soluble laminin) involved in sickle RBC adhesion, and antibodies to this integrin dramatically inhibit sickle RBC adhesion.
- Hypoxia also decreases nitric oxide production (nitric oxide is a potent vasodilator), thereby adding to the adhesion of sickle cells to the vascular endothelium.
- Continuing active hemolysis of RBCs leads to liberation of free Hb in the plasma. Free Hb is an avid scavenger of nitric oxide, thus contributing to vasoconstriction.
- In addition to leukocyte recruitment, inflammatory activation of endothelium may have an indispensable role in enhanced sickle RBC-endothelium interactions.
- Sickle RBC adhesion in postcapillary venules can cause increased microvascular transit times and initiate vaso-occlusion.
- Sickle RBCs also adhere to macrophages. This property may contribute to erythrophagocytosis and the hemolytic process.
- The microvascular perfusion at the level of the pre-arterioles is influenced by RBCs containing Hb S polymers. This occurs at arterial oxygen saturation, before any morphologic change is apparent.
- Hemolysis is a constant finding in sickle cell syndromes. Approximately one-third of RBCs undergo intravascular hemolysis, possibly due to loss of membrane filaments during oxygenation and deoxygenation. The remainder hemolyze by erythrophagocytosis by macrophages. This process can be partially modified by Fc (crystallizable fragment) blockade, suggesting that the process can be mediated by immune mechanisms.
- Sickle RBCs have increased immunoglobulin G (IgG) on the cell surface. Vaso-occlusive crisis is often triggered by infection. The levels of fibrinogen, fibronectin, and D-dimer are elevated in these patients. Plasma clotting factors likely participate in the microthrombi in the pre-arterioles.

- In addition, under inflammatory conditions, increased leukocyte recruitment in combination with adhesion of sickle RBCs may further contribute to stasis.
- Sickle RBCs adhere to endothelium because of increased stickiness. The endothelium participates in this process, as do neutrophils, which also express increased levels of adhesive molecules.
- Deformable sickle cells express CD18 and adhere abnormally to endothelium up to ten times more than normal cells, while ISCs do not. As paradoxical as it might seem, individuals who produce large numbers of ISCs have fewer vaso-occlusive crises than those with more deformable RBCs.
- The clinical course of sickle cell anemia is variable even within the afflicted family members.
- The continual premature destruction of the sickled red blood cells leads to chronic anemia.
- The sickling of red blood cells leads to occlusion of the fine capillaries. The bones are particularly affected, leading to recurrent frequent and severe bone pain which is the usual presentation during a sickle cell crisis.
- Long term, recurrent episodes of vaso-occlusive crisis leads to damage to the internal organs, in particular the kidneys, heart, and lungs.
- Sickle cell anemia usually presents in infancy with:
  - Repeated infections
  - Failure to thrive
  - Dactylitis (painful hand-foot syndrome), characterized by sudden onset of a painful swelling of the dorsum of the hands and or feet (Fig. 2.20)
  - Anemia
  - Splenomegaly (Fig. 2.21)
- Children with sickle cell anemia have an increased susceptibility to infections due to *Streptococcus pneumonia*, *Salmonella*, and *Haemophilus influenza*.
- Pneumococcal pneumonia and septicemia are the most devastating complications of sickle cell anemia and a common cause of death in infants and children.

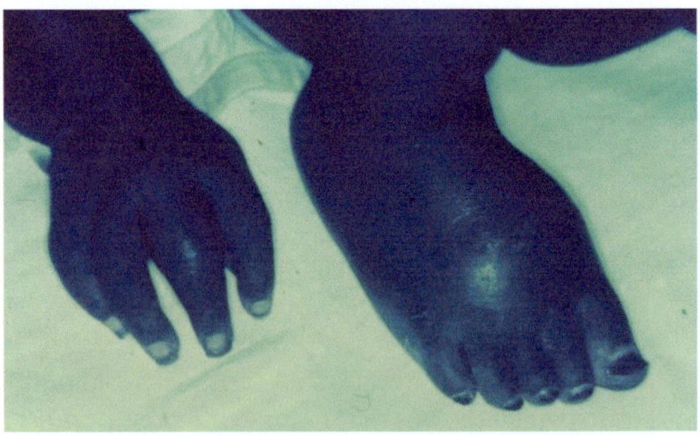

Fig. 2.20 A clinical photograph showing dactylitis (the hand-foot syndrome) in a child with sickle cell anemia

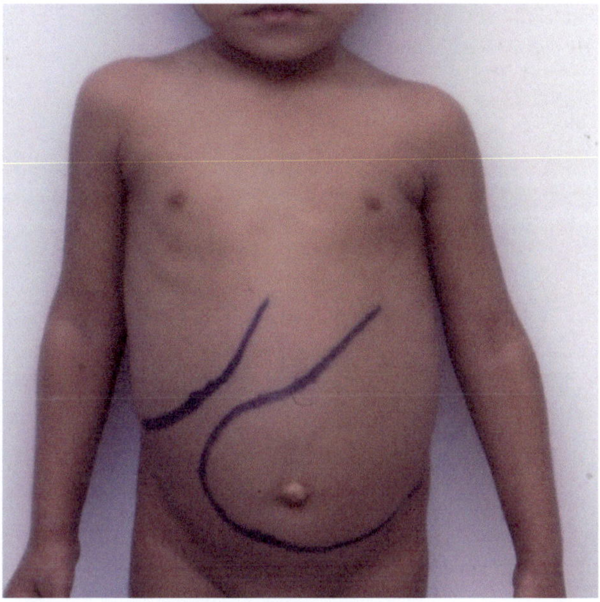

Fig. 2.21 A clinical photograph showing persistent splenomegaly in a child with sickle cell anemia

- Approximately half the individuals with homozygous HbS disease experience vaso-occlusive crises. The frequency of crises is extremely variable. Some individuals have as many as six or more episodes annually, whereas others may have episodes only at great intervals or none at all.
- Many individuals with HbSS experience chronic low-level pain, mainly in bones and joints. Intermittent vaso-occlusive crises may be superimposed, or chronic low-level pain may be the only expression of the disease.

Presentations of Sickle Cell Anemia During Infancy

- Anemia
- Repeated infections
- Failure to thrive
- Dactylitis (hand-foot syndrome)
- Splenomegaly

- After recurrent episodes of sickling, membrane damage occurs and the cells are no longer capable of resuming the biconcave shape upon reoxygenation. Thus, they become irreversibly sickled cells (ISCs). From 5 to 50 % of RBCs permanently remain in the sickled shape.
- When RBCs sickle (Figs. 2.22 and 2.23):
  - They gain Na+ and lose K+.
  - The red blood cells membrane permeability to Ca^{++} increases, possibly due, in part, to impairment in the Ca^{++} pump that depends on adenosine triphosphatase (ATPase).

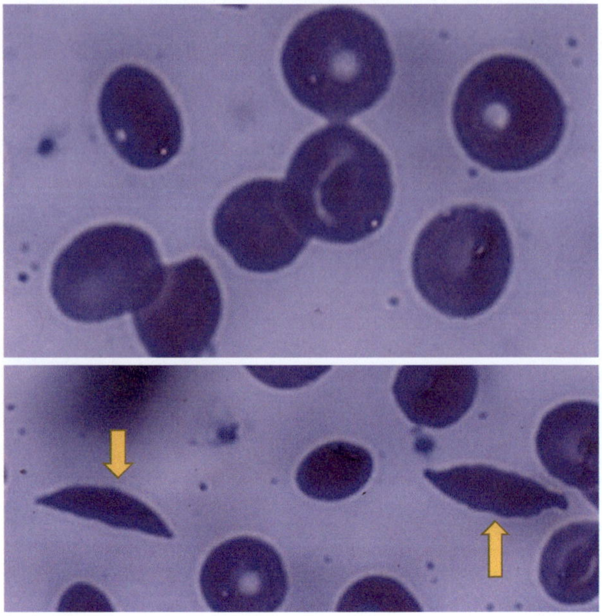

Figs. 2.22 and 2.23 Microscopic photographs showing normal red blood cells and sickle red blood cells

   - The intracellular Ca^{++} concentration rises to four times the reference level.
   - The membrane becomes more rigid, possibly due to changes in cytoskeletal protein interactions; however, these changes are not found consistently. In addition, whether calcium is responsible for membrane rigidity is not clear.
- Membrane vesicle formation occurs, and the lipid bilayer is perturbed. The outer leaflet has increased amounts of phosphatidylethanolamine and contains phosphatidylserine. The latter may play a role as a contributor to thrombosis, acting as a catalyst for plasma clotting factors. Membrane rigidity can be reversed in vitro by replacing HbS with HbA, suggesting that HbS interacts with the cell membrane.

Further Readings

Hebbel RP. Ischemia-reperfusion injury in sickle cell anemia: relationship to acute chest syndrome, endothelial dysfunction, arterial vasculopathy, and inflammatory pain. Hematol Oncol Clin North Am. 2014;28(2):181–98.

Hebbel RP, Yamada O, Moldow CF, Jacob HS, White JG, Eaton JW. Abnormal adherence of sickle erythrocytes to cultured vascular endothelium: possible mechanism for microvascular occlusion in sickle cell disease. J Clin Invest. 1980;65:154–60.

Hofstra TC, Kalra VK, Meiselman HJ, Coates TD. Sickle erythrocytes adhere to polymorphonuclear neutrophils and activate the neutrophil respiratory burst. Blood. 1996;87:4440–7.

Manwani D, Frenette PS. Vaso-occlusion in sickle cell disease: pathophysiology and novel targeted therapies. Hematology Am Soc Hematol Educ Prog. 2013a;20132013:362362–99.

Manwani D, Frenette PS. Vaso-occlusion in sickle cell disease: pathophysiology and novel targeted therapies. Blood. 2013b;122(24):3892–8.

Rodgers GP. Overview of pathophysiology and rationale for treatment of sickle cell anemia. Semin Hematol. 1997;34(3 Suppl 3):2–7.

Sakamoto TM, Lanaro C, Ozelo MC, Garrido VT, Olalla-Saad ST, Conran N, Costa FF. Increased adhesive and inflammatory properties in blood outgrowth endothelial cells from sickle cell anemia patients. Microvasc Res. 2013;90:173–9.

Steinberg MH, Rodgers GP. Pathophysiology of sickle cell disease: role of cellular and genetic modifiers. Semin Hematol. 2001;38(4):299–306.

Variants of Sickle Cell Anemia

3

3.1 Introduction

- The normal hemoglobin is made up of two parts (Fig. 3.1):
  - Heme
  - Globin
- The heme is composed of iron plus a protoporphyrin molecule.
- The globin part is made up of four polypeptide chains, two alpha chains, and two beta chains.
- Each of the two alpha chains is made up of 141 amino acids.
- Each of the two beta chains is made up of 146 amino acids.
- The two alpha chains are derived from genes in the alpha gene cluster on chromosome 16.
- The two beta chains are derived from genes in the beta gene cluster on chromosome 11.

3.2 Normal Hemoglobins

- Hemoglobin A
  - This is the normal hemoglobin that exists after birth.
  - Hemoglobin A is a tetramer made up of two alpha chains and two beta chains (a_2b_2).
- Hemoglobin A2
  - This is a minor component of the hemoglobin found in red blood cells after birth.
  - Hemoglobin A2 consists of two alpha chains and two delta chains (a_2d_2).
  - Hemoglobin A2 generally comprises less than 3 % of the total red cell hemoglobin.

A. Al-Salem, *Medical and Surgical Complications of Sickle Cell Anemia*,
DOI 10.1007/978-3-319-24762-5_3

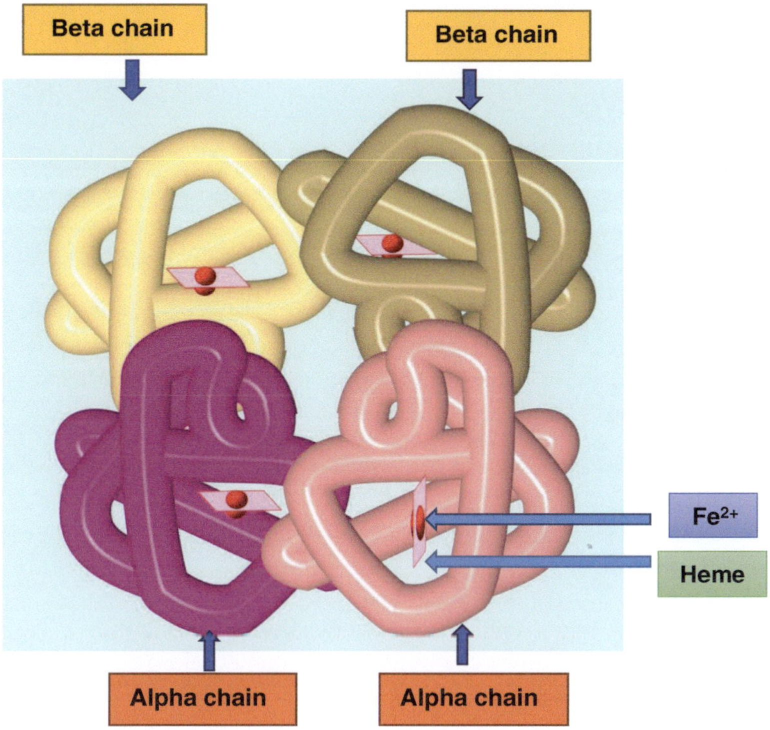

Fig. 3.1 Diagrammatic representation of the normal hemoglobin which is made up of heme and globin (2 alpha chains and 2 beta chains)

- Hemoglobin F
  - Hemoglobin F is the predominant hemoglobin during fetal development.
  - Hemoglobin F is a tetramer made up of two alpha chains and two gamma chains (a_2g_2).
  - The genes for hemoglobin F and hemoglobin A are closely related, existing in the same gene cluster on chromosome 11.
  - Hemoglobin F production falls dramatically after birth, although some people continue to produce small amounts of hemoglobin F for their entire lives.
- In healthy adults, 95 % of the Hb is Hb A ($\alpha_2\beta_2$) with small amounts (<3.5 %) of Hb A_2 ($\alpha_2\delta_2$) and HbF ($\alpha_2\gamma_2$) present.

Hemoglobin	Adults	Fetal
Hb A (2alpha and 2 beta)	96–98 %	15–20 %
Hb A2 (2 alpha and 2 gamma)	Undetectable	2.5 %–3.5 %
Hb F (2 alpha and 2 lambda)	< 1 %	80–85 %

Normal Hemoglobins
- Hemoglobin A: two alpha chains and two gamma chains (a_2g_2)
- Hemoglobin A2: two alpha chains and two delta chains (a_2d_2)
- Hemoglobin F: two alpha chains and two gamma chains (a_2g_2)

Normal Hemoglobins in Adults
- Hb A: 95–98 %
- Hb A2: 2–3 %
- HbF: 0.8–2 %
- Hb S: 0 %
- Hb C: 0 %

Homozygous HBS
HbA: absent unless transfused
HbS: over 50 %
HbF: up to 10 %. Higher for infants
HbA2: 2–4 %

Sickle Cell Trait
HbA: typically 50–65 %
HbS: typically 35–45 %
HbA2: normal (1.5–4 %)
HbF: higher for infants

3.3 Abnormal Hemoglobins

- There are hundreds of hemoglobin variants that involve genes both from the alpha and beta gene clusters.
- Hemoglobin variants
- Hb S
- Hb C
- Hb E
- Hb D-Punjab
- Hb O-Arab
- Hb G-Philadelphia
- Hb Constant Spring
- Hb Hasharon
- Hb Korle-Bu
- Hb Lepore
- Hb M
- Hb Kansas
- Hemoglobin S:
  - This is the predominant hemoglobin in people with sickle cell disease.
  - This results from a single change of one amino acid, where glutamic acid at the sixth position of the 146 amino acids of the beta chain of hemoglobin is replaced by valine.
  - The molecule structure is $a_2b^S{}_2$.
  - People who have one sickle mutant gene and one normal beta gene have sickle cell trait which is considered benign.
- Hemoglobin C:
  - Hemoglobin C results from a mutation in the beta globin gene.
  - This results from a single change of one amino acid, where glutamic acid at the sixth position of the 146 amino acids of the beta chain of hemoglobin is replaced by lysine.
  - It is the predominant hemoglobin found in people with hemoglobin C disease.
  - The molecule structure is $a_2b^C{}_2$.
  - Hemoglobin C disease is relatively benign, producing a mild hemolytic anemia and splenomegaly.
  - Hemoglobin C trait is a benign disease.
- Hemoglobin E:
  - This variant results from a single mutation in the hemoglobin beta chain.
  - This results from a single change of one amino acid, where glutamic acid at the 26th position of the 146 amino acids of the beta chain of hemoglobin is replaced by lysine.
  - Hemoglobin E is most prevalent in Southeast Asia (Thailand, Myanmar, Cambodia, Laos, Vietnam).
  - People with hemoglobin E disease have a mild hemolytic anemia and mild splenomegaly.
  - Hemoglobin E trait is a benign disease.

- Hemoglobin Constant Spring:
  - Hemoglobin Constant Spring is a variant in which a mutation in the alpha globin gene produces an alpha globin chain that is abnormally long.
  - It is an abnormal hemoglobin having an extended polypeptide chain (31 additional amino acyl residues) on the α chain (thus, the α chain is 172 amino acids long instead of 141).
  - Approximately 20 % of the patients with Hb H disease also have this defect.
  - The designation hemoglobin Constant Spring derives its name from the isolation of the hemoglobin variant in a family of ethnic Chinese background from the Constant Spring district of Jamaica.
- Hemoglobin H:
  - Hemoglobin H is a beta-4 tetramer which occurs when there are excess beta chains produced in the presence of defective alpha chain synthesis.
  - In hemoglobin H, only one gene for the production of alpha chain production has been inherited.
- Hemoglobin Barts (Hb Barts):
  - Hemoglobin Barts develops in fetuses with four-gene deletion alpha thalassemia.
  - Hemoglobin Barts consists of four gamma chains.
  - Most individuals with four-gene deletion thalassemia and consequent hemoglobin Barts die in utero (hydrops fetalis).
  - The abnormal hemoglobin seen during fetal development in individuals with four-gene deletion alpha thalassemia was characterized at St. Bartholomew's Hospital in London. The hospital has the fond sobriquet, St. Barts, and the hemoglobin was named "hemoglobin Barts."
- Although hemoglobinopathies and thalassemias are two genetically distinct disease groups, the clinical manifestations of both include anemia of variable severity and variable pathophysiology.
- The hemoglobinopathies, or structural Hb variants, are attributable to amino acid substitution in either α or non-α chain.
- More than 700 hemoglobinopathies have been described to date, the majority of which are clinically benign.
- The clinically significant hemoglobinopathies are attributable to amino acid substitutions, primarily in the non-α chain.

Abnormal Hemoglobins

- Hemoglobin S: a single change of one amino acid, where glutamic acid at the sixth position of the 146 amino acids of the beta chain of hemoglobin is replaced by valine ($a_2b^S{}_2$).
- Hemoglobin C: a single change of one amino acid, where glutamic acid at the sixth position of the 146 amino acids of the beta chain of hemoglobin is replaced by lysine ($a_2b^C{}_2$).

- Hemoglobin E: a single change of one amino acid, where glutamic acid at the 26th position of the 146 amino acids of the beta chain of hemoglobin is replaced by lysine ($a_2b^E{}_2$).
- Hemoglobin Constant Spring: an abnormal hemoglobin having an extended polypeptide chain (31 additional amino acyl residues) on the α chain (thus, the α chain is 172 amino acids long instead of 141).
- Hemoglobin H: a beta-4 tetramer which occurs when there are excess beta chains produced in the presence of defective alpha chain synthesis. It is a form of alpha thalassemia with only one (out of four) alpha chain genes being present.
- Hemoglobin Barts (Hb Barts): hemoglobin Barts develops in fetuses with four-gene deletion alpha thalassemia. It consists of four gamma chains.

- Compound heterozygous conditions:
  - These results from inheriting two different variant genes from the alpha globin gene cluster or two different variant genes from the beta globin gene cluster.
  - The nature of two genes inherited determines whether a clinically significant disease state develops.

Abnormal Hemoglobins

- Hb D-Punjab: an abnormal Hb with a single β chain substitution, glutamine for glutamic acid (Glu >Gln) in the beta globin chain (molecular formula $\alpha_2A\beta_2121Glu \rightarrow Gln$).
- Hb O-Arab: hemoglobin O Arab is a beta globin chain mutation ($\alpha_2\beta_2{}^{121\,Glu \rightarrow Lys}$).
- Hb G-Philadelphia: this is a common alpha globin chain variant [α68(E17) Asn >Lys].
- Hb Hasharon: Hb Hasharon is a hemoglobin variant with an alpha globin mutation. Hemoglobin Hasharon (α_2 47 Asp → His β_2).
- Hb Korle-Bu: the amino acid aspartic acid at the 73rd position of the beta chain is replaced by asparagine.
- Hb Lepore: the Hb Lepore variant, consisting of two normal alpha globin chains (HBA) and two delta beta globin fusion chains which occur due to a "crossover" between the delta (HBD) and beta globin (HBB) gene loci during meiosis.
- Hb M: a group of abnormal hemoglobins in which amino acid substitutions take place in either the alpha or beta chains but near the heme iron. This results in facilitated oxidation of the hemoglobin to yield excess methemoglobin. Specific types include Hb M_{Iwate}, $\alpha^{87His \rightarrow Tyr}$ (α chain, position 87, histidine replaced by tyrosine); Hb $M_{Hyde\ Park}$, $\beta^{92His \rightarrow Tyr}$; Hb M_{Boston}, $\alpha^{58His \rightarrow Tyr}$; Hb $M_{Saskatoon}$, $\beta^{63His \rightarrow Tyr}$; and Hb $M_{Milwaukee-1}$, $\beta^{67Val \rightarrow Glu}$.
- Hb Kansas: in Hb Kansas, threonine replaces asparagine in position 102 of the β chain.

3.4 Sickle Syndromes

- The sickle syndromes are a group of hemoglobinopathies with the common feature of having at least one gene that produces hemoglobin S.
- Sickle cell disease (SCD) and its variants are genetic disorders resulting from the presence of a mutated form of hemoglobin, hemoglobin S (HbS).
- SCD denotes all genotypes containing at least one sickle gene, in which HbS makes up at least half the hemoglobin present.
- In this book, the term sickle cell disease is used to denote all hemoglobinopathies having at least one gene that produces hemoglobin S.
- The term sickle cell disease should not be used to denote sickle cell anemia.
- Sickle cell anemia denotes homozygous sickle cell (HbSS).
- There are many different types of sickle cell disease, but hemoglobin SS, hemoglobin SC, and sickle beta-thalassemia are the most common types of sickle cell disease.
- Hemoglobin SS is a homozygous sickle cell disease. The hemoglobin S gene is inherited from both parents.
- Hemoglobin SC is heterozygous sickle cell disease. Hemoglobin S is inherited from one parent and hemoglobin C is inherited from the other parent.
- Sickle beta-thalassemia is a heterozygous sickle cell disease. Hemoglobin S is inherited from one parent and the beta-thalassemia gene is inherited from the other parent.
- Sickle cell anemia:
- This term is used to refer to a hemoglobinopathy in which a person has inherited two genes for hemoglobin S, one from each parent (homozygous SS).
- This is the most common type of the sickle syndromes.
- The severity of sickle cell anemia varies tremendously.
- Some patients have almost no symptoms, while others are virtually incapacitated. The reason for this is not fully understood.
- Sickle beta-thalassemia:
  - In this condition, the patient has inherited a gene for hemoglobin S from one parent and a gene for beta-thalassemia from the other parent.
  - The severity of the condition is determined to a large extent by the quantity of normal hemoglobin produced by the beta-thalassemia gene.
  - Thalassemia genes produce normal hemoglobin but in variably reduced amounts.
  - If the gene produces no normal hemoglobin, b^0-thalassemia, the condition is virtually identical to sickle cell disease (sickle – b^0 – thalassemia).
  - Some patients have a gene that produces a small amount of normal hemoglobin, called b^+-thalassemia.
  - The severity of the condition is determined to a large extent by the quantity of normal hemoglobin produced by the beta-thalassemia gene (sickle- b^+-thalassemia).
  - Sickle beta-thalassemia is the most common sickle syndrome seen in people of Mediterranean descent (Italian, Greek, and Turkish).
  - Hemoglobin electrophoresis of blood from a patient with sickle/b^0-thalassemia shows no hemoglobin A.

  - Patients with sickle/b^{+}-thalassemia have an amount of hemoglobin A that depends on the level of function of the b^{+}-thalassemia gene.
  - Those with HbS beta 0-thalassemia usually have a severe form of SCD.
  - People with HbS beta+–thalassemia tend to have a milder form of SCD.
- Hemoglobin SC disease:
  - Patients with hemoglobin SC disease inherit a gene for hemoglobin S from one parent and a gene for hemoglobin C from the other.
  - In general, patients with hemoglobin SC disease have milder symptoms than do those with sickle cell disease, but some of them have a condition equal in severity to those with sickle cell anemia.
  - The predominant red cell abnormality on the peripheral smear is an abundance of target cells.
  - Folded (pita bread, clamshell) cells, irreversibly sickled cells, "billiard ball" cells, and crystal-containing cells also may be seen.
  - Individuals with HbSC disease are at risk for the same life-threatening complications as HbSS but at a decreased frequency.
  - The diagnosis of HbSC disease is made by hemoglobin electrophoresis, which demonstrates approximately equal amounts of HbS and HbC (or slightly more HbS than HbC), with no HbA present.
- Hemoglobin E:
  - This is one of the most common variant hemoglobin on earth.
  - The gene is most common in people of South East Asian ancestry (Cambodian, Vietnamese, and Thai).
  - The combination of hemoglobin E and hemoglobin A is benign.
  - People with two hemoglobin E genes have a mild anemia and few other manifestations.
  - The combination of hemoglobin E and beta-thalassemia produces a clinically severe condition with marked anemia. The condition is much like thalassemia intermediate.
- Hemoglobin E/beta-thalassemia:
  - The combination of hemoglobin E and beta-thalassemia produces a condition more severe than is seen with either hemoglobin E trait or beta-thalassemia trait.
  - The disorder manifests as a moderately severe thalassemia that falls into the category of thalassemia intermediate.
  - Hemoglobin E/beta-thalassemia is most common in people of South East Asian background.
- Alpha thalassemia/hemoglobin Constant Spring.
  - This syndrome is a compound heterozygous state of the alpha globin gene cluster.
  - The alpha globin gene cluster on one of the two chromosomes 16 has both alpha globin genes deleted.
  - On the other chromosome 16, the alpha1 gene has the Constant Spring mutation.
  - The compound heterozygous condition produces a severe shortage of alpha globin chains.
  - The excess beta chains associate into tetramers to form hemoglobin H.

- Sickle cell trait (SCT) (HbAS)
  - People who have SCT inherit one sickle cell gene ("S") from one parent and one normal gene ("A") from the other parent.
  - This is called sickle cell trait (SCT).
  - Sickle cell trait or the carrier state is the heterozygous form characterized by the presence of around 40 % HbS.
  - People with SCT usually do not have any of the signs of the disease and live a normal life, but they can pass the trait onto their children.
  - Some patients with sickle cell trait may under certain conditions of low oxygen tension such as mountain climbing or traveling in unpressurized aircrafts develop sickle cell-related complications.

3.5 The Alpha Thalassemia (α-Thalassemia) Syndromes

- The hemoglobin is made up of heme and globin.
- The globin part is made up of two alpha (141 amino acids) and two beta (146 amino acids) chains.
- The genes that regulate both the synthesis and the structure of different globins are organized into two separate clusters.
- The alpha globin genes are encoded on chromosome 16, and the gamma, delta, and beta globin genes are encoded on chromosome 11.
- Healthy individuals have four alpha globin genes, two on each chromosome 16 (αα/αα).
- Alpha thalassemia syndromes are caused by deficient expression of one or more of the four alpha globin genes on chromosome 16 and are characterized by absent or reduced synthesis of alpha globin chains.
- Abnormal production of alpha globin chains results in a relative excess of gamma-globin chains in fetuses and newborns and of beta globin chains in children and adults.
- The alpha thalassemia (α-thalassemia) syndromes are a group of hereditary anemias of varying clinical severity.
- They result from decreased production of $alpha_2$ globin or $alpha_1$ globin gene products.
- Alpha thalassemias are broadly classified according to whether the loss of alpha globin genes is complete or partial into two types:
  - Alpha (0) thalassemia
  - Alpha (+) thalassemia
- Alpha (0) thalassemia:
  - This is characterized by absence production of alpha globin.
  - It is also called hydrops fetalis, alpha thalassemia major, or hemoglobin Barts.
  - Hydrops fetalis is incompatible with extrauterine life.
  - Fetuses with this condition die either in utero or shortly after birth because of severe anemia.

- Alpha (+) thalassemia:
  - There are more than 15 different genetic mutations that result in decreased production of alpha globin, usually through functional deletion of one or more of the 4 alpha globin genes.
  - Alpha (+) thalassemia is subclassified into the following three general forms on the basis of the number of inherited alpha genes.
  - Silent carrier:
    - People who are silent carriers inherit three normal alpha globin genes (–α/αα).
    - This is also called alpha thalassemia minima, alpha thalassemia-2 trait, and heterozygosity for alpha (+) thalassemia minor.
    - The affected individuals are asymptomatic with no clinical abnormalities.
    - Hematologically they are also normal or have mild reductions in RBC mean corpuscular volume (MCV) and mean corpuscular hemoglobin (MCH).
  - Alpha thalassemia trait:
    - People with alpha thalassemia trait inherit two normal alpha globin genes through either heterozygosity for alpha (0) thalassemia (αα/--) or homozygosity for alpha (+) thalassemia (–α/-α).
    - This is also called alpha thalassemia minor or alpha thalassemia-1 trait.
    - The affected individuals are asymptomatic and clinically normal.
    - They frequently have mild anemia and reduced MCV and MCH.
    - The RBC count is usually increased, typically exceeding 5.5×10^{12}/L.
  - Hemoglobin H disease:
    - People with hemoglobin H disease (HbH disease) inherit one normal alpha globin gene (–α/--).
    - The loss of three alpha globin genes results in abundant formation of HbH, which is characterized by a high ratio of beta globin to alpha globin and a twofold to fivefold excess in beta globin production.
    - The excess beta chains aggregate into tetramers, which account for 5–30 % of the hemoglobin level in patients with HbH disease.
    - HbH has a high affinity for oxygen and has no Bohr effect or heme-heme interaction; therefore, it is an ineffective supplier of oxygen to the tissues.

3.6 Sickle –Alpha Thalassemia

- Alpha thalassemia results from impaired production of alpha globin chains, which leads to a relative excess of beta globin chains.
- Concurrent alpha thalassemia with sickle cell anemia has a beneficial effect upon the pathobiology of sickle cell anemia because unbalanced globin chain synthesis leads to a deficiency in the amount of hemoglobin per cell.
- The number of dense cells is lower, the red cell deformability is better, and anemia is significantly milder in patients with concurrent alpha thalassemia.

- Sickle cell-alpha thalassemia is associated with milder anemia, fewer reticulocytes, and sickled cells.
- The peripheral blood smear shows more hypochromia and microcytosis, less polychromasia, and fewer sickle forms.
- HbA2 levels are increased according to the number of alpha globin gene deletions, while HbF levels are not consistently affected.

3.7 The Sickle Beta-Thalassemia Syndromes

- Thalassemia refers to a spectrum of diseases characterized by reduced or absent production of one or more globin chains.
- Beta-thalassemia is due to impaired production of beta globin chains, which leads to a relative excess of alpha globin chains.
- These excess alpha globin chains are unstable, incapable of forming soluble tetramers on their own, and precipitate within the cell, leading to a variety of clinical manifestations.
- Sickle cell-beta-thalassemia is divided into two main types:
  - Sickle cell-beta0 thalassemia
  - Sickle cell-beta + thalassemia
- This classification is based upon the complete absence of beta globin or the presence of reduced amounts of beta globin, respectively, which in turn determines the level of HbA.
- Sickle cell-beta0 thalassemia is characterized by complete absence of beta globin.
- The percentage of HbA produced in individuals with sickle cell-beta + thalassemia varies from 5 to 30 %, depending upon the molecular defect of the mutation.
- Compound heterozygous sickle cell-beta0 thalassemia results in the production of no normal beta chains and therefore no HbA.
- The hematologic and clinical severity of sickle cell-beta-thalassemia depends on the quantity of HbA produced.
- Patients with sickle cell-beta0 thalassemia (i.e., no HbA production) have a clinical course that resembles homozygous sickle cell anemia.
- Patients with sickle cell-beta + thalassemia (i.e., low HbA production) generally have a more benign clinical course than those with sickle cell-beta0 thalassemia or sickle cell anemia because individuals with sickle cell-beta + thalassemia have more HbA.
- Diagnosis:
  - The electrophoresis findings are similar in sickle cell anemia and sickle cell-beta0 thalassemia, as nearly all the hemoglobin consists of HbS, and there is no HbA present.
  - Differences in the HbF and HbA2 levels may be useful in distinguishing these syndromes.
  - The presence of microcytosis is a useful indicator of sickle cell-beta0 thalassemia.

The Sickle Beta-Thalassemia Syndromes

- $S\beta^{+}$-thal: HbS and beta plus thalassemia
  - HbS: always dominates, typically 60–80 %
  - HbA: 15–30 %
  - HbA2: elevated to 3–8 %
  - HbF: 2–20 %, higher for age in infants
- $S\beta^{o}$-thal: HbS and beta null thalassemia
  - HbS: 75–90 %
  - HbA: absent unless transfused
  - HbA2: 5–8 %
  - HbF: 5–20 % in adults, higher for age in infants

- Sickle cell-beta+thalassemia and sickle cell trait both have substantial amounts of HbA and HbS.
- Sickle cell trait is not associated with anemia or microcytosis and has an HbA fraction that exceeds 50 %.
- Sickle cell-beta+thalassemia is associated with anemia, microcytosis, and an HbA fraction that ranges between 5 and 30 %.
- In the neonatal period, the diagnosing sickle beta+thalassemia may be more difficult. The high HbF and the low levels of HbS and HbA may make it unclear which one is in greater amount.
- Neonates with sickle beta+thalassemia may have so little HbA present that the diagnosis of sickle beta0 thalassemia is given.
- Family studies and more definitive testing are important to diagnose questionable cases.

3.8 Sickle-Hereditary Persistence of Fetal Hb

- Normally, the physiologic switch from the production of fetal hemoglobin (HbF, two alpha and two gamma chains) to the adult form of hemoglobin (HbA, two alpha and two beta chains) is usually accomplished by 2 years of age, resulting in a normal adult level of HbF of less than 1 %.
- It was found that increased levels of HbF can ameliorate the clinical severity of sickle cell anemia and the HbF level is an important prognostic factor for both sickle cell pain and mortality.
- HbF is a potent inhibitor of HbS polymerization.
- It has been suggested that an HbF level of 10–20 % is important in decreasing the clinical severity of sickle cell anemia.
- In those with hereditary persistence of fetal hemoglobin (HPFH), expression of the gamma-globin gene of HbF persists at high levels in adults with normal red blood cell indices and morphology.

- Hemoglobin electrophoresis in those with sickle-HPFH reveals only HbS, F, and A2, which resembles sickle cell anemia, sickle cell-beta0 thalassemia, and sickle cell-delta beta0 thalassemia.
- Notable differences between these, however, are the markedly increased percentage of HbF (10–40 %) and HbA2 levels <2.5 %.

3.9 Sickle-HbD Disease

- The most common hemoglobin D variant, HbD Los Angeles, is caused by a glutamic acid to glutamine substitution at codon 121 of the beta globin gene.
- Although asymptomatic in the heterozygous form, inheritance together with an HbS allele (HbSD disease) can result in a severe disease with clinical manifestations similar to sickle cell anemia.
- HbSD disease was first reported as an unusual variant of sickle cell anemia.
- HbD can be distinguished from HbS by acid electrophoresis or isoelectric focusing.
- There is moderately severe hemolytic anemia, and the peripheral smear shows marked anisocytosis and poikilocytosis, target cells, and irreversibly sickled cells.
- Some children have severe disease similar to that of sickle cell anemia. However, persistent splenomegaly is more common.

3.10 Sickle-HbO Arab Disease

- Hemoglobin O Arab is caused by a glutamic acid to lysine substitution at 121 of the beta globin gene.
- It was first described in an Israeli Arab family but its distribution is widespread.
- Sickle cell-HbO Arab resembles HbSC on alkaline electrophoresis, but HbO Arab can be distinguished from HbC by either acid electrophoresis or isoelectric focusing.
- The syndrome is characterized by moderately severe hemolytic anemia, and the peripheral smear shows anisocytosis, poikilocytosis, and irreversibly sickled cells.
- Oxygen affinity is reduced in sickle cell-HbO Arab compared with sickle cell anemia.
- The clinical manifestations are severe and resemble those of homozygous sickle cell anemia.

3.11 Sickle-HbE Disease

- HbE is a beta thalassemic hemoglobinopathy found predominantly in Southeast Asia.
- HbE is caused by a glutamic acid to lysine substitution at 26 of the beta globin gene.

- The mutant hemoglobin has an electrophoretic mobility similar to HbC under alkaline conditions but can be resolved by acid electrophoresis or isoelectric focusing.
- HbE comprises only 30 % of the total hemoglobin in patients with compound heterozygosity for the sickle cell and HbE genes.
- Heterozygotes and homozygotes for HbE are asymptomatic with minimal anemia and microcytosis.
- HbSE disease may cause only mild hemolysis, no vaso-occlusive complications, and no remarkable abnormality of red blood cell morphology in those 18 years of age or less.
- There are, however, several case reports of more severe manifestations including:
  - Hematuria
  - Massive splenic infarct during air travel
  - Acute chest syndrome
  - Reversible bone marrow necrosis associated with parvovirus B19 infection

Further Readings

Ballas SK, Lewis CN, Noone AM, et al. Clinical, hematological, and biochemical features of Hb SC disease. Am J Hematol. 1982;13:37.

Bunn HF. Pathogenesis and treatment of sickle cell disease. N Engl J Med. 1997;337:762.

Embury SH, Dozy AM, Miller J, et al. Concurrent sickle-cell anemia and alpha-thalassemia: effect on severity of anemia. N Engl J Med. 1982;306:270.

Embury SH, Clark MR, Monroy G, Mohandas N. Concurrent sickle cell anemia and alpha-thalassemia. Effect on pathological properties of sickle erythrocytes. J Clin Invest. 1984;73:116.

Gonzalez-Redondo JM, Kutlar A, Kutlar F, et al. Molecular characterization of Hb S(C) beta-thalassemia in American blacks. Am J Hematol. 1991;38:9.

Higgs DR, Aldridge BE, Lamb J, et al. The interaction of alpha-thalassemia and homozygous sickle-cell disease. N Engl J Med. 1982;306:1441.

Lane PA, O'Connell JL, Lear JL, et al. Functional asplenia in hemoglobin SC disease. Blood. 1995;85:2238.

Lawrence C, Fabry ME, Nagel RL. The unique red cell heterogeneity of SC disease: crystal formation, dense reticulocytes, and unusual morphology. Blood. 1991;78:2104.

Marcus SJ, Kinney TR, Schultz WH, et al. Quantitative analysis of erythrocytes containing fetal hemoglobin (F cells) in children with sickle cell disease. Am J Hematol. 1997;54:40.

Masiello D, Heeney MM, Adewoye AH, et al. Hemoglobin SE disease: a concise review. Am J Hematol. 2007;82:643.

Michlitsch J, Azimi M, Hoppe C, et al. Newborn screening for hemoglobinopathies in California. Pediatr Blood Cancer. 2009;52:486.

Murray N, Serjeant BE, Serjeant GR. Sickle cell-hereditary persistence of fetal haemoglobin and its differentiation from other sickle cell syndromes. Br J Haematol. 1988;69:89.

Ngo DA, Aygun B, Akinsheye I, et al. Fetal haemoglobin levels and haematological characteristics of compound heterozygotes for haemoglobin S and deletional hereditary persistence of fetal haemoglobin. Br J Haematol. 2012;156:259.

Orringer EP, Fowler Jr VG, Owens CM, et al. Case report: splenic infarction and acute splenic sequestration in adults with hemoglobin SC disease. Am J Med Sci. 1991;302:374.

Piel FB, Weatherall DJ. The a-thalassemias. N Engl J Med. 2014;371(20):1908–16.

Seward DP, Ware RE, Kinney TR. Hemoglobin sickle-Lepore: report of two siblings and review of the literature. Am J Hematol. 1993;44:192.

Steinberg MH, Rosenstock W, Coleman MB, et al. Effects of thalassemia and microcytosis on the hematologic and vasoocclusive severity of sickle cell anemia. Blood. 1984;63:1353.

Zimmerman SA, O'Branski EE, Rosse WF, Ware RE. Hemoglobin S/O(Arab): thirteen new cases and review of the literature. Am J Hematol. 1999;60:279.

Clinical Features of Sickle Cell Anemia

4

4.1 Introduction

- Sickle cell anemia (SCA) is an autosomal recessive disorder that results from an abnormal gene found on the short arm of chromosome 11. This leads to the production of a mutated form of hemoglobin, hemoglobin S (HbS), where a single amino acid, glutamic acid, is replaced by valine at the 6th position of the 146 amino acids of hemoglobin beta chain.
- A single change of one amino acid causes significant morbidity and mortality (Fig. 4.1).
- Approximately 50 % of patients with SCA develop vaso-occlusive crises. The frequency of these crises is however extremely variable. Some patients have as many as six or more attacks of vaso-occlusive crises per year, whereas others may have episodes only at great intervals or none at all.
- SCA usually manifests early in childhood. For the first 6 months of life, infants with sickle cell anemia are protected largely by elevated levels of HbF. Once the level of HbF level decreases, the disease becomes evident.
- Early diagnosis, close follow-up, and improved management and supportive care are important in reducing both morbidity and mortality of patients with sickle cell anemia.
- As a result of this, screening for sickle cell anemia at birth should be mandatory in areas where sickle cell is common.

4.2 Epidemiology

- Sickle cell anemia affects millions of people worldwide in Africa; Greece, Turkey, and Italy; the Arabian Peninsula; India; and Spanish-speaking regions in South America, Central America, and parts of the Caribbean.

A. Al-Salem, *Medical and Surgical Complications of Sickle Cell Anemia*,
DOI 10.1007/978-3-319-24762-5_4

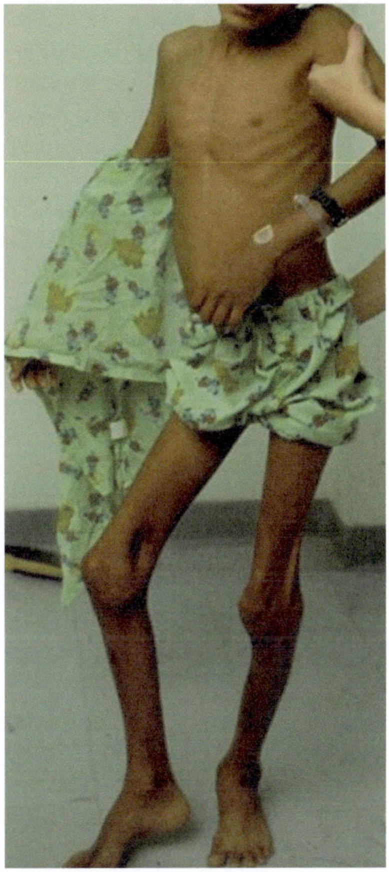

Fig. 4.1 A clinical photograph showing a child with severe sickle cell anemia

- The highest frequency of sickle cell anemia is found in tropical regions, particularly sub-Saharan Africa, tribal regions of India, and the Middle East.
- Sickle cell anemia occurs more commonly among people whose ancestors lived in tropical and sub-tropical sub-Saharan regions where malaria is or was common.
- Patients with sickle cell trait (heterozygous AS) living in these regions have a protective effect, and they develop less severe symptoms when compared with those with sickle cell anemia (homozygous SS).
- Around 2 % of newborns in Nigeria were affected by sickle cell anemia, giving a total of 150,000 affected children born every year in Nigeria alone.
- The carrier frequency ranges between 10 % and 40 % across equatorial Africa, decreasing to 1–2 % on the North African coast and <1 % in South Africa.

- Sickle cell anemia is the most common inherited blood disorder in the United States, affecting 70,000–80,000 Americans. The prevalence of sickle cell anemia in the United States is approximately 1 in 5000 African-American children and one in every 36,000 Hispanic-American children. Sickle cell trait on the other hand occurs among about 1:12 African-Americans and 1:100 Hispanic-Americans.
- In France, sickle cell anemia has become the most common genetic disease in the country, with an overall birth prevalence of 1/2,415 in mainland France.
- In the United Kingdom, it is estimated that between 12,000 and 15,000 people have sickle cell anemia with an estimate of 250,000 carriers of the gene in England alone.
- In Saudi Arabia about 4.2 % of the population carries the sickle cell trait and 0.26 % has sickle cell disease. The highest prevalence is in the Eastern province where approximately 17 % of the population carries the gene and 1.2 % has sickle cell disease.
- In India, sickle cell anemia is common in the tribal people of central India, where the prevalence has ranged from 9.4 to 22.2 % in endemic areas of Madhya Pradesh, Rajasthan, and Chhattisgarh.
- In Jamaica, 10 % of the population carries the sickle cell gene, making it the most prevalent genetic disorder in the country.

4.3 Clinical Manifestations

- The signs and symptoms of sickle cell anemia usually begin in early childhood, but the severity of symptoms varies from one patient to another and also in affected members of the same family.
- Some people have mild symptoms, while others are frequently hospitalized for more serious complications.
- Although the disease can be diagnosed at birth, clinical manifestations usually do not occur before age 6 months, when the level of HbF decreases and functional asplenia develops.
- Functional asplenia results in susceptibility to overwhelming infection with encapsulated bacteria. Patients with sickle cell anemia and as a result of repeated attacks of splenic vaso-occlusive crisis develop splenic infarcts. These repeated splenic infarcts lead to the development of autosplenectomy.
- Anemia is a common manifestation of sickle cell anemia and results from premature rupture of red blood cells. Depending on the severity of anemia, it can cause shortness of breath, fatigue, and delayed growth and development in children.
- The rapid breakdown of red blood cells may also cause jaundice.
- Painful episodes (painful vaso-occlusive crisis) occur in patients with sickle anemia, and these are one of the causes of frequent emergency room visits and hospital admissions of patients with sickle cell anemia.

- These attacks are secondary to occlusion of small blood vessels by sickled red blood cells.
- A serious complication of sickle cell anemia is pulmonary hypertension.
- Affected patients with sickle cell anemia present with a wide range of clinical manifestations that result from vascular obstruction and ischemia.
- Hemolysis is a constant feature of patients with sickle cell anemia.
  - Approximately one-third of RBCs undergo intravascular hemolysis, possibly due to loss of membrane filaments during oxygenation and deoxygenation.
  - The remainder gets hemolyzed as a result of erythrophagocytosis by macrophages.
- Currently, the diagnosis of sickle cell anemia is made early as a result of neonatal screening, but the symptoms usually do not develop until the age of 6–12 months.
- This is attributed to the high levels of circulating fetal hemoglobin which exerts a protective effect in these patients.
- Subsequently, the clinical manifestations of sickle cell anemia are attributed to:
  - Hemolytic anemia
  - Painful vaso-occlusive crisis
  - Multi-organ damage from sickle cell anemia-related complications
- Sickle cell anemia affects every organ in the body and results in several complications.
- The clinical severity, however, widely varies, and patients may exhibit some or all of the symptoms described.
- Hemolytic anemia:
  - Sickle cell anemia patients suffer from chronic mild to severe anemia.
  - This is secondary to repeated hemolysis and phagocytosis of sickled RBCs.
  - Normal red blood cells last about 120 days, but sickled cells expire after an average of 16 days. This rapid deterioration of red blood cells contributes to anemia.
  - Repeated episodes of deoxygenation and sickling of RBCs lead to irreversible damage of red blood cell membranes and their hemolysis.
  - The bone marrow tries to compensate by increasing red blood cell production but is unable to compensate for the high rate of hemolysis. This will lead to production of premature RBCs (reticulocytosis).
  - Patients with chronic anemia readily adjust and may exhibit only few symptoms of anemia on exertion.
  - Patients with sickle cell anemia can also develop acute anemic episodes secondary to:
    - Aplastic crisis
    - Acute splenic sequestration crisis
    - Hyperhemolysis
    - Delayed transfusion reactions from alloantibodies
    - Hepatic sequestration crisis

- Aplastic crisis:
  - This is seen following infection with parvovirus B-19.
  - This infection normally causes a benign childhood disorder associated with fever, malaise, anemia, and a mild rash.
  - This however is not the case in patients with sickle cell anemia.
  - The virus has trophism for erythroid progenitor cells and impairs cell division for a few days during the infection. This will lead to a shutdown in erythroid production for a few days, and because of the continuous hemolysis, there will be a marked drop in hemoglobin and hematocrit leading to severe anemia.
  - In these patients and in spite of the severe anemia, there is no reticulocytosis.
  - Aplastic anemia usually coincides with painful crises.
  - Treatment of aplastic anemia is supportive, with blood transfusions to maintain an acceptable hematocrit until marrow activity is restored.

Causes of Anemia in Patients with Sickle Cell Anemia

- Hemolytic anemia (acute and chronic)
- Aplastic crisis
- Acute splenic sequestration crisis
- Hyperhemolysis
- Delayed transfusion reactions from alloantibodies
- Hepatic sequestration crisis
- Severe infection and multi-organ damage

- Splenic complications:
  - The spleen is normally enlarged during the first decade of life but does undergo progressive atrophy as a result of repeated vaso-occlusive crisis leading to autosplenectomy (Fig. 4.2).

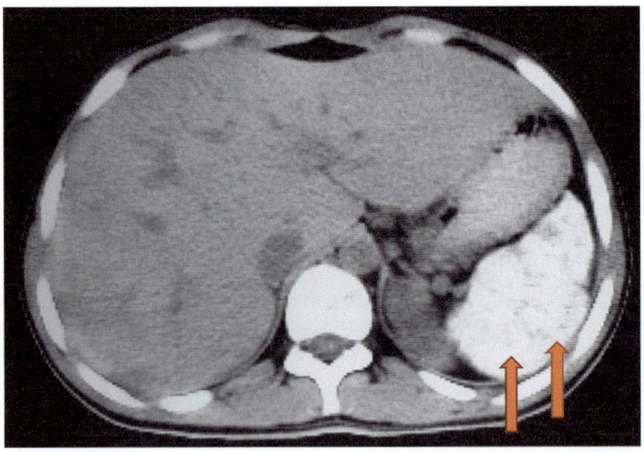

Fig. 4.2 Abdominal CT scan showing an atrophied calcified spleen in a patient with sickle cell anemia

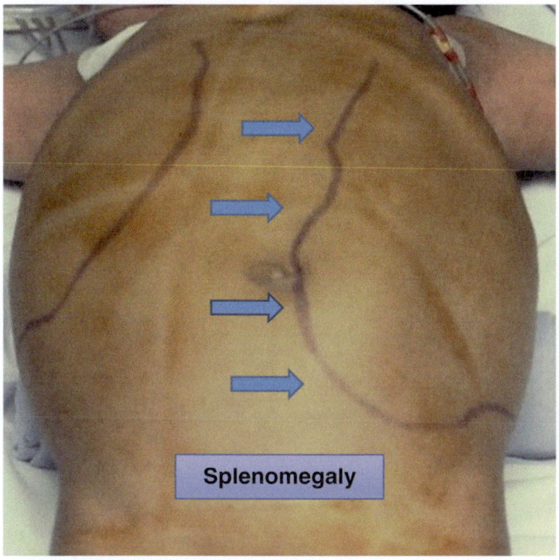

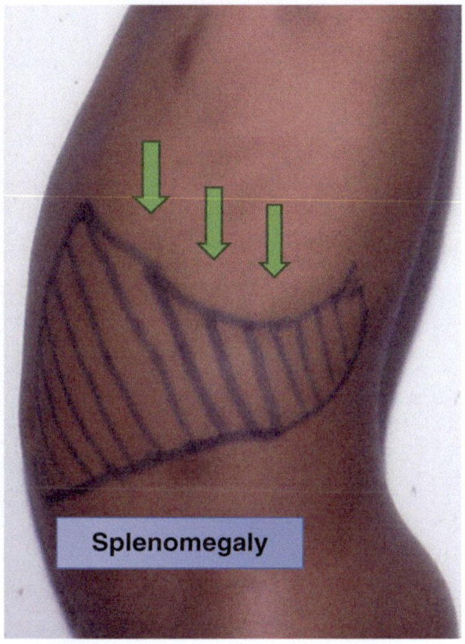

Figs. 4.3 and 4.4 Clinical photographs showing persistent splenomegaly in two patients with sickle cell anemia

- Persistence of splenomegaly in these patients is known to be associated with complications necessitating splenectomy (Figs. 4.3, 4.4, 4.5 and 4.6).
- These complications include:
  - Persistent splenomegaly with a non-functioning spleen
  - Acute splenic sequestration crisis (minor and major attacks)
  - Splenic abscess
  - Hypersplenism
  - Massive splenic infarction

Splenic Complications of Sickle Cell Anemia
- Persistent splenomegaly
- Acute splenic sequestration crisis (minor and major attacks)
- Splenic abscess
- Hypersplenism
- Massive splenic infarction

- Splenic sequestration crisis:
  - This occurs with highest frequency during the first 5 years of life in children with sickle cell anemia.
  - Splenic sequestration crisis can also occur at an older age group in those with persistent splenomegaly.

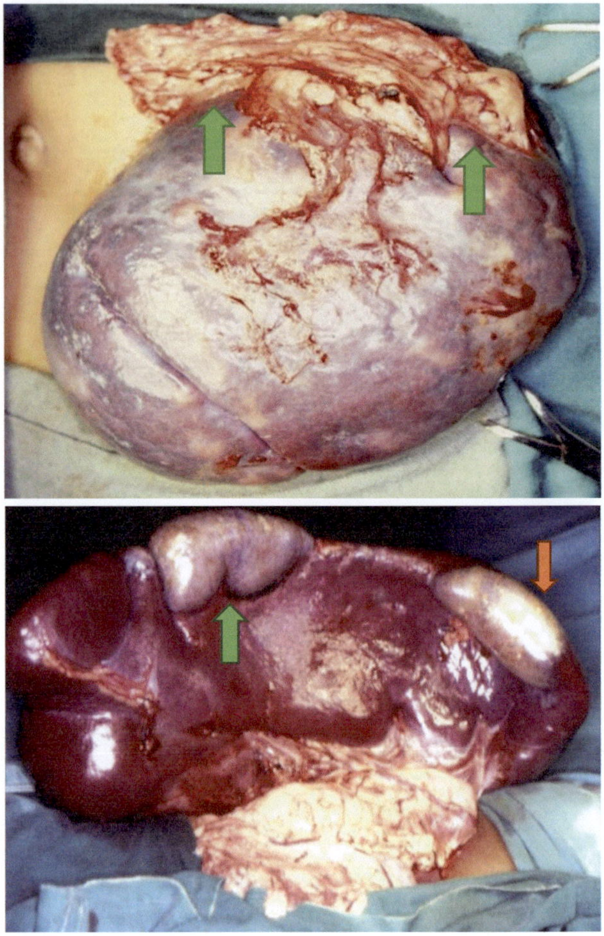

Figs. 4.5 and 4.6 Intra-operative photographs showing enlarged spleens with splenic infarcts. Note the omentum adherent to the splenic infarcts

- Acute splenic sequestration crisis and depending on the degree of anemia is divided into major and minor attacks.
- Acute splenic sequestration crisis is characterized by:

- The onset of life-threatening anemia especially in those with major splenic sequestration crisis where the hemoglobin level can drop to as low as 2 g/dl
- Sudden enlargement of the spleen
- High reticulocyte count
- Regression of the spleen size after blood transfusion
  - Acute splenic sequestration crisis is a medical emergency and considered the second leading cause of death following infection in children younger than 5 years of age.

- To obviate this, it is important to teach the mothers how to palpate the spleen and report to the hospital if there is sudden enlargement of the spleen.
- Treatment of acute splenic sequestration crisis requires early recognition, careful monitoring, and aggressive blood transfusion support.
- Because these episodes tend to recur, some advocate long-term blood transfusion to prevent recurrence.
- Others advocate splenectomy if the child develops one major or two minor sequestration crises.

Characteristics of Acute Splenic Sequestration Crisis

- Sudden onset of life-threatening anemia
- Sudden enlargement of the spleen
- High reticulocyte count
- Regression of the spleen size after blood transfusion

- Infection:
  - Children with sickle cell anemia are susceptible to recurrent attacks of infection.
  - This is because these patients develop functional asplenia early as a result of splenic vaso-occlusive crisis.
  - Add to this a defective immune response in these patients.
  - The increased risk of severe bacterial infections is also attributed to loss of functioning spleen as a result of autosplenectomy.
    - These infections are typically caused by encapsulated organisms such as *Streptococcus pneumoniae* and *Haemophilus influenzae.*
    - To obviate this, daily penicillin prophylaxis is commonly used during childhood.
    - Add to this the routine vaccination for *S. pneumoniae*, *H. influenzae*, *and* meningococci.
  - A variety of organisms cause infection in patients with sickle cell anemia, but organisms that pose the greatest danger include *Streptococcus pneumonia*, *Haemophilus influenza*, *and Salmonella.*
  - The mortality rate of such infections has been reported to be as high as 10–30 %.
  - *Staphylococcus* and *Salmonella* are the two most likely organisms responsible for osteomyelitis and septic arthritis in patients with sickle cell anemia. This is important when considering empirical antibiotic treatment.
  - Meningitis is 200 times more common in children with sickle cell anemia.

Major Infections in Patients with Sickle Cell Anemia

- Septicemia
- Pneumonia
- Meningitis
- Osteomyelitis
- Septic arthritis
- Splenic abscess

  - Treatment of infections in patients with sickle cell anemia depends on the site of infection and the likely organisms. Treatment includes:
    - Early recognition.
    - Aggressive diagnostic evaluation including CBC count, urinalysis, chest radiographs, and blood cultures.
    - Prompt administration of intravenous antibiotics. The antibiotic cover should be broad to cover *S. pneumonia* and other organisms.
    - Close observation.
    - Children younger than 12 months with a temperature higher than 39°C who appear toxic, with an infiltrate on chest radiograph and an elevated WBC count, should be admitted to the hospital.
    - Empirical antibiotics should be started early and should cover all possible organisms depending on the site of infection.

Causative Organisms of Major Infections in Patients with Sickle Cell Anemia

- *Streptococcus pneumoniae*
- *Haemophilus influenzae*
- *Meningococci*
- *Staphylococcus*
- *Salmonella*

- Acute chest syndrome:
  - Acute chest syndrome is a serious complication of sickle cell anemia and one of the causes of mortality (Figs. 4.7 and 4.8).
  - It is defined as a combination of respiratory symptoms, new lung infiltrates on chest X-ray, and fever.
  - The appearance of the lung infiltrate may be delayed and these patients should be followed up closely.
  - The lung infiltrate in patients with acute chest syndrome is usually progressive despite treatment with antibiotics.
  - Children have a higher incidence of acute chest syndrome but a lower mortality rate than adults.
  - In children, acute chest syndrome is usually due to infection. Other etiologies include pulmonary infarction and secondary fat embolism due to sickling with bone infarction.

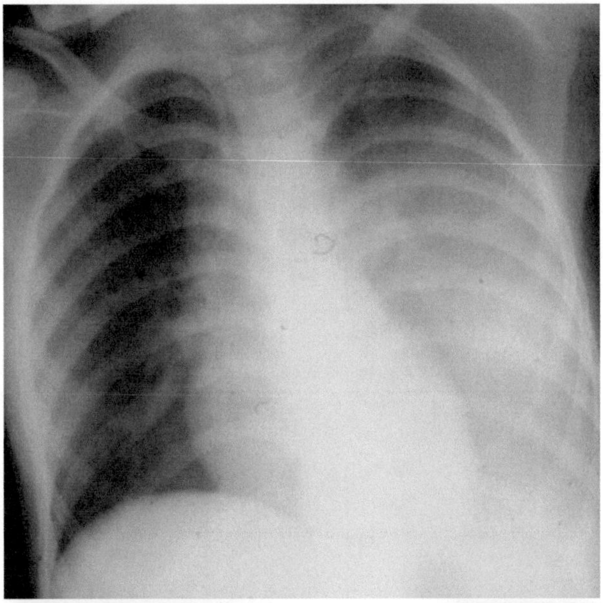

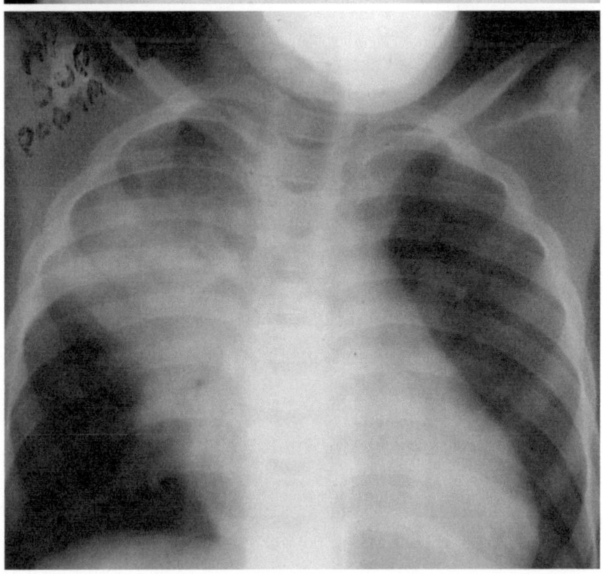

Figs. 4.7 and 4.8 Chest X-rays showing acute chest syndrome. Note the extent of the acute chest syndrome in the first and second chest X-ray

– Treatment of acute chest syndrome includes:
  - Close monitoring for hypoxemia.
  - Oxygen therapy.
  - Empiric treatment with intravenous antibiotics after appropriate cultures are obtained.
  - The antibiotics should be active against *S. pneumoniae* and chlamydial and mycoplasmal organisms.
  - The antibiotics are changed based on response to therapy and results of cultures and sensitivities.

- Patients with moderate or severe acute chest syndrome should be admitted to ICU for close monitoring and observation.
- Analgesics including acetaminophen and nonsteroidal anti-inflammatory drugs (NSAIDs) can be used. Narcotic agents may be used for more severe pain.
- Simple packed RBC transfusion can be used, and this may help prevent the progress of acute chest syndrome and respiratory deterioration.
- Exchange blood transfusion or erythrocytapheresis can be used in the more severe cases.
- Careful intravenous hydration to avoid volume overload, which may contribute to pulmonary infiltrates and exacerbate hypoxia.
- The role of corticosteroids in nonasthmatic patients with acute chest syndrome remains controversial.
- Respiratory decompensation can develop quickly in these patients and this requires mechanical ventilation.
- Acute chest syndrome is known to be recurrent, and one way to prevent this is to give chronic blood transfusion therapy to patients with recurrent acute chest syndrome.

- Stroke:
  - This results from progressive narrowing and occlusion of intracranial blood vessels.
  - This may lead to cerebral infarction in children and cerebral hemorrhage in adults.
  - Silent stroke also occur in patients with sickle cell anemia and usually causes no immediate symptoms but can cause brain damage.
    - Silent stroke is probably five times as common as symptomatic stroke.
    - About 10–15 % of children with SCA suffer strokes.
    - Silent strokes predominantly occur in younger patients.
- Cholelithiasis and biliary sludge (Figs. 4.9, 4.10, and 4.11):
  - Cholelithiasis results from excessive bilirubin production and precipitation due to prolonged hemolysis.
  - Cholelithiasis is common in patients with sickle cell anemia.
  - The frequency of cholelithiasis is variable but increases with age.
  - An overall of 19.7 % frequency of gallstones was reported in children with SCA. This frequency increased from 8.7 % in those less than 10 years of age to 36 % in those 15–18 years of age.
  - It is estimated that an overall 70 % of patients with SCA will develop gallstones at one stage of their life.
  - Laparoscopic cholecystectomy is advocated for those with cholelithiasis even if they are asymptomatic.

Complications of Cholelithiasis

- Choledocholithiasis
- Obstructive jaundice
- Acute and chronic cholecystitis
- Ascending cholangitis
- Acute pancreatitis

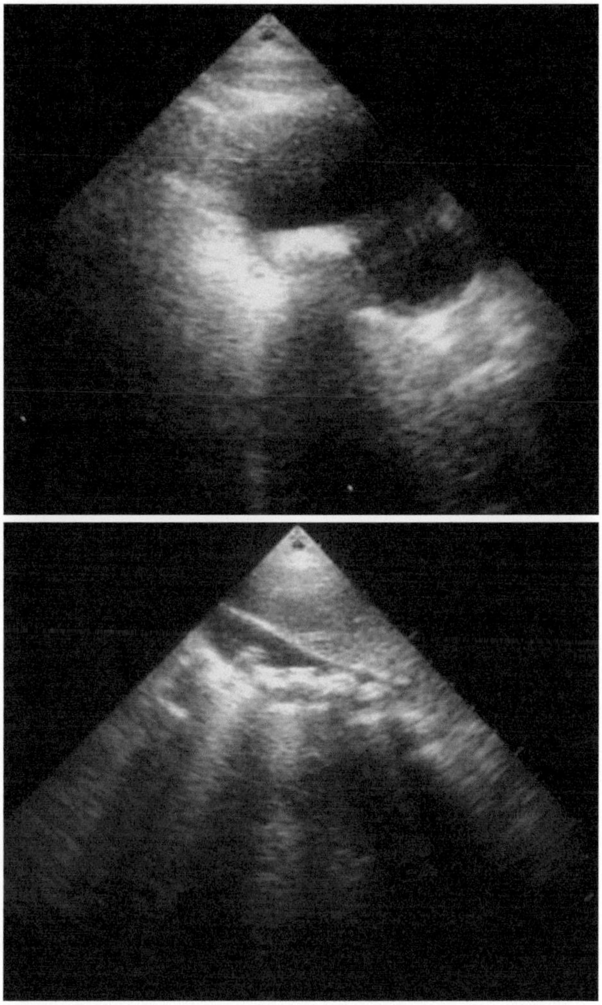

Figs. 4.9 and 4.10 Abdominal ultrasound showing a single and multiple gallstones in patients with sickle cell anemia

- Cholelithiasis can lead to:
  - Choledocholithiasis with or without obstructive jaundice (Figs. 4.12, 4.13 and 4.14)
  - Acute and chronic cholecystitis
  - Ascending cholangitis
  - Acute pancreatitis
- Biliary sludge is another common complication of sickle cell anemia.
- Biliary sludge is a mixture of calcium bilirubinate and cholesterol crystals within viscous bile that contains a high concentration of mucus and proteins.
- It can be seen in the gallbladder or sometimes in the bile ducts (Figs. 4.15, 4.16 and 4.17).
- A large number of sickle cell anemia patients with biliary sludge will develop gallstones, and these patients should be followed up closely.

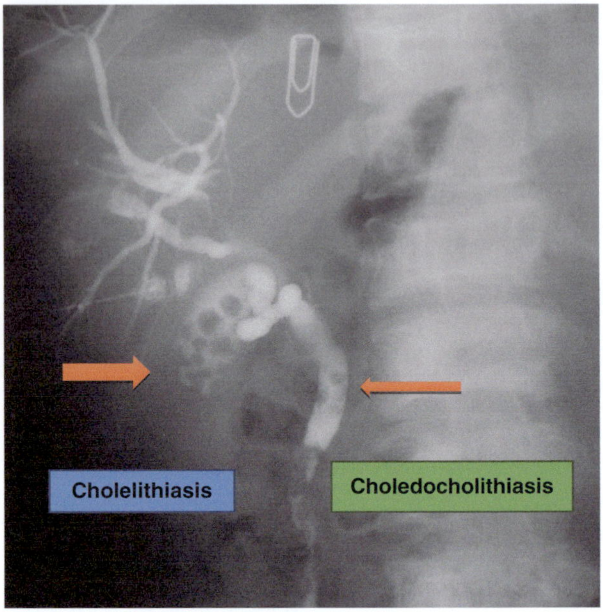

Fig. 4.11 A PTC (percutaneous transhepatic cholangiogram) showing cholelithiasis and choledocholithiasis

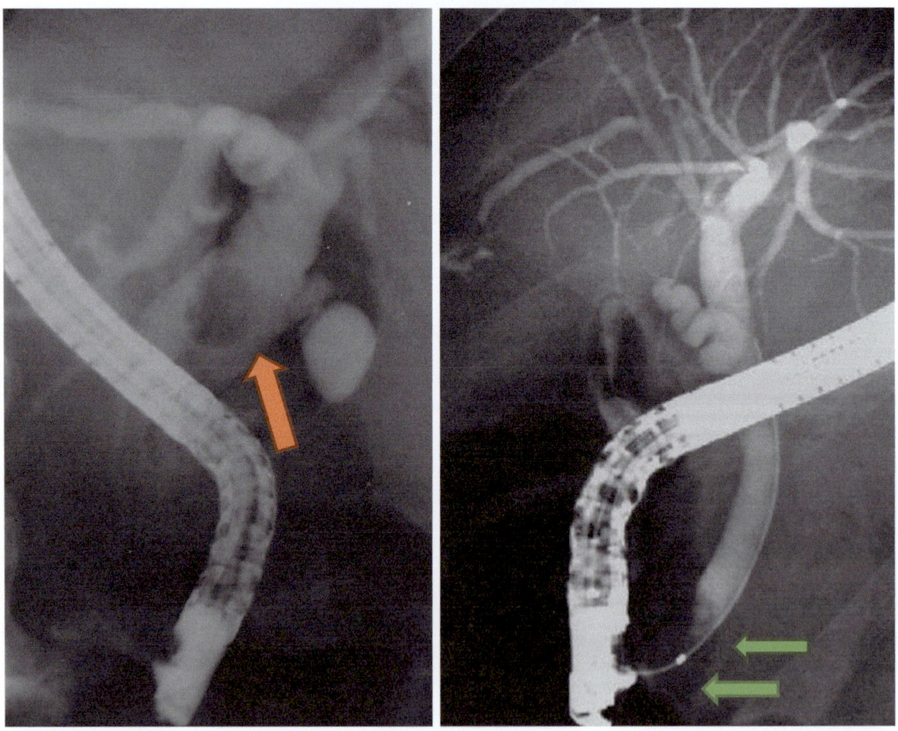

Figs. 4.12 and 4.13 Endoscopic retrograde cholangiopancreatography (EDCP) showing choledocholithiasis in two patients with sickle cell anemia

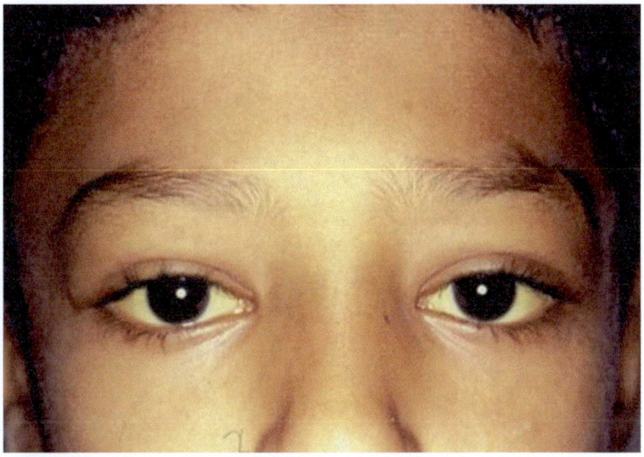

Fig. 4.14 A clinical photograph showing a child with sickle cell anemia and obstructive jaundice

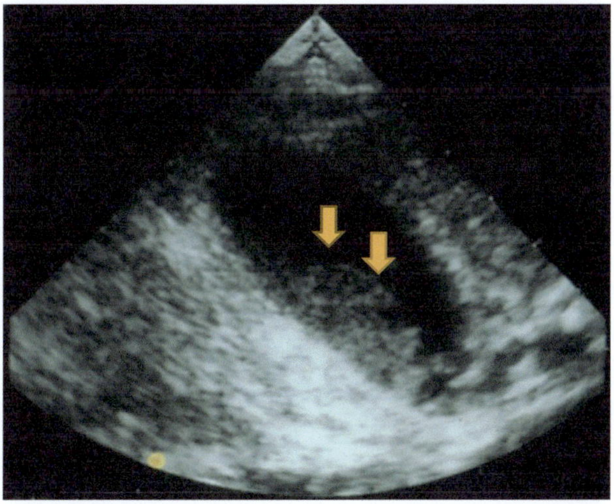

Fig. 4.15 Abdominal ultrasound showing biliary sludge in the gallbladder

- Avascular necrosis (Figs. 4.18, 4.19 and 4.20):
  - Avascular necrosis of the hip and other major joints may occur as a result of vaso-occlusive ischemia (Figs. 4.9 and 4.10).
  - This one of the severe complications of sickle cell anemia.
  - The hip joint is the most commonly affected joint.
  - Both hips can be affected simultaneously but the degree of affection is variable. Sometimes, one joint is affected more than the other one.
  - Other joints can be affected also including the shoulder, elbow, and spine.

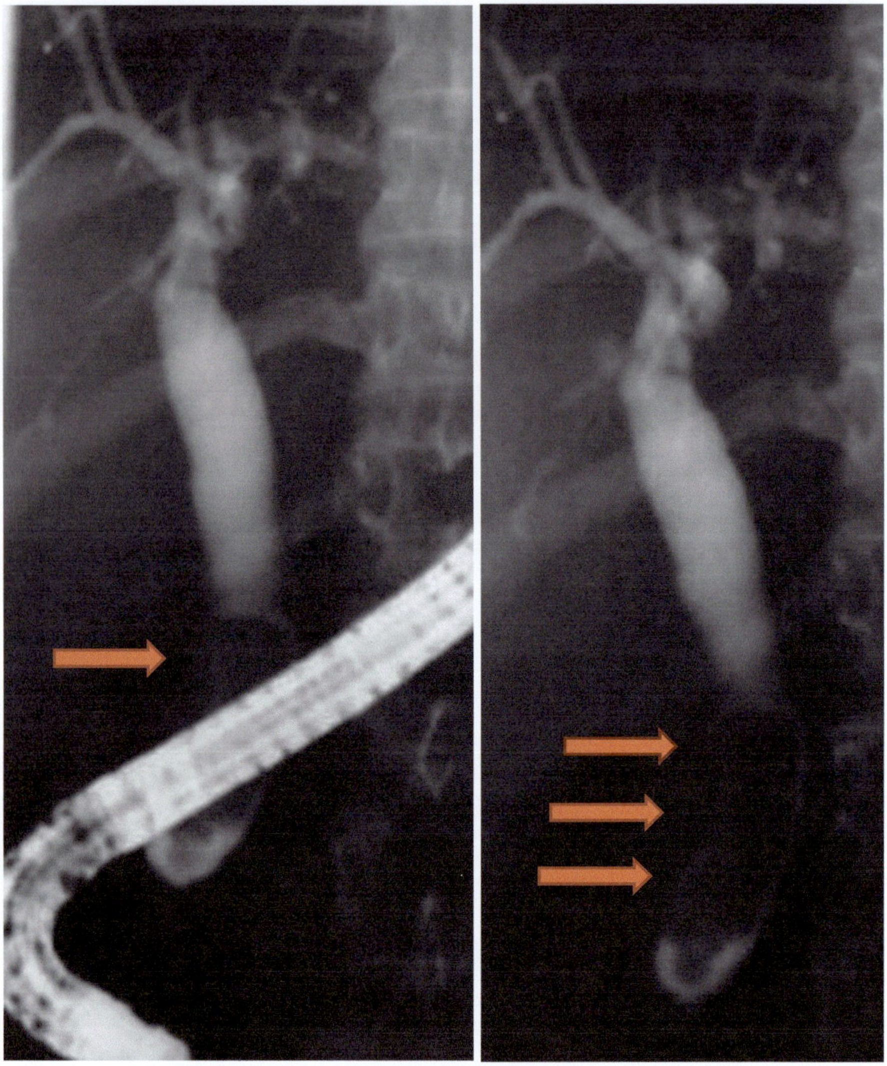

Figs. 4.16 and 4.17 ERCP (endoscopic retrograde cholangiopancreatography) showing biliary sludge in the common bile duct

- Priapism:
  - Priapism is defined as sustained painful erection without sexual desire (Figs. 4.21 and 4.22).
  - Early recognition and appropriate treatment of priapism in males with SCA is critical, as prolonged and/or repeated attacks of priapism can lead to ischemia and fibrosis in the corpora cavernosa of the penis.
  - This ultimately leads to impaired sexual function and impotence.

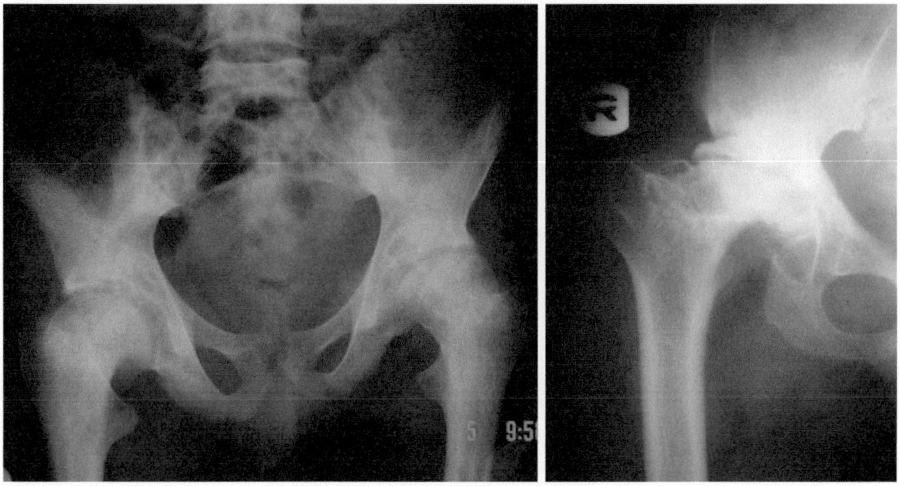

Figs. 4.18 and 4.19 X-rays showing avascular necrosis of the femoral head

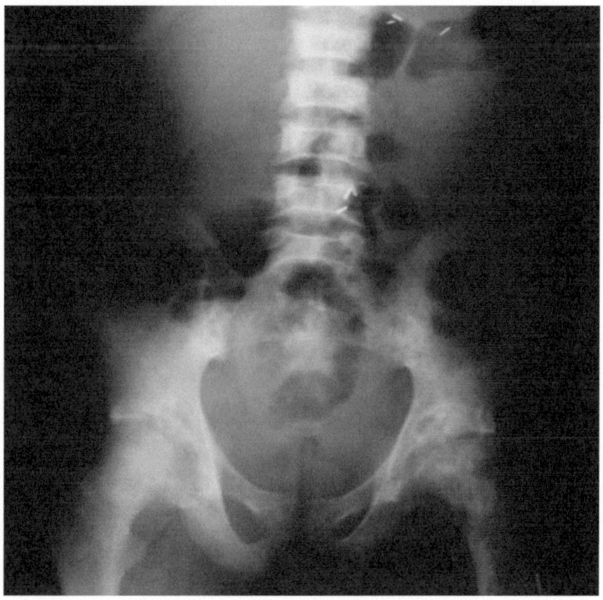

Fig. 4.20 Plain X-ray showing bilateral avascular necrosis of the hip joint. Note the left hip joint is affected more than the right joint

- Osteomyelitis and septic arthritis (Figs. 4.23, 4.24 and 4.25):
  - Osteomyelitis and septic arthritis are common complications of sickle cell anemia.
  - This is predisposed to by avascular necrosis and in the presence of bacteremia.
  - Normally, *Staphylococcus aureus* is the causative organism of osteomyelitis.

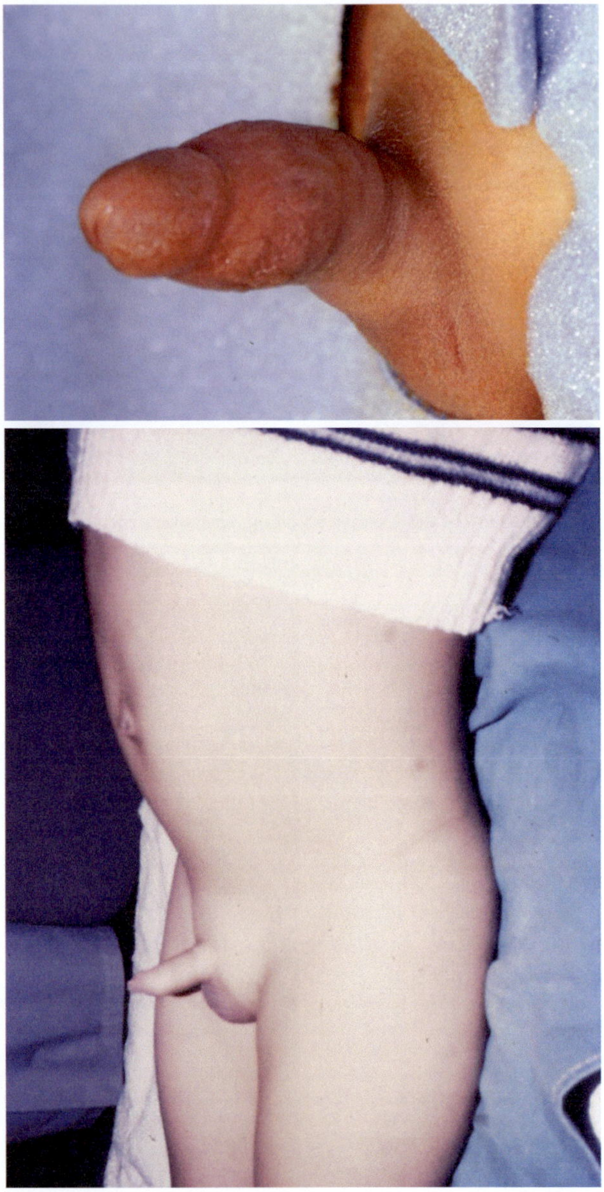

Figs. 4.21 and 4.22 Clinical photographs showing priapism in two children with sickle cell anemia

– The most common cause of osteomyelitis in SCA is *Salmonella* (especially the atypical serotypes *Salmonella typhimurium*, *Salmonella enteritidis*, *Salmonella choleraesuis*, and *Salmonella paratyphi* B), followed by *Staphylococcus aureus* and Gram-negative enteric bacilli.

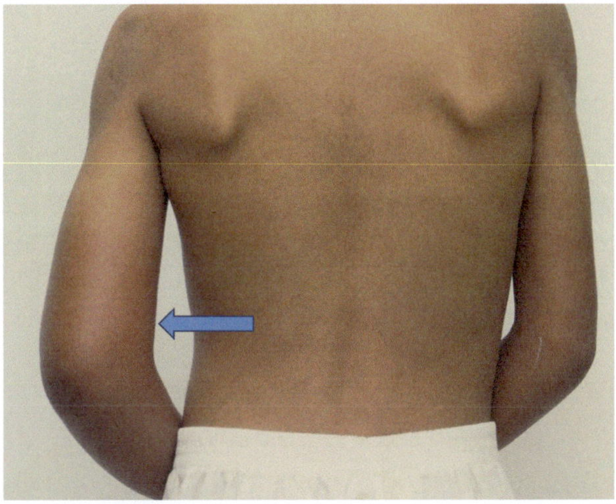

Fig. 4.23 A clinical photograph showing a child with sickle cell anemia and septic arthritis

Causative Organisms of Osteomyelitis and Septic Arthritis

- *Salmonella*
  - *Salmonella typhimurium*
  - *Salmonella enteritidis*
  - *Salmonella choleraesuis*
- *Salmonella paratyphi* B
- *Staphylococcus aureus*
- *Gram-negative enteric bacilli*

  - The reason for this predisposition to *Salmonella* and Gram-negative osteomyelitis and septic arthritis is not known exactly, but intravascular sickling of the bowel leads to patchy ischemic infarction and migration of organisms leading to bacteremia. In the presence of areas of bony avascular necrosis, osteomyelitis and septic arthritis may develop.
- Leg ulcers (Figs. 4.26 and 4.27):
  - Leg ulcers are a relatively common complication in patients with sickle cell anemia.
  - They are considered as markers of disease severity.
  - The incidence of leg ulcers is variable worldwide. It is commonly seen in African and Jamaican.
  - Leg ulcers are rarely seen before age of 10 years and commonly affect areas with less subcutaneous fat, thin skin, and decreased blood flow
- Eyes complications include:
  - Background retinopathy
  - Proliferative retinopathy

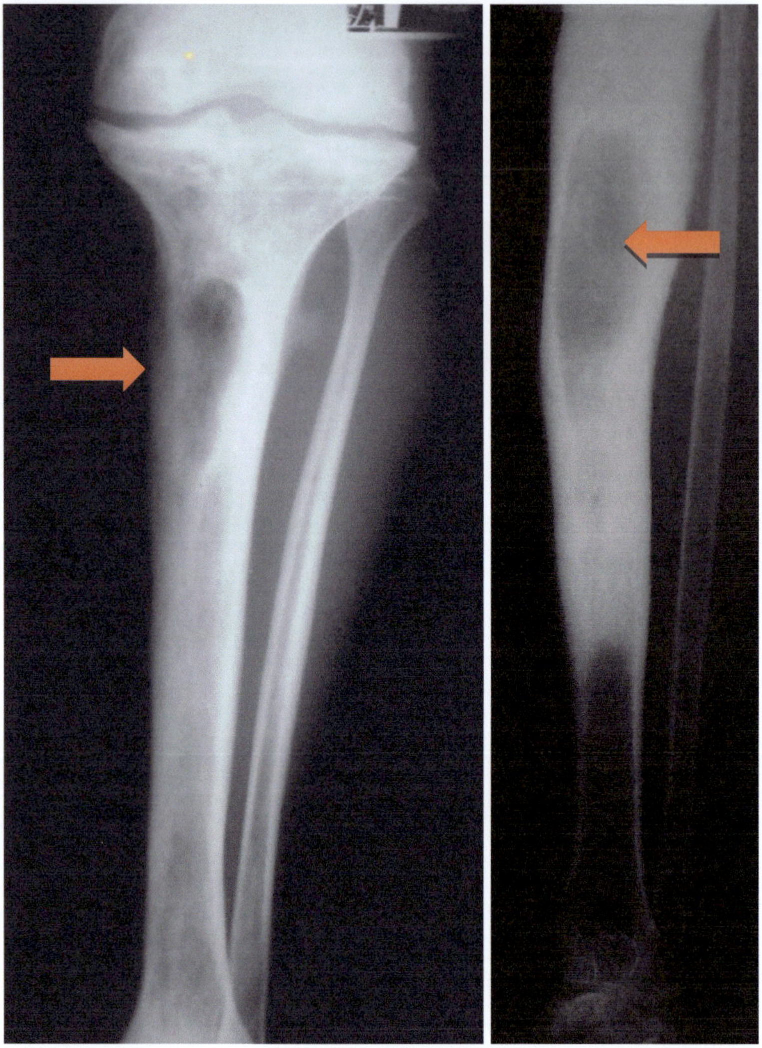

Figs. 4.24 and 4.25 A bony X-ray showing chronic osteomyelitis in a patient with sickle cell anemia. Note the cavity in the upper tibia

  - Vitreous hemorrhages
  - Retinal detachments
  - Blindness
- In patients with sickle cell anemia, pregnancy can be complicated by intrauterine growth retardation, spontaneous abortion, and preeclampsia.
- Many patients with sickle cell anemia complain of chronic pain even in the absence of acute vaso-occlusive crisis.
- Pulmonary hypertension is a well-known complication of sickle cell anemia.

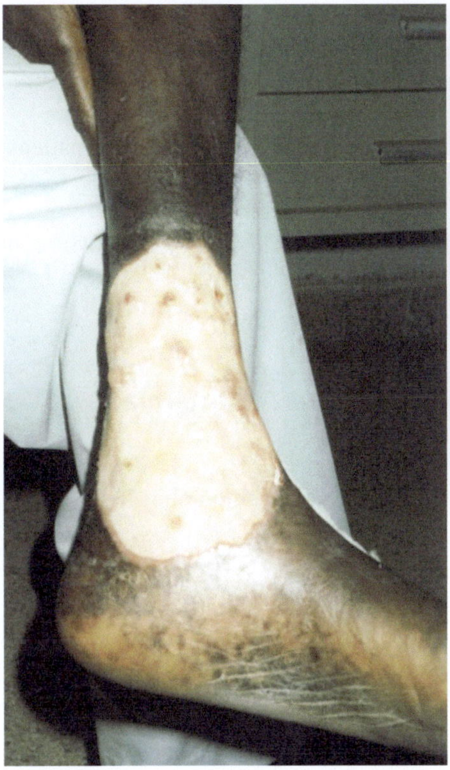
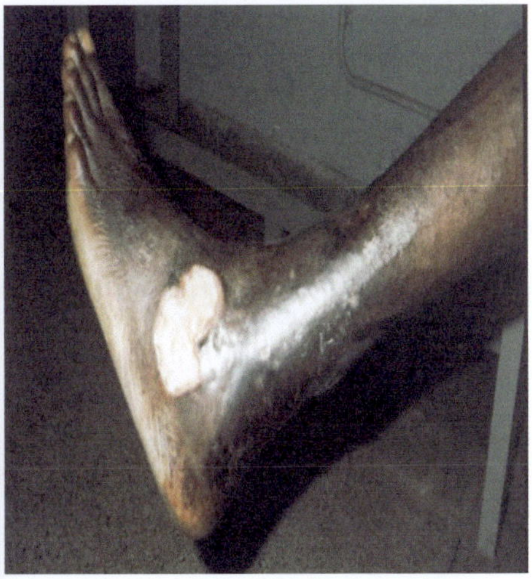

Figs. 4.26 and 4.27 Clinical photographs showing leg ulcers in patients with sickle cell anemia

- It is estimated that about 20 % of children and 30 % of adults with sickle cell anemia have evidence of pulmonary hypertension.
- This can lead to strain on the right ventricle and a risk of heart failure.
- The typical symptoms include shortness of breath, decreased exercise tolerance, reduced walking distance, and episodes of syncope.
- Pulmonary hypertension is known to be associated with increased mortality.

- Renal complications:
  - Acute papillary necrosis in the kidneys.
  - Sickle cell nephropathy can lead to chronic renal failure.
  - This manifests as hypertension, proteinuria, hematuria, and worsened anemia.
  - If it progresses to end-stage renal failure, it carries a poor prognosis.
- Cardiac and vascular complications:
  - Cardiac complications are common among patients with sickle cell anemia.
  - They are an important cause of the morbidity and mortality in patients with sickle cell anemia.
  - The anemia associated with sickle cell anemia results in an increase in cardiac output.

- As a result, the left ventricular stroke volume increases with significant dilation and hypertrophy of the left ventricle.
- The end result is an increase in LV mass and impaired LV filling and diastolic dysfunction.
- Vascular obstruction is a major cause of morbidity and mortality in patients with sickle cell anemia (Figs. 4.28 and 4.29).
- Vascular intimal hyperplasia, alone or associated with superimposed thrombosis, is an important cause of peripheral vascular occlusion in patients with SCA.

4.4 Investigations of Patients with Sickle Cell Anemia

- CBC:
  - The full blood count reveals chronic anemia with hemoglobin levels in the range of 6–8 g/dL.
  - A high reticulocyte count as a result of bone marrow compensation for the premature destruction of sickle cells.
  - Thrombocytosis may suggest hyposplenism or asplenia as a result of autosplenectomy.
  - A blood film may show target cells and Howell-Jolly bodies indicative of hyposplenism.
  - Elevated WBCs with increased neutrophils may suggest infection.
  - Sickling test:
    - Sickling of the red blood cells, on a blood film, can be induced by the addition of sodium metabisulfite.
    - The presence of sickle hemoglobin can also be demonstrated with the "sickle solubility test." A mixture of hemoglobin S (Hb S) in a reducing solution (such as sodium dithionite) gives a turbid appearance, whereas normal Hb gives a clear solution.
- Hemoglobin electrophoresis:
  - Abnormal hemoglobin forms can be detected on hemoglobin electrophoresis, a form of gel electrophoresis on which the various types of hemoglobin move at varying speeds.
  - Sickle cell hemoglobin (HgbS) and hemoglobin C with sickle cell anemia (HgbSC) can be identified.
  - The diagnosis can also be confirmed with high-performance liquid chromatography (HPLC).
  - Hemoglobin electrophoresis should be done on umbilical cord blood samples at birth to provide sickle cell anemia screening for all neonates at risk.
  - After infancy, hemoglobin electrophoresis will show approximately 90 % hemoglobin S (HbS), 2–10 % hemoglobin F (HbF), and a normal amount of minor fraction of adult hemoglobin (HbA2). Adult hemoglobin (HbA) is usually absent and starts to appear after the first 3 months of age.

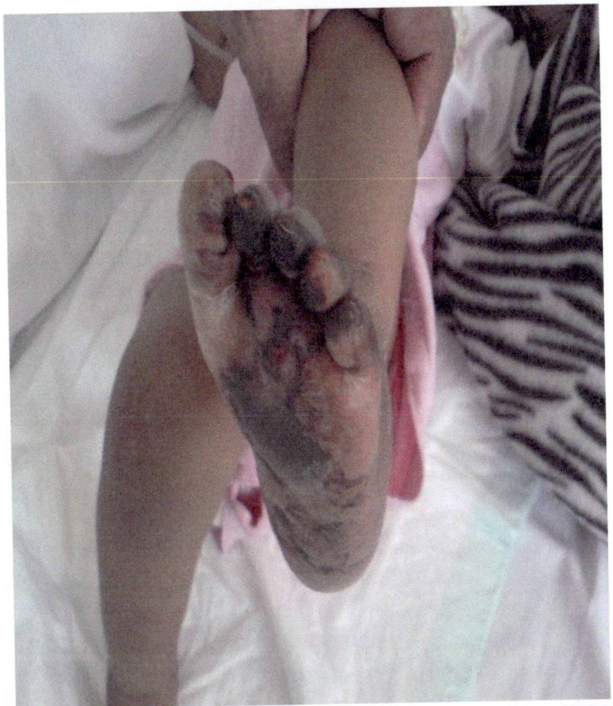

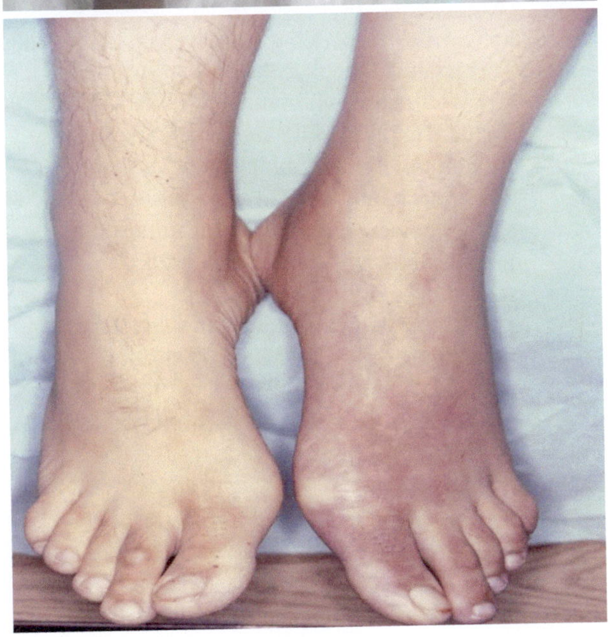

Figs. 4.28 and 4.29 Clinical photographs showing ischemia and gangrene in two patients with sickle cell anemia as a result of vascular occlusions

- Urine analysis and culture and sensitivity:
  - A urinalysis and culture and sensitivity to detect an occult urinary tract infection
  - Chest X-ray:
    - Chest X-ray to look for occult pneumonia
- Iron level:
  - The serum iron level is elevated.
  - This must be kept in mind especially in those receiving frequent blood transfusions.
  - Liver biopsy is a more accurate way of detecting iron overload.
- Genetic counseling:
  - Genetic counseling is important in those with sickle cell anemia to understand the risk of having a child with sickle cell anemia. This is also important in those planning to get married whether they have sickle cell anemia or sickle cell trait. The risks for future children being carriers or having sickle cell anemia should be explained to them. This is important and one way to decrease the frequency of sickle cell anemia by diluting the sickle cell gene.
  - In vitro fertilization using preimplantation genetic diagnosis is an alternative procedure that improves the chances that parents who both carry the sickle cell gene will have a child with normal hemoglobin. Fertilized eggs free of the sickle cell gene can be implanted into the mother for normal development. However, this procedure is expensive and not always successful.
- Brain:
  - Transcranial Doppler ultrasonography (TCD), MRI with or without angiography, and neuropsychometric (NPM) studies have been used extensively to evaluate children with sickle cell anemia.
  - An abnormally high blood flow velocity determined with TCD in the middle cerebral or internal carotid arteries is associated with an increased risk of stroke; however, blood flow results should be interpreted cautiously because they depend on the technique used.
  - Recommendations:
    - TCD screening of children with sickle cell anemia at the age 2 years and continued annually if TCD results are normal or every 4 months if TCD results are marginal.
    - Abnormal results should prompt a repeat TCD within 2–4 weeks.
  - A transfusion program reduces the risk of strokes in patients with abnormal TCD results.
  - Children with sickle cell anemia who have "silent" cerebral infarcts revealed with MRI have a higher rate of abnormal NPM findings and a higher risk of overt strokes.
  - Children with abnormal MRI or NPM findings may be evaluated more frequently and carefully and considered for therapeutic measures.
  - Newer techniques for noninvasive assessment of the brain have also been used to identify children with asymptomatic brain disease.

  - Transcranial near-infrared spectroscopy or cerebral oximetry is increasingly being used as a screening tool for low cerebral venous oxygen saturation in children with sickle cell anemia.
- Lungs:
  - Chest X-rays are valuable for the diagnosis and follow-up of patients with acute chest syndrome.
  - Children with sickle cell anemia frequently have abnormal pulmonary function test (PFT) results.
  - PFTs should be performed regularly in those with a history of recurrent acute chest syndrome or low oxygen saturation.
  - Because lung function declines with age, it is important to identify those who require close monitoring and treatment.
- Heart:
  - Echocardiography is an important investigation in those with suspected pulmonary hypertension based on tricuspid regurgitant jet velocity.
  - Patients with sickle cell anemia may also have an array of abnormalities of systolic and diastolic cardiac function.
- Abdominal ultrasonography:
  - This is important to visualize gallstones, common bile duct stones, and biliary sludge and to detect signs of possible cholecystitis.
  - Abdominal ultrasound is also important to assess spleen size and splenic complications of sickle cell anemia including splenic abscess and massive splenic infarction.

4.5 Management

- Children born with sickle cell anemia should be evaluated by a hematologist and kept undergo close observation.
- These patients should receive folic acid (1 mg) daily for life.
- To obviate infection, sickle cell anemia patients should be covered with daily penicillin from birth to 5 years of age.
- Patients with sickle cell anemia living in malarial endemic areas should receive antimalarial chemoprophylaxis for life.
- Anemia
  - Folic acid (1 mg/d) is commonly prescribed for patients with sickle cell anemia to prevent development of megaloblastic anemia due to increased folate requirements caused by RBC hemolysis.
  - Acute splenic sequestration crisis:
    - For those with acute splenic sequestration crisis, it is important to give red blood cell transfusions early to avoid progression and development of shock.
    - It is also important not to over transfuse them since the spleen may disgorge trapped cells, which can increase blood viscosity leading to complications.
    - An Hb around 10 g/dl is an acceptable posttransfusion level in these patients.

- Aplastic crisis is a self-limiting complication, but blood transfusion may be necessary in those with severe anemia causing dyspnea and signs of hypovolemia.
- Infection:
  - Penicillin prophylaxis is important in these patients and significantly reduces the incidence of *S. pneumoniae* infection and may decrease the mortality rate.
    - Penicillin prophylaxis should be started at age 2–4 months with 125 mg bid.
    - The dose is increased at 3 years of age to 250 mg bid.
    - Penicillin prophylaxis is continued till 5 years of age.
    - These patients are also given protein-conjugated pneumococcal vaccines (PCVs).
    - The 7-serotype PCV (PCV7) in combination with penicillin prophylaxis and PPV23 booster vaccination offers the best hope for improved prevention against *S. pneumoniae* infection in these patients.
    - Children with sickle cell anemia should also receive *H. influenzae* and meningococcal vaccines.
    - Antibiotic coverage should be started early in those with suspected infection.
- The goals of management of patients with sickle cell anemia are:
  - Symptomatic treatment
  - Management and prevention of SCA-related complications
- Treatment strategies include:
  - Management of vaso-occlusive crisis
  - Management of patients with chronic pain
  - Management of hemolytic anemia
  - Prevention and treatment of infections
  - Prevention of stroke
  - Detection and treatment of pulmonary hypertension
  - Management of the complications includes:
    - Acute chest syndrome
    - Acute splenic sequestration crisis
    - Priapism
    - Avascular necrosis
    - Osteomyelitis and septic arthritis
    - Leg ulcers
    - Ophthalmological complications
    - Splenic abscess
    - Massive splenic infarction
    - Cholelithiasis, choledocholithiasis, biliary sludge, acute cholecystitis, ascending cholangitis, and acute pancreatitis
    - Acute appendicitis, abdominal vaso-occlusive crisis, and ischemic colitis
    - Hepatic crisis
    - Cerebrovascular crisis

- Pain management:
  - Pain, resulting from vascular occlusion and ischemia, is the most common presentation of sickle cell anemia.
  - This can affect any part of the body.
  - Bone pain is often due to bone marrow infarction.
  - During the first 18 months of life, the metatarsals and metacarpals can be involved, presenting as dactylitis or hand-foot syndrome.
  - As the child grows older, pain often involves the long bones of the extremities.
  - During adolescence, pain often involves the vertebral bodies, especially in the lumbar region.
  - Abdominal pain can result from referred pain from other sites or intra-abdominal solid organs or soft tissue infarction.
  - Abdominal vaso-occlusive crisis can lead to reactive ileus, intestinal distention, and pain.
  - Painful vaso-occlusive crisis can be triggered by several factors including:
    - Hypoxemia secondary to acute chest syndrome or accompanying respiratory complications.
    - Dehydration and hemoconcentration.
    - Acidosis results in a shift of the oxygen dissociation curve (Bohr effect), causing hemoglobin to desaturate more readily.
    - Hypothermia leads to peripheral vasoconstriction.
  - Hydroxyurea may decrease the frequency and severity of painful vaso-occlusive crisis.
  - These patients should wear warm clothes to avoid hypothermia.
  - Chronic transfusion therapy designed to maintain the HbS concentration at less than 30 % may decrease the frequency of this painful vaso-occlusive crisis.
  - Pain is a common manifestation of patients with sickle cell anemia.
  - Mild attacks of pain can be treated at home with simple nonsteroidal anti-inflammatory medications. Mild narcotic analgesics can be used for pain that does not respond to lesser measures.
  - Moderate and severe pain will not respond to the above measures, and these patients should be hospitalized.
  - These patients should be treated with morphine or other major narcotic analgesics in doses sufficient to provide a reasonable degree of pain relief.
  - Continuous morphine infusion is considered effective in reducing the pain with a lesser dose of morphine.
  - A starting dose of morphine (0.05–0.01 mg/kg/h) is suggested following a bolus dose to provide a reasonable degree of pain relief. The dose is adjusted according to patient response, and overdose should be avoided as it can cause respiratory depression.
  - Patient-controlled analgesia and low-dose continuous intravenous (IV) infusion of morphine are effective and well accepted by patients.
  - Fentanyl and nalbuphine have also been used as continuous IV infusion.

  - Ketorolac can be given along with opioid analgesics and typically reduces the opioid dose required to achieve the desired effect.
  - Well-controlled and careful dosage of opioids does not cause dependency or addiction. The duration of sickle pain is usually short lasting 5–7 days, and a carefully designed analgesic regimen should avoid the problem of addiction.
- Acute chest syndrome:
  - The management of patients with acute chest syndrome depends on the severity of the attack, but the management includes:
    - The course of these patients is unpredictable, and so patient with acute chest syndrome should be admitted to the hospital for close observation, and if their condition deteriorates, they should be admitted to intensive care unit.
    - Antibiotics coverage.
    - Oxygen supplementation for those with hypoxia.
    - Close observation.
    - If the pulmonary infiltrate worsens or the oxygen requirements increase, these patients should receive simple blood transfusion or even exchange blood transfusion in severe cases.
  - Patients with moderate and severe acute chest syndrome should be admitted to ICU.
  - Obtain appropriate cultures.
  - Start empirical antibiotic treatment that covers *Streptococcus pneumoniae* and *Mycoplasma pneumoniae*.
  - Administer oxygen if saturation is less than 94 %.
  - Simple blood transfusion can be given in mild cases, but to those with severe acute chest syndrome, exchange blood transfusion should be given.
  - Avoid raising hematocrit to more than 36 % and aim to reduce the HbS level to 30 % in those receiving erythrocytapheresis or exchange transfusion.
  - These patients must be kept under close observation as acute chest syndrome can progress rapidly to respiratory failure necessitating ventilatory support.
  - Acute chest syndrome tends to be recurrent, and these patients should have chronic blood transfusion which was shown to reduce the recurrence of acute chest syndrome.
  - Hydroxyurea also reduces recurrence of acute chest syndrome.
- Stroke:
  - It has been estimated that approximately 11 % of patients with sickle cell anemia develop strokes before they reach age 20 years.
  - The deficit associated with these strokes is variable depending on the site of stroke, but convulsions and hemiparesis are the usual presentation.
  - Hemoconcentration secondary to rapid and excessive blood transfusion increases blood viscosity and can lead to stroke.
  - Silent brain infarcts occur in 17 % of patients with sickle cell anemia and may affect the cognitive function, with effects on learning and behavior in these patients.

  - Transcranial Doppler ultrasound (TCD) is used to identify children at high risk for stroke before they have suffered a clinical stroke.
  - Chronic blood transfusion therapy was shown to decrease the risk of stroke in children with abnormal TCD blood flow patterns, but once transfusion was stopped, an unacceptably high rate of TCD reversion to high risk was noted, as were actual strokes.
  - Chronic blood transfusion therapy has been shown to reduce the recurrence of stroke in patients with sickle cell anemia who already developed a stroke.
  - Many advocate lifelong blood transfusions to completely eliminate the risk of recurrences.
  - Hemorrhagic stroke is often caused by rupture of aneurysms that might be a result of sickle cell vasculopathy, and this tends to occur later in life.
  - Hemorrhagic stroke is associated with a mortality rate of more than 30 %.
  - Stroke is also known to be recurrent in patients with sickle cell anemia, and one way to prevent this is to subject these patients to chronic blood transfusion.
  - Unless long-term blood transfusion therapy is provided, 70–90 % of children who experience a single stroke have subsequent stroke.
  - The ultimate goal of chronic blood transfusion is to maintain the HbS level at less than 30 %.
  - A proliferation of small fragile vessels similar to moyamoya can be found in sickle cell anemia patients with stenotic lesions. This can also lead to cerebral hemorrhage.
- Cholelithiasis and cholecystitis:
  - Cholelithiasis is common in patients with sickle cell anemia.
  - In patients with sickle cell anemia, cholelithiasis develops a result of chronic hemolysis and increased bilirubin production.
  - The frequency of cholelithiasis in patients with sickle cell anemia is variable, but it increases with age.
  - It has been estimated that about 70 % of patients with sickle cell anemia develop cholelithiasis at one stage of their life.
  - Cholelithiasis can be complicated by acute or chronic cholecystitis or choledolithiasis and obstructive jaundice with the risk of ascending cholangitis.
  - Patients with cholelithiasis and acute cholecystitis should be treated with intravenous fluids and antibiotics, and once the patient improves, elective laparoscopic cholecystectomy should be done.
  - Laparoscopic cholecystectomy is now the procedure of choice to treat cholelithiasis in patients with sickle cell anemia even those with asymptomatic cholelithiasis.
  - Cholecystectomy is beneficial in these patients. Not only it will relief their symptoms but will also simplify their future management when they present with abdominal pain as the possibility of acute cholecystitis is eliminated.
- Avascular necrosis of the femoral or humeral head:
  - Avascular necrosis results from vascular occlusion and can affect commonly the femoral and humeral heads, but other sites can be affected also.

  - It has been estimated that about 30 % of all patients with sickle cell anemia will have avascular necrosis of the femoral head by age 30 years.
  - In patients aged 12 years or younger, treatment of avascular necrosis of the femoral head includes analgesics, NSAIDs, and protected weight bearing. This usually results in healing and remodeling of the involved capital epiphysis.
  - In adolescents and adults, conservative treatment is usually not successful and leads to progressive flattening and collapse of the femoral head with secondary degenerative arthritis.
  - These patients can be treated with core decompression and osteotomy in those who have precollapse femoral head involvement or hip replacement in those with already collapsed femoral head.
- Priapism:
  - Priapism is defined as a sustained, painful, and unwanted erection.
  - This is a well-recognized complication of sickle cell anemia, and if not recognized and treated early, it can lead to impotence.
  - The mean age at which priapism occurs is 12 years, and by the age 20 years, as many as 89 % of males with sickle cell anemia have experienced one or more episodes of priapism.
  - Priapism can be classified as:
    - Prolonged if it lasts for more than 3 h.
    - Stuttering if it lasts for more than a few minutes but less than 3 h and resolves spontaneously.
    - Stuttering episodes may recur or develop into more prolonged episodes.
  - Prolonged priapism is an emergency that requires immediate conservative and/or surgical treatment.
  - This should be taken seriously and treated aggressively.
  - The initial management includes:
    - Instruct the patients to drink extra fluids, use oral analgesics, and attempt to urinate.
    - A nightly dose of pseudoephedrine (30 mg orally [PO]) may prevent priapism in some cases.
    - For episodes that last more than 2 h, the patients should be admitted to the hospital for intravenous hydration and parenteral analgesia.
    - If priapism does not resolve within 1 h after admission (within 4–6 h of priapism onset), surgical intervention should be performed.
    - This includes penile aspiration followed by irrigation of the corpora with a 1:1,000,000 solution of epinephrine in saline.
    - Red blood cell exchange transfusions to reduce the HbS level to less than 30 % may also be considered, especially if irrigation fails.
  - In those who fail to respond to irrigation or if there is recurrence, a shunt procedure should be considered.
  - The Winter shunt is the commonly used procedure where a shunt is created between the glans penis and the distal corpora cavernosa. This allows blood from the distended corpora cavernosa to drain into the uninvolved corpus spongiosa.

  - Complications of priapism and treatment include:
    - Bleeding from the aspiration sites or shunt procedure
    - Infection
    - Skin necrosis
    - Damage or strictures of the urethra
    - Urethral fistulas
    - Impotence
  - If impotence persists for 12 months, the patient may wish to consider implantation of a penile prosthesis.
  - Recurrent episodes of priapism can result in fibrosis and impotence, even when adequate treatment is attempted.
  - Failure of conservative treatment calls for early surgical interventions including aspiration and irrigation or shunt procedure.
  - Chronic blood transfusion is advocated for those with recurrent priapism.
- Pulmonary hypertension:
  - This is a serious complication of sickle cell anemia.
  - It is an underestimated complication but being increasingly recognized with an estimated incidence as high as 25–35 %.
  - Pulmonary hypertension is characterized by a regurgitant pulmonary jet velocity of more than 2.5 m/s by echocardiography.
  - Pulmonary hypertension is known to be associated with a high mortality. This is especially more common in adults than in children.
- Hydroxyurea:
  - Hydroxyurea increases the production of fetal hemoglobin.
  - Hydroxyurea was shown to decrease the number and severity of attacks in patients with sickle cell anemia.
  - Hydroxyurea was also shown to decrease the frequency of hospital admissions, decrease the frequency of blood transfusions, and increase survival time.
- Transfusion therapy:
  - Blood transfusions are considered an important part in the management of patients with sickle cell anemia.
  - Blood transfusions are used to treat acute events of sickle cell anemia and also to prevent SCA-related complications.
  - Blood transfusion was shown to be beneficial in sickle cell anemia patients complaining of acute chest syndrome, acute splenic sequestration crisis, priapism, and stroke.
  - Prophylactic chronic red blood cell transfusion therapy has been shown to be beneficial in reducing the risk of first stroke or silent stroke when transcranial Doppler (TCD) ultrasonography shows abnormally increased cerebral blood flow velocities.
  - In those who have sustained a prior stroke, prophylactic chronic red blood cell transfusion therapy also reduces the risk of recurrent stroke and additional silent strokes.

  - Prophylactic chronic red blood cell transfusion therapy is also beneficial to reduce recurrent attacks of acute chest syndrome, splenic sequestration crisis, and recurrent priapism.
- Bone marrow and stem cell transplants:
  - Bone marrow transplants are the only cure available for patients with sickle cell anemia.
  - It has proven to be effective in children with sickle cell anemia.
  - Bone marrow transplants have limitations:
    - Bone marrow transplant is expensive.
    - It is not readily available and only specialized centers have this facility.
    - It is difficult to find a donor for bone marrow transplant because of the specific HLA typing.
    - Ideally, a twin family member or a close relative would donate the bone marrow necessary for transplantation which may not be easy.
    - Bone marrow transplant is also associated with a high incidence of complications and even mortality.
  - Stem cell transplantation is considered curative for patients with sickle cell anemia, but it is complex, expensive, and not readily available.
  - Another limitation is that donors must be human leukocyte antigen (HLA) compatible and candidates should be limited to patients younger than 16 years of age.
  - The current results are encouraging and report an event-free survival rate of approximately 84 % and a mortality rate of less than 6 %.
  - Candidates for stem cell transplantation should have evidence of disease severity demonstrated by the following:
    - Stroke
    - Recurrent acute chest syndrome
    - Recurrent severe painful crisis (>2 episodes/y for several years)
    - Recurrent priapism
    - Impaired neuropsychological function with evidence of cerebral infarction
    - Sickle cell nephropathy
    - Bilateral proliferative retinopathy and major visual impairment in at least one eye
    - Osteonecrosis of multiple joints
    - Red cell alloimmunization with more than two antibodies during long-term transfusion therapy
- Gene therapy:
  - In 2001 it was reported that sickle cell anemia had been successfully treated in mice using gene therapy.
  - The researchers used a viral vector to make the diseased mice produce fetal hemoglobin (HbF).
  - In humans, hydroxyurea is used to stimulate production of HbF. This is effective but only temporarily alleviates sickle cell anemia symptoms.

- The researchers demonstrated that this gene therapy method is a more permanent way to increase therapeutic HbF production.
- Clinical trials of gene therapy for sickle cell anemia in humans started in 2014 and are still going on.

4.6 Prognosis

- About 90 % of patients survive to age 20, and close to 50 % survives beyond the fifth decade.
- In 2001, according to one study performed in Jamaica, the estimated mean survival for sickle cell patients was 53 years old for men and 58 years old for women with homozygous SCD.
- The improved survival of patients with sickle cell anemia is attributed to several factors including:
  - Early diagnosis and better understanding of the pathophysiology of sickle cell anemia
  - Improved care given to these patients including immunization and antibiotic coverage
  - Development of new modalities of treatment both for acute management and prevention of complications including:
    - Blood transfusions
    - Hydroxyurea
  - Increased availability of bone marrow and stem cell transplantation

Further Readings

Adams RJ, McKie VC, Hsu L, et al. Prevention of a first stroke by transfusions in children with sickle cell anemia and abnormal results on transcranial Doppler ultrasonography. N Engl J Med. 1998;339(1):5–11.

Castro O, Brambilla DJ, Thorington B, et al. The acute chest syndrome in sickle cell disease: incidence and risk factors. The cooperative study of sickle cell disease. Blood. 1994;84(2):643–9.

Charache S, Terrin ML, Moore RD, et al. Effect of hydroxyurea on the frequency of painful crises in sickle cell anemia. Investigators of the multicenter study of hydroxyurea in sickle cell anemia. N Engl J Med. 1995;332(20):1317–22.

Gladwin MT, Sachdev V, Jison ML, et al. Pulmonary hypertension as a risk factor for death in patients with sickle cell disease. N Engl J Med. 2004;350(9):886–95.

Heeney MM, Ware RE. Hydroxyurea for children with sickle cell disease. Pediatr Clin North Am. 2008;55(2):483–501.

Hulbert ML, Scothorn DJ, Panepinto JA, et al. Exchange blood transfusion compared with simple transfusion for first overt stroke is associated with a lower risk of subsequent stroke: a retrospective cohort study of 137 children with sickle cell anemia. J Pediatr. 2006;149(5):710–2.

Onyekwere OC, Campbell A, Teshome M, et al. Pulmonary hypertension in children and adolescents with sickle cell disease. Pediatr Cardiol. 2008;29(2):309–12.

Platt OS, Brambilla DJ, Rosse WF, et al. Mortality in sickle cell disease. Life expectancy and risk factors for early death. N Engl J Med. 1994;330(23):1639–44.

Steinberg MH. Sickle cell anemia, the first molecular disease: overview of molecular etiology, pathophysiology, and therapeutic approaches. ScientificWorldJournal. 2008;8:1295–324.
Strouse JJ, Lanzkron S, Beach MC, et al. Hydroxyurea for sickle cell disease: a systematic review for efficacy and toxicity in children. Pediatrics. 2008;122(6):1332–42.
Stuart MJ, Nagel RL. Sickle-cell disease. Lancet. 2004;364(9442):1343–60.
Vichinsky EP, Haberkern CM, Neumayr L, et al. A comparison of conservative and aggressive transfusion regimens in the perioperative management of sickle cell disease. The preoperative transfusion in sickle cell disease study group. N Engl J Med. 1995;333(4):206–13.
Walters MC, Patience M, Leisenring W, et al. Bone marrow transplantation for sickle cell disease. N Engl J Med. 1996;335(6):369–76.
Wang WC, Helms RW, Lynn HS, et al. Effect of hydroxyurea on growth in children with sickle cell anemia: results of the HUG-KIDS study. J Pediatr. 2002;140(2):225–9.

The Spleen and Sickle Cell Anemia

5

5.1 Introduction

- The word spleen comes from the Greek σπλήν (*splḗn*) and is the idiomatic equivalent of the heart in English, i.e., to be good-spleened (εὔσπλαγχνος, *eúsplankhnos*) means to be good-hearted or compassionate.
- The spleen is considered part of the lymphatic system and resembles a large lymph node.
- It is the largest lymphoid tissue of the human body, accounting for 25 % of total body lymphocytes.
- The spleen is a valuable organ and should not be removed unless it becomes pathological (Figs. 5.1 and 5.2).
- The spleen, in healthy adults, is approximately 11 cm (4.3 in) in length.
- The spleen weight normally ranges from 150 g (5.3 oz.) to 200 g (7.1 oz.).
- The role of $1 \times 3 \times 5 \times 7 \times 9 \times 11$. This is an easy way to remember the anatomy of the spleen.
  - 1, 3, 5: the spleen is 1″ by 3″ by 5″ in size.
  - 7: the spleen weighs approximately 7 oz.
  - 9, 11: the spleen lies between the 9th and 11th ribs on the left side.
- The spleen is one of the commonly organs to be affected in patients with SCA.
- It enlarges early and then undergoes progressive atrophy as a result of repeated attacks of vaso-occlusive crisis leading to autosplenectomy. The spleen becomes shrunken and nonfunctional. The spleen may disappear completely or form a small fibrotic nodule. Sometimes the remnant of the spleen becomes calcified and takes different shapes (Figs. 5.3, 5.4, and 5.5).
- Splenomegaly however persists in some of these patients to an older age group and sometimes to adults.
- The reason for this is not known, but an elevated level of HbF is known to contribute to the persistence of splenomegaly in these patients (Figs. 5.6 and 5.7).
- Persistence of splenomegaly in these patients is known to be associated with complications necessitating splenectomy.

A. Al-Salem, *Medical and Surgical Complications of Sickle Cell Anemia*,
DOI 10.1007/978-3-319-24762-5_5

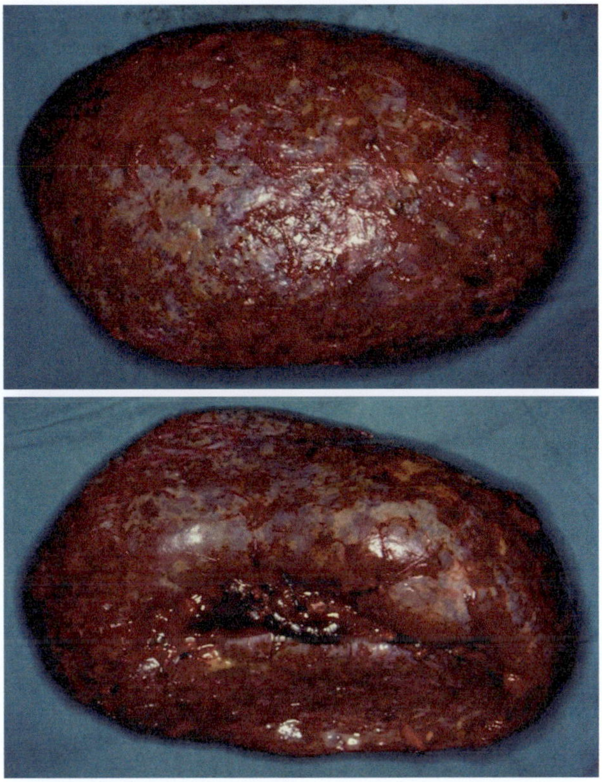

Figs. 5.1 and 5.2 Clinical photographs showing a pathological spleen in a patient with sickle cell anemia that was removed

- These complications include:
  - Acute splenic sequestration crisis
  - Splenic abscess
  - Massive splenic infarction
  - Hypersplenism

5.2 Embryology

- Normally, the gastrointestinal tract is derived from endoderm. The spleen is unique as it is derived from mesenchymal tissue.
- The spleen however shares the same blood supply where it receives its blood supply from the celiac trunk via the splenic artery and also the short gastric blood vessels.
- Embryologically, the spleen develops within and from the dorsal mesentery.
- The spleen appears about the 5th week of intrauterine life as a localized thickening of the mesoderm in the dorsal mesogastrium above the tail of the pancreas.

Figs. 5.3, 5.4, and 5.5 CT scan showing a small calcified spleen in patients with SCA

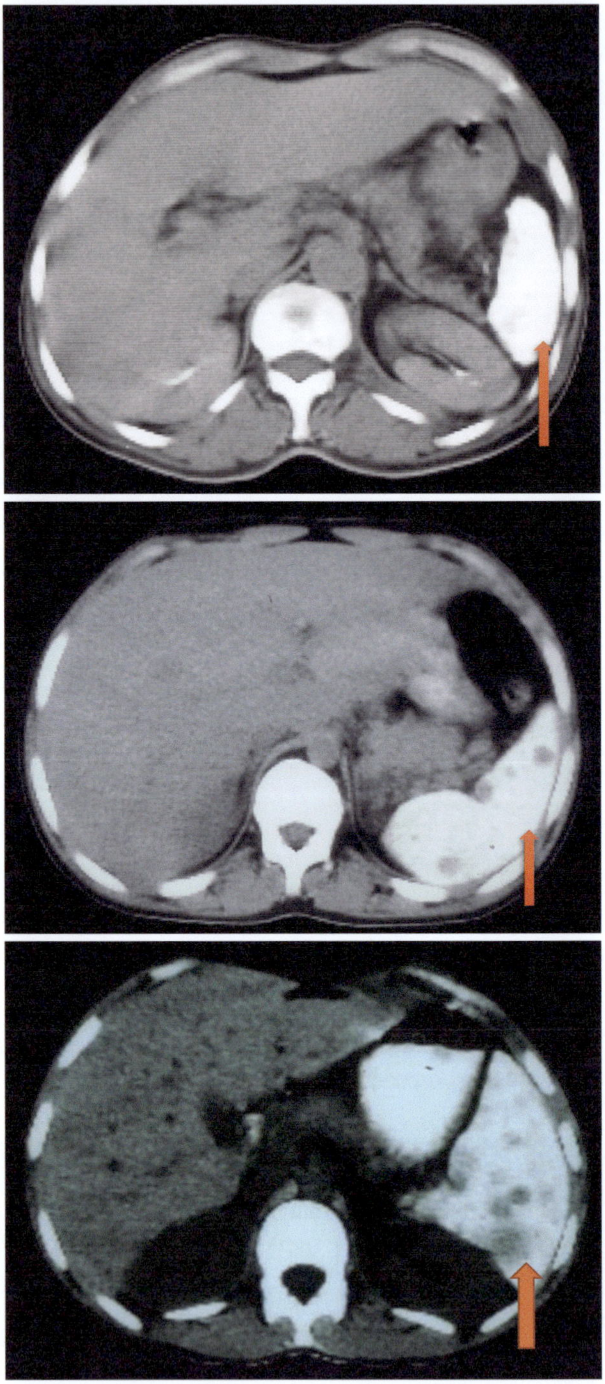

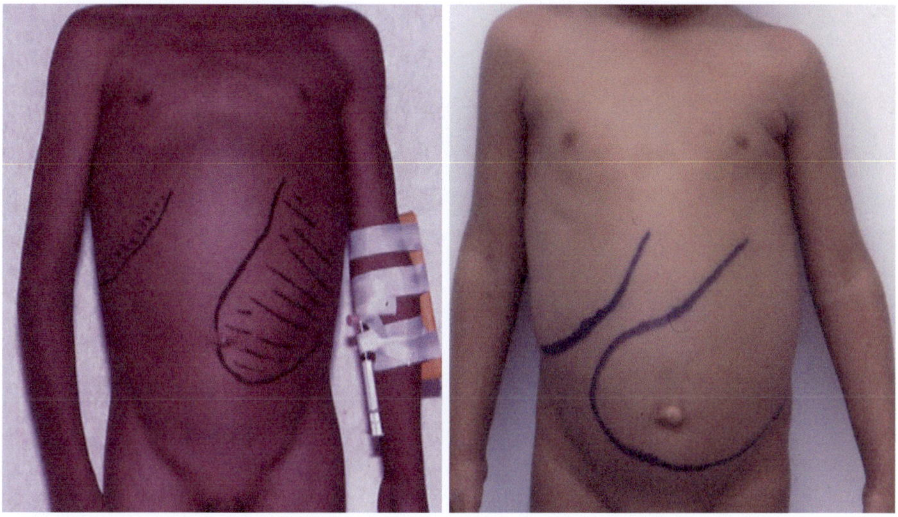

Figs. 5.6 and 5.7 Clinical photographs showing persistent splenomegaly in two patients with SCA

- As the stomach changes its position, the spleen moves to the left and comes to lie behind the stomach and in contact with the left kidney.
- The part of the dorsal mesogastrium which intervened between the spleen and the greater curvature of the stomach forms the gastrosplenic ligament.
- Histologically, the spleen is made of two parts:
  - The red pulp
  - The white pulp separated by the marginal zone
- Each part of the spleen has separate and important functions.
- Splenectomy should always be avoided, and every attempt should be made to preserve the spleen even traumatic rupture of the spleen.

5.3 Functions of the Spleen

- The red pulp:
  - This is made up of thin-walled venous sinusoids which are lined by special endothelial cells with a discontinuous wall allowing the passage of red blood cells between the sinuses and splenic cords.
  - The sinuses are separated by splenic cords (cords of Billroth) which contain macrophages.
  - The red pulp has the following important functions:
    - It filters red blood cells and ingests old RBC, damaged RBCs such as sickle cells or spherocytes, and antibody-coated RBCs.
    - It removes Heinz bodies and other RBC inclusions such as Howell-Jolly bodies.

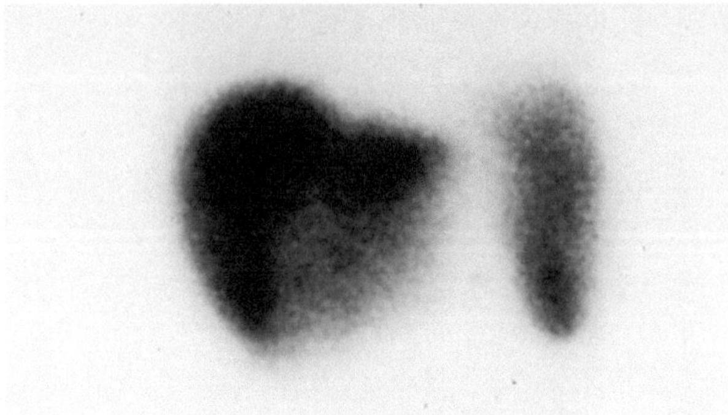

Fig. 5.8 A technetium sulfur colloid scan showing a normally functioning spleen in a patient with sickle cell anemia

- The white pulp:
  - This is made up of sheaths of lymphoid cells located around arteries (periarteriolar lymphatic sheath).
  - These sheaths are composed of T cells and lymphoid follicles (B cells) which traps antigens for processing.
  - The white pulp has the following functions:
    - It is responsible for the active immune response through both humoral- and cell-mediated pathways.
- Other functions of the spleen:
  - Production of opsonins, properdin, and tuftsin.
  - Natural antibodies are required for phagocytosis. These are immunoglobulins that facilitate phagocytosis either directly or by complement deposition on the capsule. They are produced by IgM memory B cells in the marginal zone of the spleen.
  - Production of red blood cells:
    - Normally, the bone marrow is the primary site of hematopoiesis, but the spleen has important hematopoietic functions up until the 5th month of gestation.
    - After birth, erythropoietic functions cease, except in some hematologic disorders.
    - As a major lymphoid organ and a central player in the reticuloendothelial system, the spleen retains the ability to produce lymphocytes and, as such, remains a hematopoietic organ.
  - Storage of red blood cells, lymphocytes, and other formed elements.
  - The red blood cells can be released when needed.
  - It has been estimated that in humans, up to a cup (236.5 ml) of red blood cells can be stored in the spleen and released in cases of hypovolemia.
  - It can store platelets in case of an emergency.
  - Up to a quarter of lymphocytes can be stored in the spleen at any one time.
  - The presence of Howell-Jolly bodies and less commonly Heinz bodies in the blood smears is an indication of decreased or absence of splenic function, but an isotope scan (technetium sulfur colloid scan) is more important to evaluate the function of the liver and spleen (Fig. 5.8).

5.4 Post-splenectomy Complications

- An increase in white blood cells.
- An increase in platelets. The post-splenectomy platelet count may rise to abnormally high levels (thrombocytosis), leading to an increased risk of potentially fatal clot formation or portal vein thrombosis.
- An increase in the number of Howell-Jolly bodies and less commonly Heinz bodies in the blood smears. Heinz bodies are usually found in cases of G6PD (glucose-6-phosphate dehydrogenase) deficiency and chronic liver disease.
- A diminished responsiveness to some vaccines.
- An increased susceptibility to infections by bacteria and protozoa; in particular, there is an increased risk of post-splenectomy sepsis from polysaccharide encapsulated bacteria such as pneumococci.

5.5 Immunizations and Splenectomy

- Splenectomy is known to be associated with an increased risk of sepsis due to encapsulated organisms (such as *S. pneumoniae* and *Haemophilus influenzae*).
- These patients especially children should receive immunization prior to splenectomy.
- These vaccines include:
  - Pneumococcal vaccine
  - Meningococcal vaccines
  - Haemophilus influenza type b vaccine
- These vaccines should be given at least 2 weeks prior to splenectomy and followed subsequently by poster doses.
- If splenectomy is done for an emergency reason, these vaccines can be given postoperatively.
- Children who undergo splenectomy should also receive prophylactic antibiotics for a minimum of 2 years depending on their age at the time of splenectomy.
- This is in the form of penicillin prophylaxis either orally or intramuscularly. Oral penicillin is preferable.
- This is because overwhelming post-splenectomy sepsis is commonly seen within the first two years post-splenectomy.

5.6 Splenic Complications of Sickle Cell Anemia

- SCA is known to affect any part of the body and poses diagnostic and therapeutic dilemmas to the treating physicians.
- The spleen is one of the most common and early organs to be affected in SCA.
- It is commonly enlarged during the first decade of life but then undergoes progressive atrophy as a result of repeated attacks of vaso-occlusion and infarction leading to autosplenectomy.

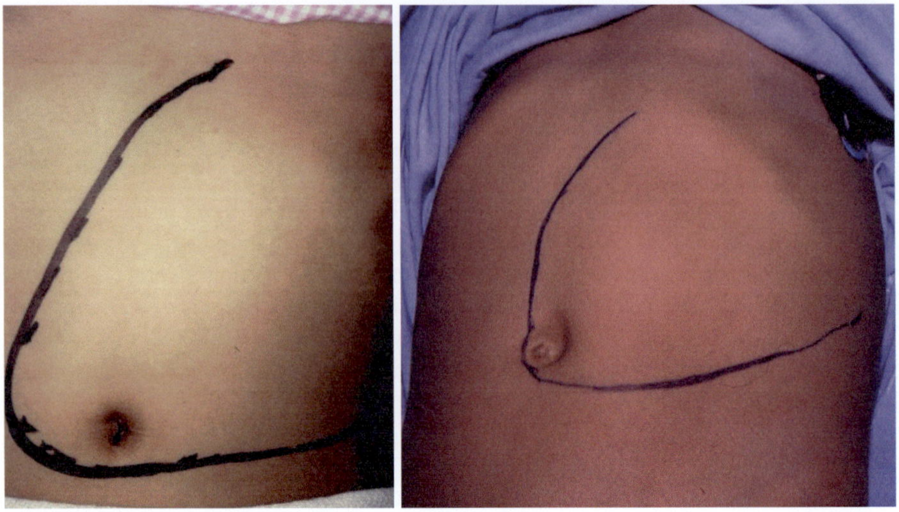

Figs. 5.9 and 5.10 Clinical photographs showing persistent splenomegaly in two patients with sickle cell anemia

- This however is not the case always, and sometimes splenomegaly persists into an older age group or even into adulthood necessitating splenectomy for a variety of reasons including (Figs. 5.9 and 5.10):
  - Acute splenic sequestration crisis
  - Hypersplenism
  - Massive splenic infarction
  - Splenic abscess
  - Splenomegaly with a nonfunctional spleen

Splenic Complications of Sickle Cell Anemia

- Acute splenic sequestration crisis (major and minor)
- Hypersplenism
- Massive splenic infarction
- Splenic abscess
- Persistent splenomegaly with a nonfunctional spleen

- Splenic complications of SCA are associated with an increased morbidity, and in some it may lead to mortality.
- To obviate this, splenectomy is an essential part of their management (Figs. 5.11 and 5.12).
- Obviously, splenectomy does not cure SCA, but it is valuable and in certain patients may be an essential part of their management.

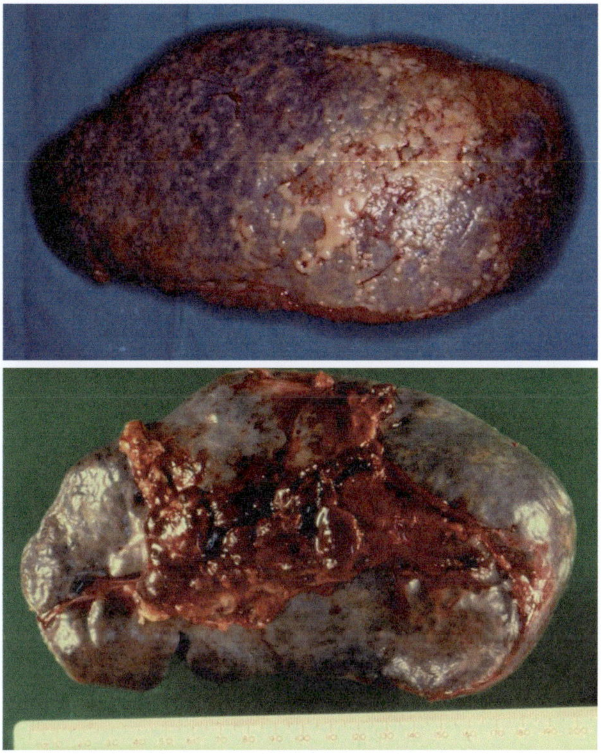

Figs. 5.11 and 5.12 A clinical photograph showing a removed spleen in a patient with sickle cell anemia. Note also the multiple infarcts

5.7 Acute Splenic Sequestration Crisis

- Acute splenic sequestration crisis (ASSC) results from the rapid sequestration of red blood cells in the spleen (Fig. 5.13, 5.14 and 5.15).
- In ASSC, there is good inflow of blood into the spleen, but the blood outflow from the spleen is obstructed as result of occlusion of the splenic vein by sickled RBCs. This will lead to pooling of blood into the spleen sinusoids leading to anemia and sometimes hypovolemia.
- It is a serious complication of SCA and considered the second leading cause of death after infection in the first decade of life.
- ASSCs are usually seen in infants and young children commonly between 5 months and 2 years of age.
- This however is not the case always, and ASSC can be seen in older patients with persistent splenomegaly. The exact reason for this is not known. One contributing factor is persistence of splenomegaly in these patients into an older age group. This is partly attributed to persistently high hemoglobin F level in these patients.

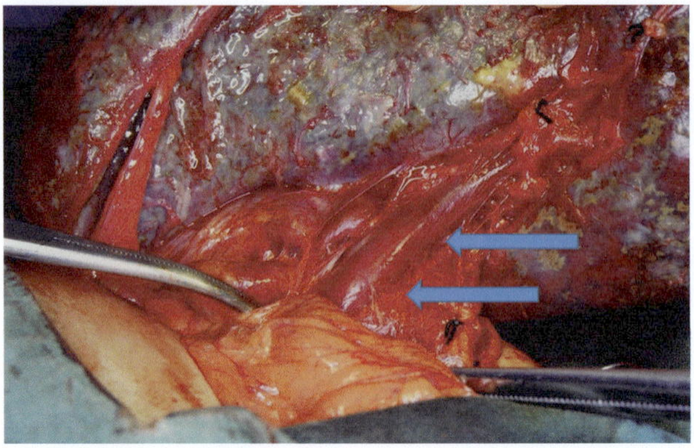

Fig. 5.13 A clinical intraoperative photograph showing enlarged spleen with multiple small infarcts in a patient with SCA and acute splenic sequestration crisis. Note the enlarged congested splenic vein

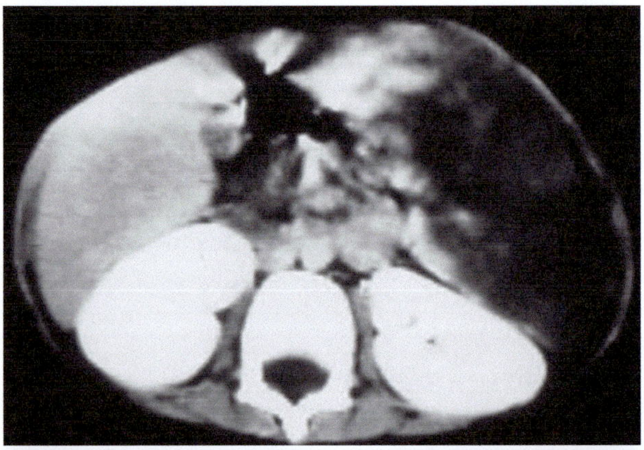

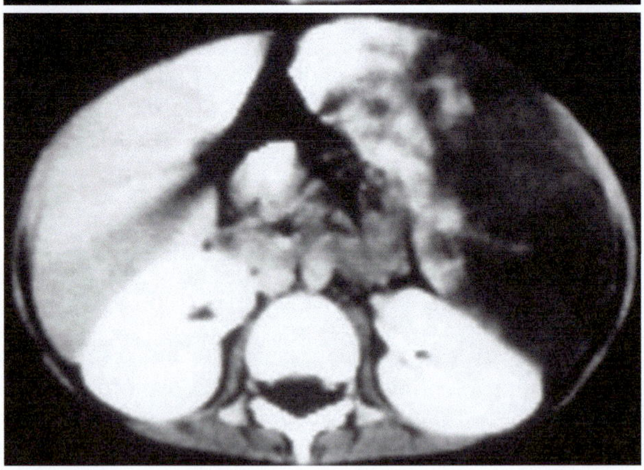

Figs. 5.14 and 5.15 CT scan showing acute splenic sequestration crisis. Note the spleen enlarged and filled with sequestered blood

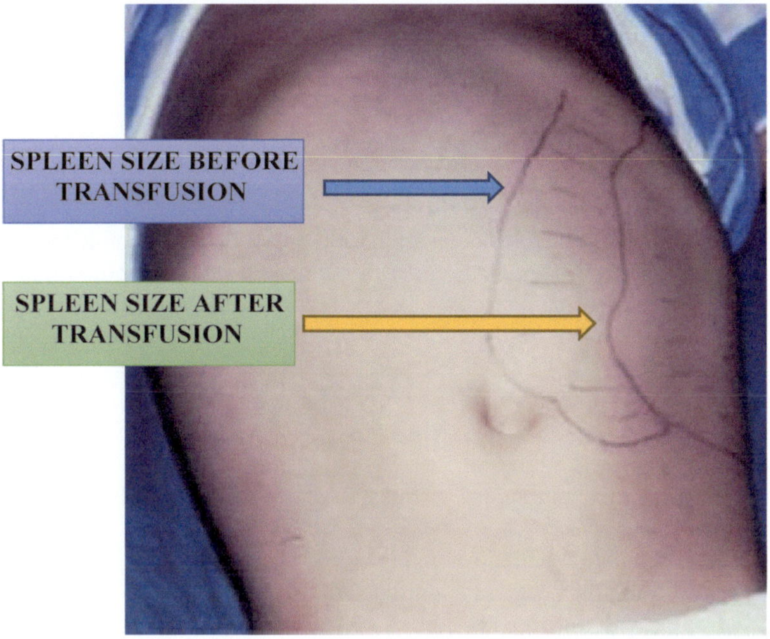

Fig. 5.16 A clinical photograph of a child with sickle cell anemia and acute splenic sequestration crisis. Note the regression of the size of the spleen following blood transfusion

- Acute splenic sequestration crisis is characterized by:
  - Sudden onset of anemia.
  - Sudden splenomegaly or an enlargement of an already enlarged spleen.
  - Evidence of active bone marrow.
  - The spleen size regresses after blood transfusion (Fig. 5.16).

Characteristics of Acute Splenic Sequestration Crisis
- Sudden onset of life-threatening anemia
- Sudden enlargement of the spleen
- High reticulocyte count
- Regression of the spleen size after blood transfusion

- This differentiates ASSC from hypersplenism where the spleen size is chronically enlarged and does not regress after blood transfusion.
- Acute splenic sequestration crisis is divided depending on the severity of the attack into:
  - Minor attack
  - Major attack
- Minor attacks are characterized by:
  - A moderate increase in the size of the spleen
  - A sudden drop of hemoglobin of 2–3 g/dl

- Major attacks are characterized by:
  - A significant sudden increase in spleen size
  - A greater drop of hemoglobin sometimes decreasing to as low as 2–3 g/dl
  - Hypovolemia
- The cause of ASSC is not known, but an association with upper respiratory tract infection suggesting a precipitating viral cause was proposed. This includes infection with human *Parvovirus* B19.
- The diagnosis of ASSC is clinical and based on sudden onset of anemia, sudden enlargement of the spleen, and regression of spleen size after blood transfusion. In these patients, it is important to keep a record of the spleen size in each visit to the clinic or hospital. This will help to recognize a sudden enlargement of the spleen.
- CBC will show anemia. The severity of anemia depends on the type of ASSC. CBC will also show reticulocytosis. The WBC and platelets may also decrease.
- The treatment of acute splenic sequestration crisis is initially supportive and includes:
  - Clinical evaluation and close monitoring.
  - Patients with major attacks should be admitted to ICU.
  - Hydration with intravenous fluids.
  - Blood transfusion with packed red blood cells. It is important to avoid over transfusing these patients as this with lead to increase in blood viscosity with its associated risks. It is also important to remember that blood is stored in the spleen and once blood transfusion is given, some of this blood will be released into the circulation which can also lead to an increase in blood viscosity. The aim should be to increase the hemoglobin level to around 10–11 g/dl.
  - It is important to teach the parents how to palpate the spleen in their affected children and recognize sudden enlargement. They should report to the hospital early if they recognize sudden enlargement.
  - These patients should be immunized with pneumococcal, meningococcal, and *H. influenzae* vaccines.

Types of Acute Splenic Sequestration Crisis

- ASSC is divided depending on the severity of the attack into:
  - Minor attack
  - Major attack
- Minor attacks are characterized by:
  - A moderate increase in the size of the spleen
  - A sudden drop of hemoglobin of 2–3 g/dl
- Major attacks are characterized by:
  - A significant sudden increase in spleen size
  - A greater drop of hemoglobin sometimes decreasing to as low as 2–3 g/dl
  - Hypovolemia

- The indication for splenectomy in major attacks is well established. Splenectomy is indicated if the child develops one major attack.
- Major ASSC is a serious complication that is associated with a high mortality. To obviate this, the parents should be taught how to palpate the spleen and report quickly to the hospital if they recognize sudden enlargement.
- The role of splenectomy in minor attacks is still controversial.
- Some advocate chronic blood transfusion as a therapy to prevent recurrent attacks. This is effective on the short term, but it is not without risks including allosensitization, hepatitis, iron overload, and other blood-borne infections. The duration of chronic blood transfusion is not known. Add to this the fact that a significant number of patients on chronic blood transfusion therapy developed ASSC when attempts were made to stop blood transfusion or shortly after completing the program. The fact that blood is not readily available, it is not without complications, and poor compliance of parents makes chronic blood transfusion unsuitable form of therapy in these patients.
- Others advocate splenectomy if the child develops two minor attacks. This is to obviate a recurrence risk of 40–50 % and a mortality rate as high as 20 %.

5.8 Hypersplenism

- Hypersplenism is arbitrarily defined as:
  - Splenomegaly with:
  - Anemia (when the transfusion requirements exceed 250 ml/kg of packed red blood cells per year)
  - Thrombocytopenia (when the platelet level is less than 100,000/mm^3)
  - Neutropenia (when the white blood cell count is less than 4000/mm^3)
  - Either singly or in combination
- Splenomegaly in hypersplenism is persistent to differentiate it from acute splenic sequestration crisis.
- These hematological changes normalize following splenectomy.
- The incidence of hypersplenism is relatively low in patients with sickle cell anemia. The reason for this low incidence of hypersplenism in is not known, but early autosplenectomy in these patients is a contributing factor.
- In the past minor ASSCs were confused with hypersplenism, but when strict definition criteria are applied, hypersplenism is relatively rare in patients with sickle cell anemia.
- Hypersplenism is more commonly seen in sickle B$^+$ thalassemia patients. This confirms the observation that patients with sickle B$^+$ thalassemia tend to behave more like thalassemia.
- To obviate the risk of overwhelming post-splenectomy infection (OPSI), a variety of treatment modalities other than total splenectomy have been proposed to treat patients with hypersplenism. These include:
  - Chronic blood transfusions
  - Partial splenectomy
  - Percutaneous intraluminal occlusion of the splenic artery
  - Embolic therapy

Hypersplenism

Splenomegaly associated with:

- Anemia: transfusion requirements exceed 250 ml/kg of packed red blood cells per year
- Thrombocytopenia: < 100,000/mm^3
- Neutropenia: < 4000/mm^3

Either singly or in combination

- Chronic blood transfusion has its own complications including:
  - Alloimmunization, which occurs in up to 20 % of multiply transfused patients.
  - Transmission of blood-borne infections including hepatitis B and C and acquired immune deficiency.
  - Iron overload.
  - The poor compliance of parents and the fact that blood is not readily available make this form of therapy unsuitable for some patients.
- Partial splenic embolization, although has been shown to be safe and reliable method of treatment of hypersplenism, is associated with complications which makes it unsuitable form of treatment for patients with SCA.
- Splenectomy in SCA patients with hypersplenism was shown to be beneficial in decreasing their transfusion requirements and eliminating the discomfort from mechanical pressure of the enlarged spleen. In post-splenectomy, there is a significant increase in the hemoglobin level, platelets, and white blood cells and a significant decrease in the levels of reticulocytes. Splenectomy however is known to be associated with an increased risk of post-splenectomy sepsis.
- Partial splenectomy is a valuable alternative to total splenectomy.
- Partial splenectomy preserves part of the spleen that protects them from overwhelming post-splenectomy sepsis.
- This however is temporary as the spleen remnant tends to grow with recurrence of hypersplenism. Add to this the fact the spleen is nonfunctional in a large number of patients with sickle cell anemia. Partial splenectomy may be valuable in children who are younger than 2 years old and require splenectomy. These children are at higher risk of post-splenectomy sepsis and partial splenectomy will be protective and buy them sometime.

5.9 Splenic Abscess

- Splenic abscess is rare accounting for 0.14–0.7 % of necropsy specimens.
- Recently, there is a change in the spectrum of splenic abscess with emergence of unusual causative organisms as well as more cases being described in immunocompromised patients.
- Several factors have been described to predispose to splenic abscess, but sepsis is the commonest predisposing factor, with infective endocarditis being the commonest.

- Splenic abscess is very rare in patients with SCA as these patients tend to have early autosplenectomy.
- Persistence of splenomegaly, however, predisposes them to the development of splenic infarction. The early development of functional asplenia makes them liable to systemic infections and in the presence of splenic infarction predisposes them to the development of splenic abscess.
- Splenic abscess remains a diagnostic challenge. This is specially so in children with SCA who frequently present with fever due to other infective causes and abdominal pain which is commonly attributed to vaso-occlusive crisis. This as well as the rarity of splenic abscess leads to the delay in diagnosis.
- Physicians caring for these patients should be aware of such a complication, and the possibility of splenic abscess should be considered in children with SCA who present with fever and abdominal pain specially if found to have a tender enlarged spleen.

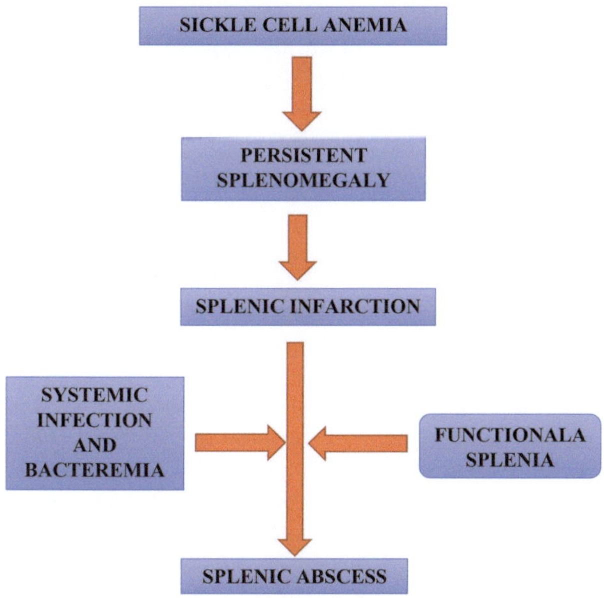

- Presentation:
  - The presentation of splenic abscess is variable, and a high index of suspicion is important for early diagnosis and treatment.
  - These patients usually present with fever and left upper quadrant abdominal pain. Most of these patients will be already on antibiotics for some other reason which may mask their fever.
  - They usually have a tender enlarged spleen.

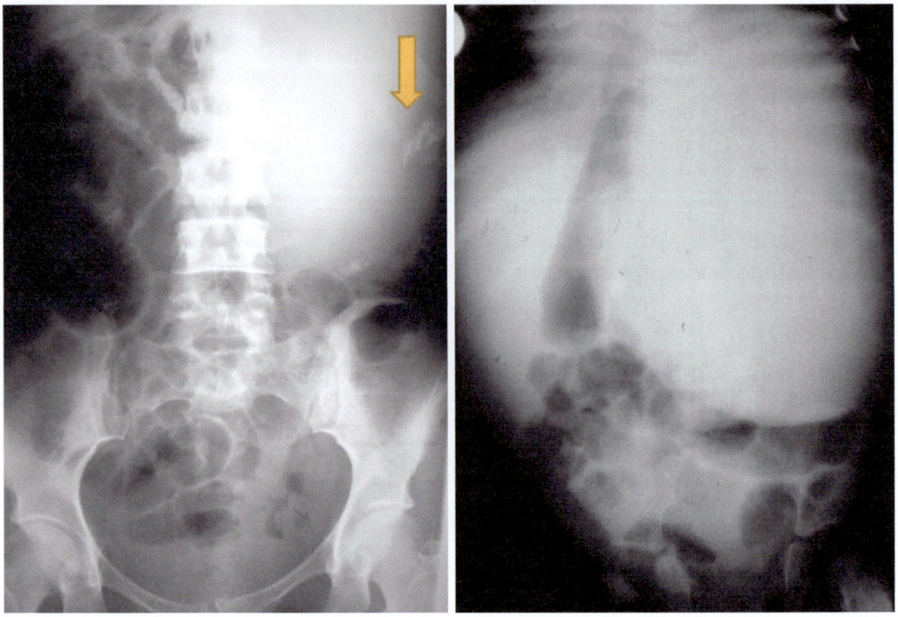

Figs. 5.17 and 5.18 Abdominal radiographs showing left upper quadrant soft tissue density in two patients with splenic abscess. Note the calcification in the first photograph

- Diagnosis:
  - Chest and abdominal X-rays:
    - These may reveal a soft tissue density in the left upper quadrant and elevated left hemidiaphragm with or without left pleural effusion (Figs. 5.17, 5.18, 5.19, 5.20, and 5.21).
  - The use of abdominal ultrasound should be liberal in these patients as it is simple, noninvasive, and easily repeatable investigation, and if in doubt, the diagnosis can be confirmed by abdominal CT scan.
  - Although abdominal ultrasound is diagnostic, CT scan is more valuable as it allows more accurate anatomical localization of site and size of the abscess (Figs. 5.22, 5.23, 5.24, 5.25, 5.26, 5.27, 5.28 and 5.29).
- The size of the splenic abscess is variable. Sometimes the whole spleen is replaced by an abscess.
- Occasionally, part of splenic tissue is found in the middle of the abscess cavity like a sequestrum (Figs. 5.30, 5.31, 5.32 and 5.33).
- *Salmonella* is known to cause a variety of infections in patients with SCA including septic arthritis, osteomyelitis, and septicemia.
- This is of paramount importance when considering antibiotic coverage as empirical antibiotic therapy should include antibiotics against *Salmonella* till the culture and sensitivity results become available.

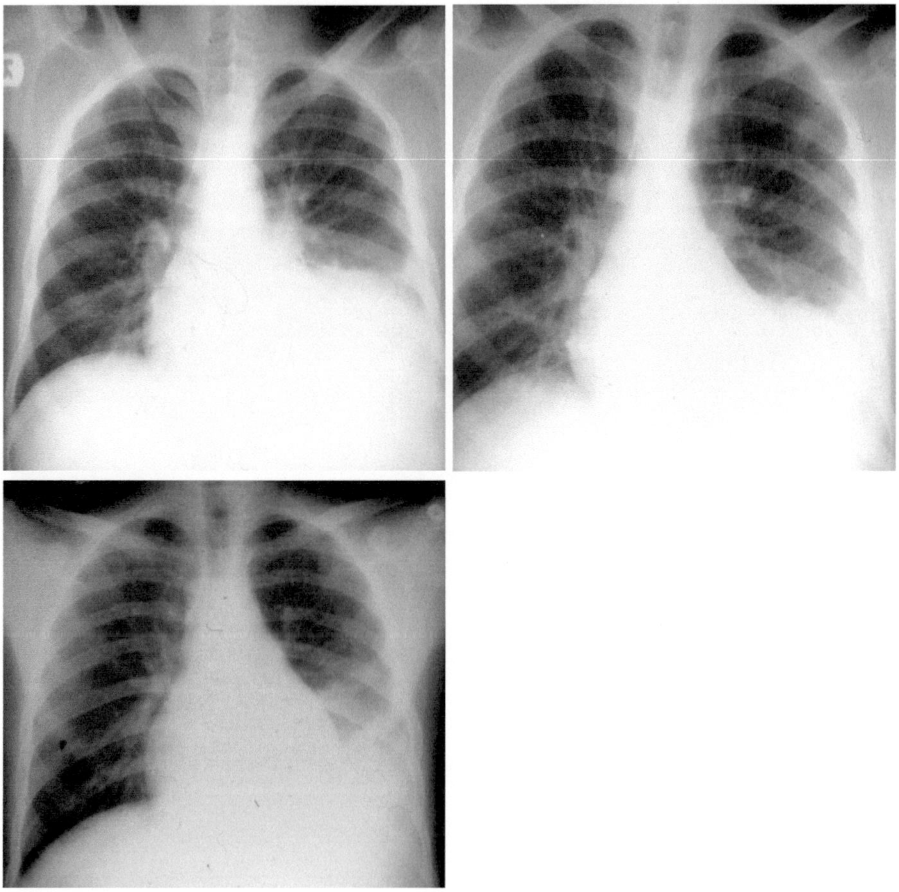

Figs. 5.19, 5.20, and 5.21 Chest X-rays in three patients with sickle cell anemia and splenic abscess. Note the elevated left hemidiaphragm and mild left pleural effusion

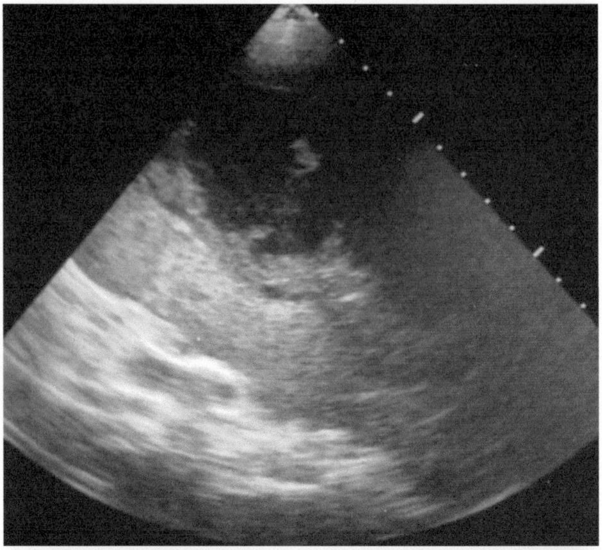

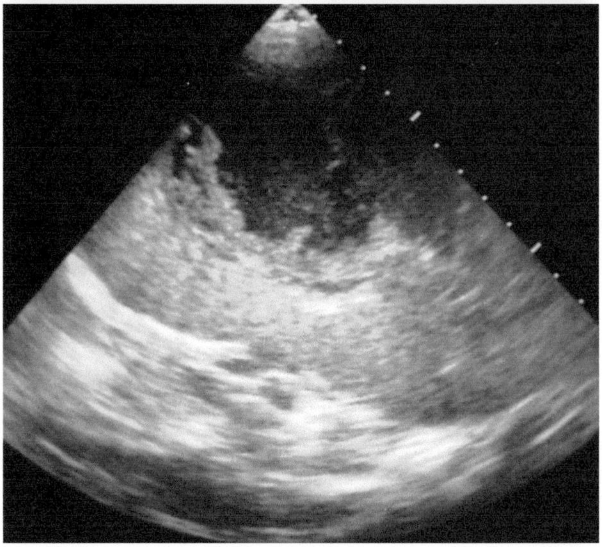

Figs. 5.22 and 5.23 Abdominal ultrasounds showing large splenic abscess

Figs. 5.24 and 5.25 Abdominal CT scans showing splenic abscess in patients with SCA. Note the splenic sequestrum in the left photographs and calcification in the right photograph

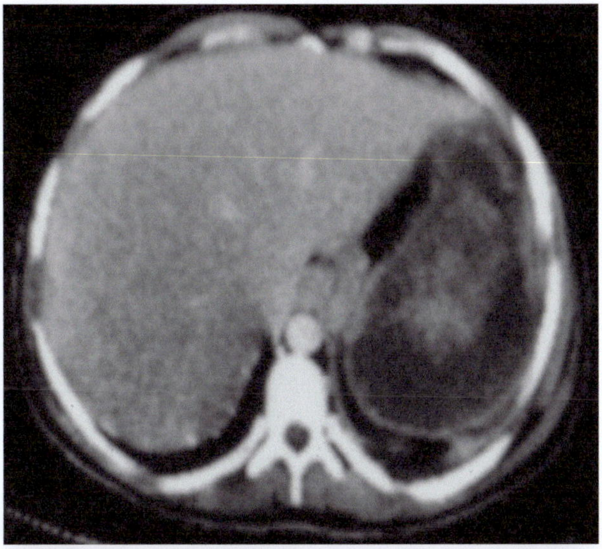

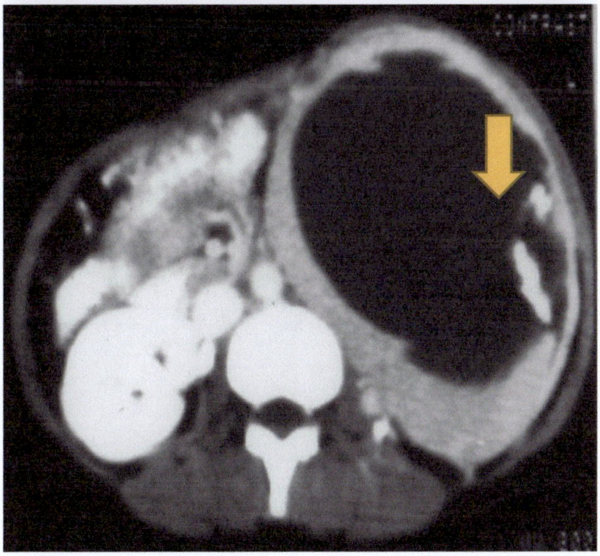

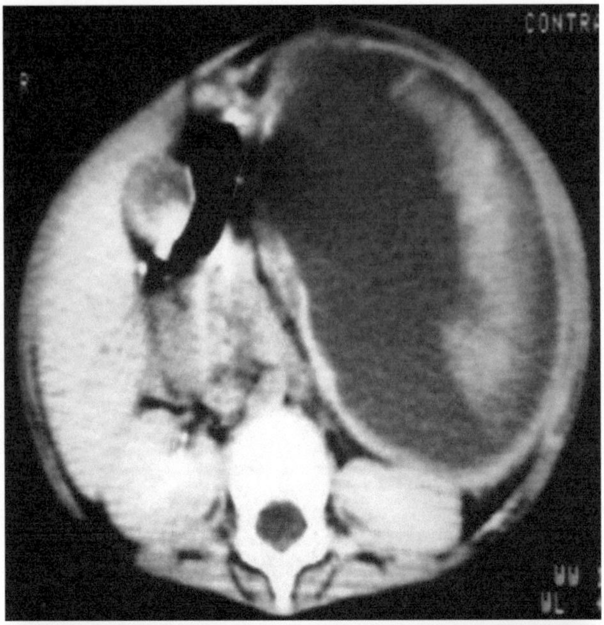

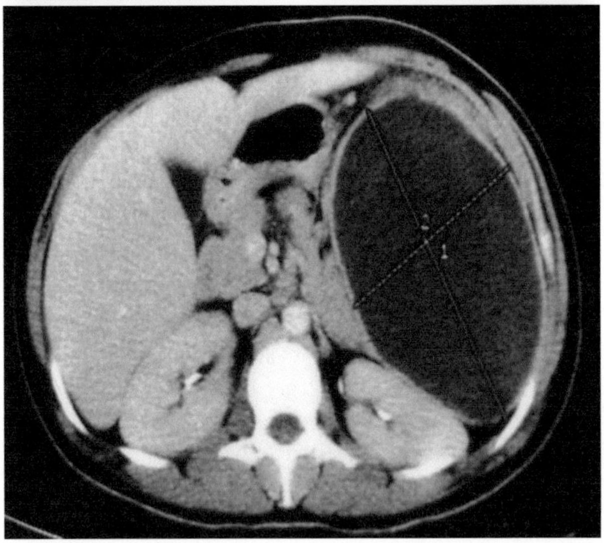

Figs. 5.26 and 5.27 Abdominal CT scans showing splenic abscess in patients with SCA. Note the splenic sequestrum in the left photographs and the large size of the abscess which is involving most of the spleen in the right photograph

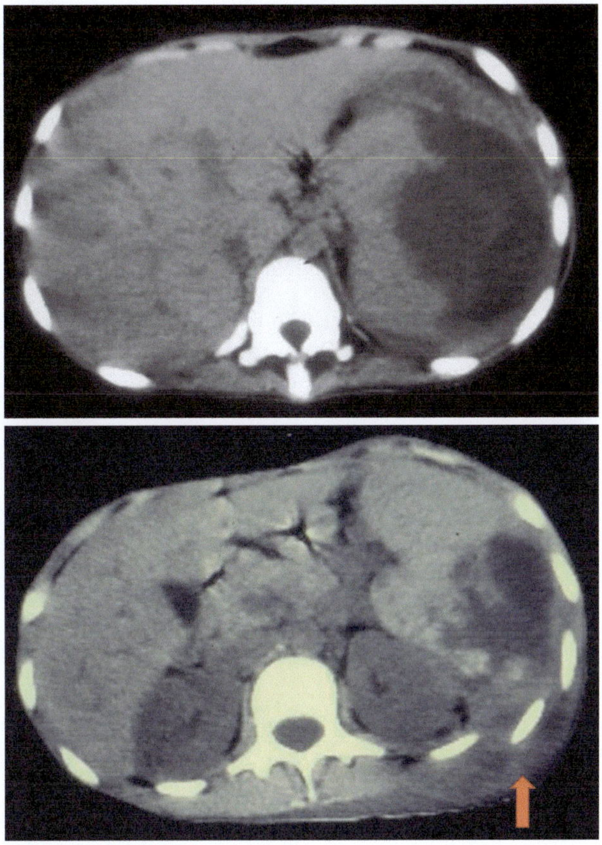

Figs. 5.28 and 5.29 Abdominal CT scan showing splenic abscess in two patients with SCA. Note the size of the splenic abscess which is involving part of the spleen. Note also the soft tissue swelling in the second photograph as a result of abscess rupture

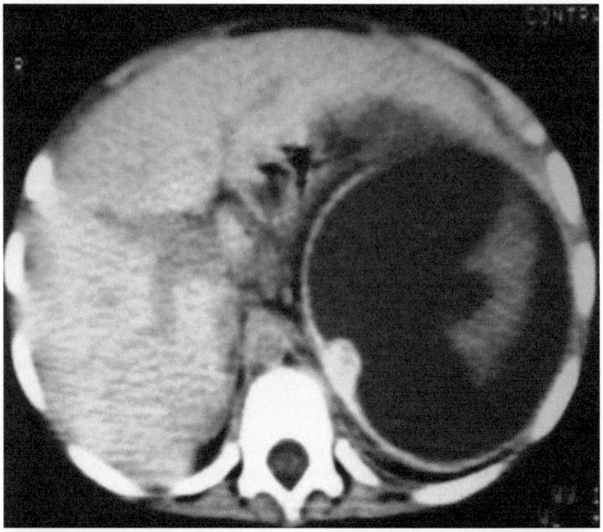

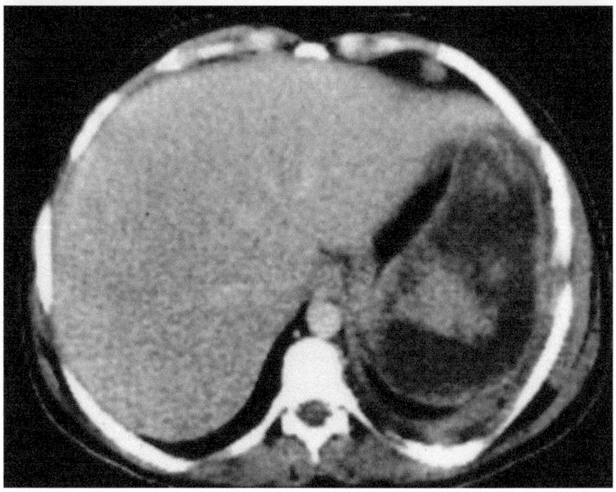

Figs. 5.30 and 5.31 Abdominal CT scan showing large splenic abscess in two patients with SCA. Note the sequestrum of splenic tissue in the middle of abscess cavity

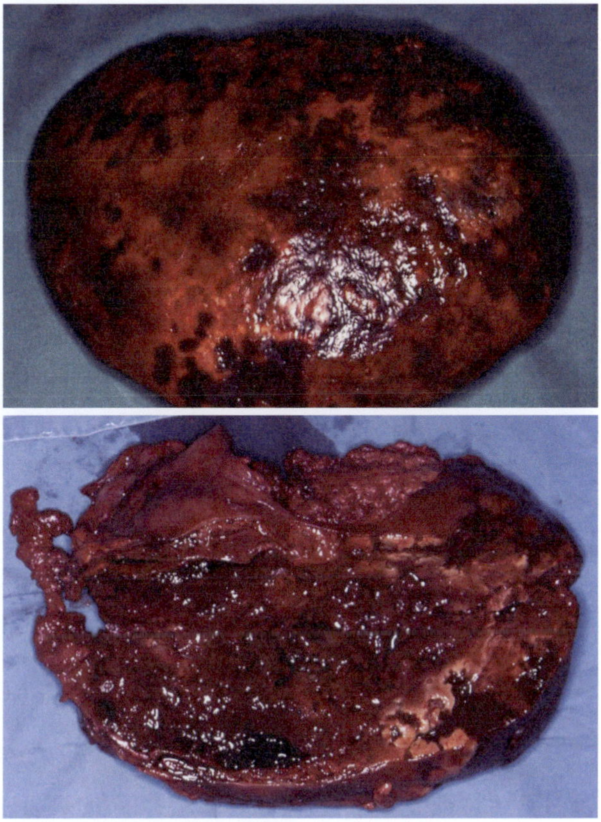

Figs. 5.32 and 5.33 Clinical photographs showing a removed spleen in a patient with SCA. Note also the splenic infarcts. The first photograph shows an intact spleen with a splenic abscess, while the second photograph shows a ruptured large splenic abscess in a patient with SCA

- A variety of organisms can cause splenic abscess including:
  - Staphylococci.
  - Streptococci.
  - Gram-negative bacilli.
  - Of interest is the finding of *Salmonella* as a causative organism in patients with sickle cell anemia (Figs. 5.34, 5.35, 5.36, 5.37 and 5.38).
- Treatment:
  - In the past, total splenectomy was the treatment of choice for splenic abscess.
  - To obviate OPSI (overwhelming post-splenectomy infection), splenic preservation was advocated even in those with splenic abscess.
  - A variety of procedures have been proposed including:
    - Partial splenectomy
    - CT-guided percutaneous catheter drainage
    - Noninterventional treatment of splenic abscess with antibiotics

Splenic Abscess: Causative Organisms

- Most frequent organisms:
  - Staphylococci
  - Streptococci
  - Gram-negative bacilli
- Other organisms include:
  - *Pseudomonas*
  - *Enterobacter*
  - *Salmonella*
  - *Serratia*
  - Fungi
- In patients with sickle cell anemia, *Salmonella* is the most common causative organism of splenic abscess.

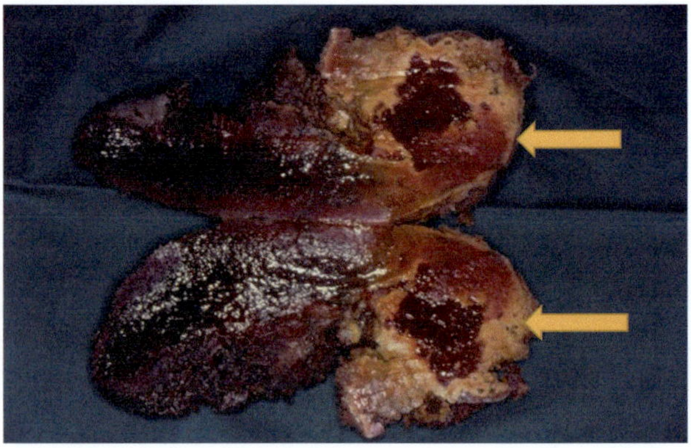

Fig. 5.34 A cut section of the spleen with splenic abscess in a patient with SCA. Note the abscess cavity

- Percutaneous abscess drainage and in the presence of personal experience in this technique can be used as a temporary measure in patients who are sick and unfit to undergo laparotomy. This a valuable option in patients who are sick and septicemic. The drainage of the abscess will help control the infection.
- Delay in diagnosing and treating splenic abscess can lead to rupture of splenic abscess leading to peritonitis. This is a serious complication which is known to be associated with morbidity and mortality (Figs. 5.39, 5.40, 5.41, and 5.42).

Splenic Abscess: Treatment Options

- Noninterventional treatment with intravenous antibiotics
- CT-guided percutaneous catheter drainage
- Ultrasound-guided percutaneous drainage
- Partial splenectomy
- Total splenectomy

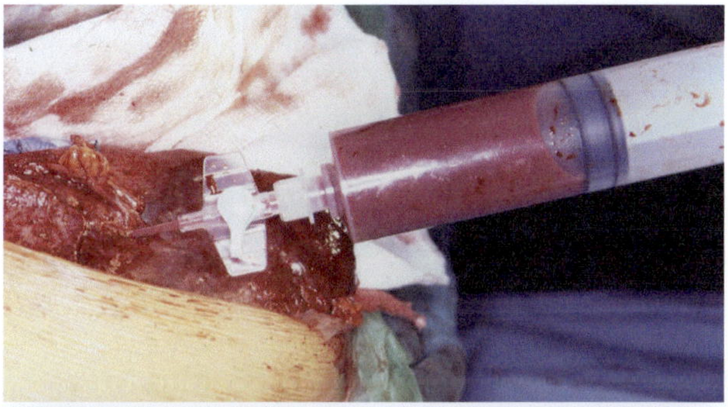

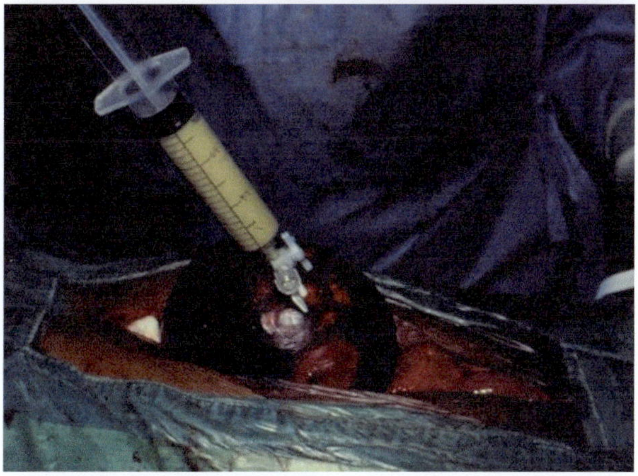

Figs. 5.35 and 5.36 Clinical intraoperative photographs showing aspiration of a large splenic abscess in two patients with SCA

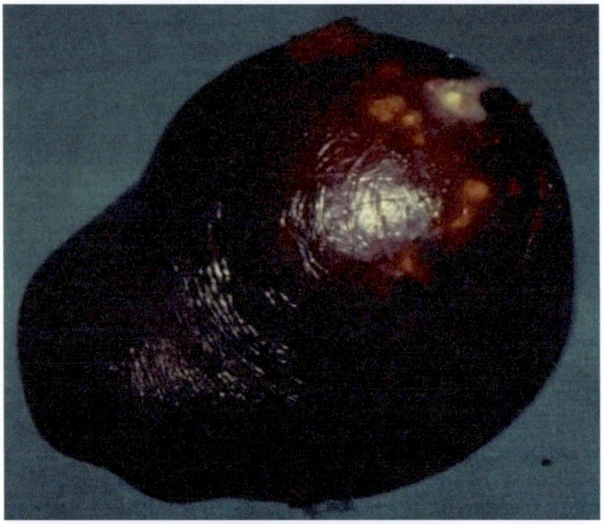

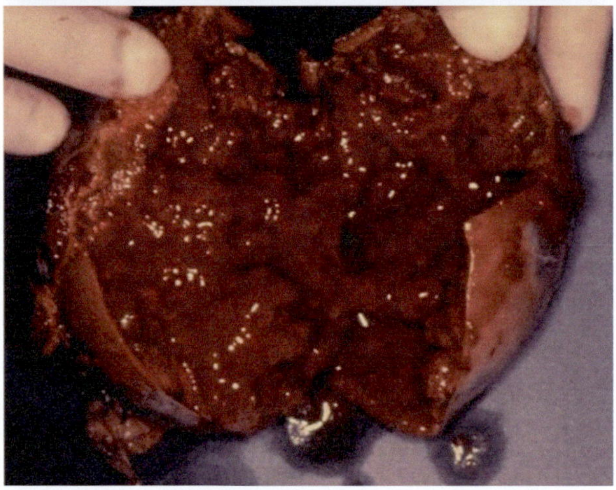

Figs. 5.37 and 5.38 Clinical photographs showing a splenic abscess. Note the large abscess cavity in the second photograph

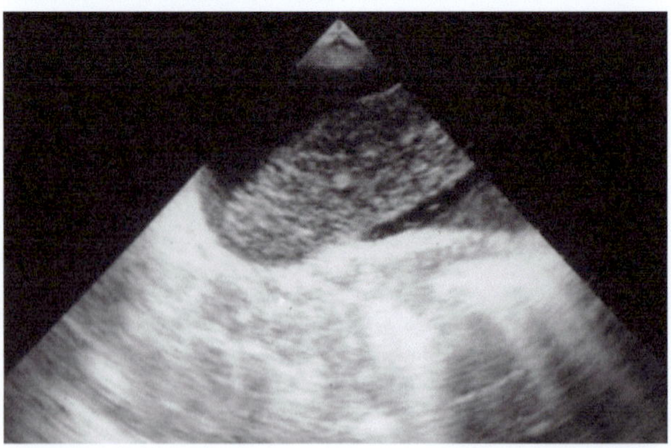

Fig. 5.39 Abdominal ultrasound of a child with sickle cell anemia and ruptured splenic abscess. Note the fluid around the spleen

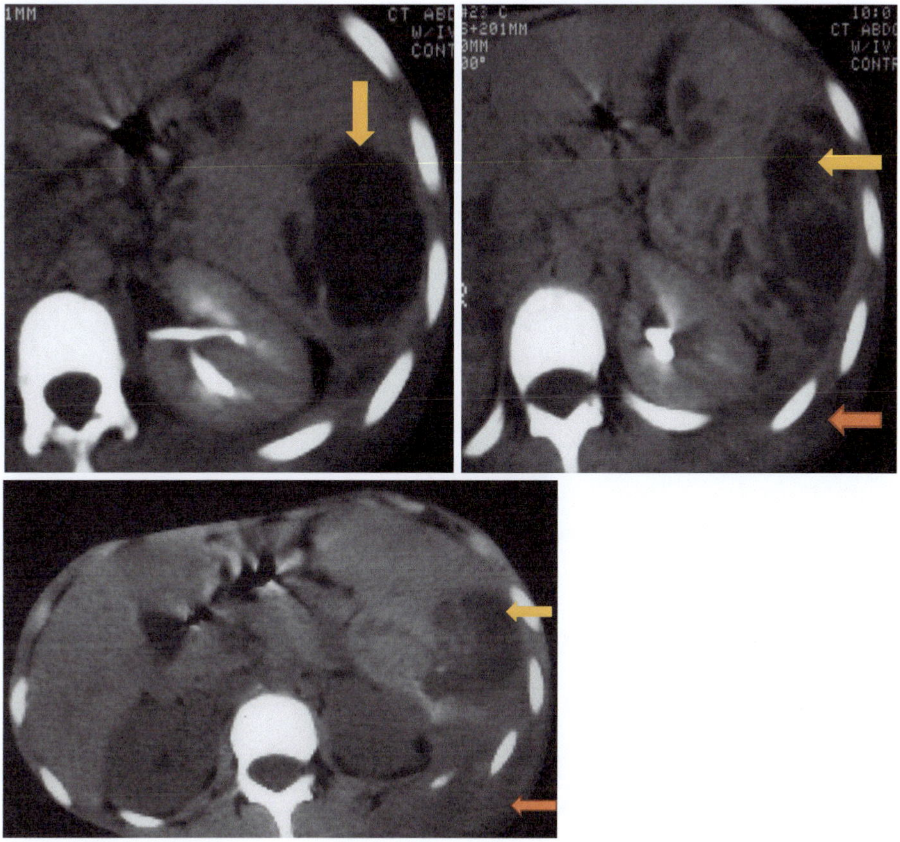

Figs. 5.40, 5.41, and 5.42 Abdominal CT scans showing ruptures of splenic abscess in patients with sickle cell anemia

5.10 Massive Splenic Infarction

- Sickle cell anemia which is an autosomal recessive inherited hemoglobinopathy can affect any part of the body.
- One of the early and commonly affected organs in sickle cell anemia is the spleen.
- The spleen is commonly enlarged during the first few years of life but then undergoes progressive atrophy as a result of multiple splenic infarcts.
- In most cases this is followed by splenic scarring leading to a small fibrosed and calcified splenic remnant (autosplenectomy).
- Sometimes the enlarged spleen becomes calcified (Figs. 5.43, 5.44, and 5.45).
- These infarcts are common and usually small, repetitive, and pass unnoticed (Figs. 5.46, 5.47, 5.48, 5.49, and 5.50).

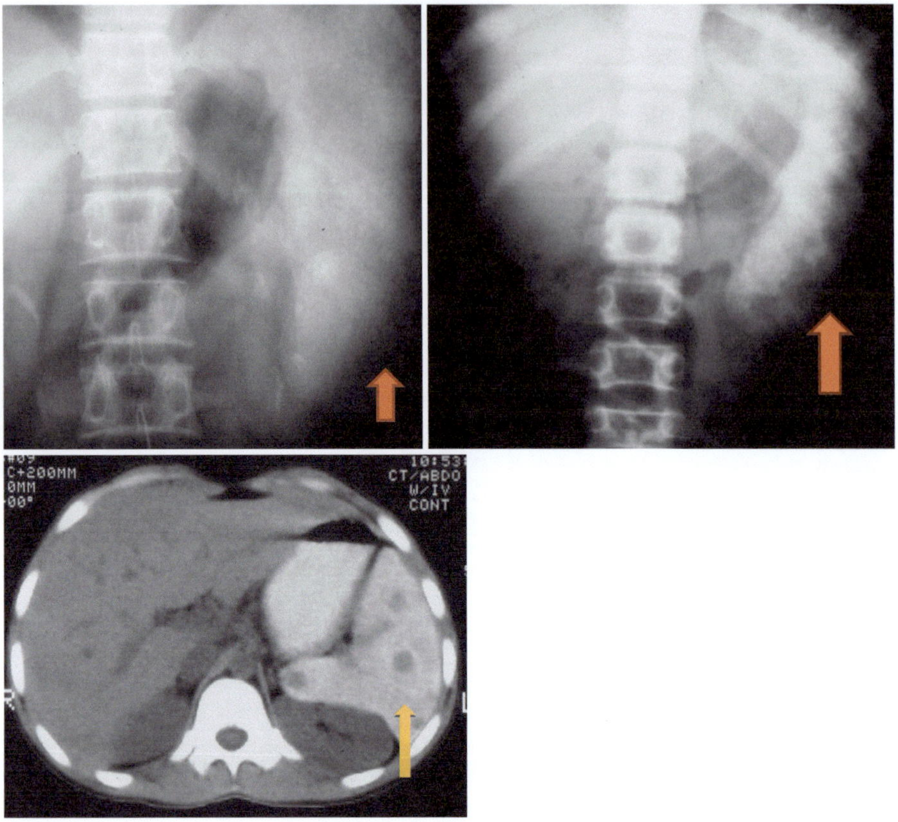

Figs. 5.43, 5.44, and 5.45 Abdominal X-rays and abdominal CT scan showing calcified spleen in three patients with sickle cell anemia

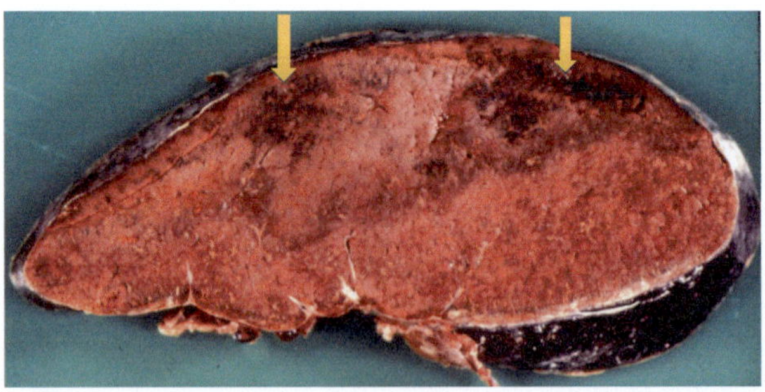

Fig. 5.46 A clinical photograph showing a cut section of a spleen from a patient with SCA. Note the splenic infarcts which are usually small and multiple

- This however is not the case always, and sometimes splenomegaly persists into an older age group or sometimes into adulthood.
- Splenomegaly persists in about 10 % of adults with sickle cell anemia in the West Indies, and such cases are usually characterized by high levels of fetal hemoglobin.
- In a prospective study from Saudi Arabia, splenomegaly was reported in the majority of patients, and only 6.6 % had autosplenectomy, while 11.8 % had massive splenomegaly (splenic index more than 120 cm^2).
- The reason for failure of these patients to undergo autosplenectomy is unknown.
- There is however a correlation between persistent splenomegaly and elevated hemoglobin F level.
- It has been suggested that hemoglobin F exhibits its favorable influence through inhibition of hemoglobin S polymerization and thus survival of hemoglobin F containing cells and less sickling.

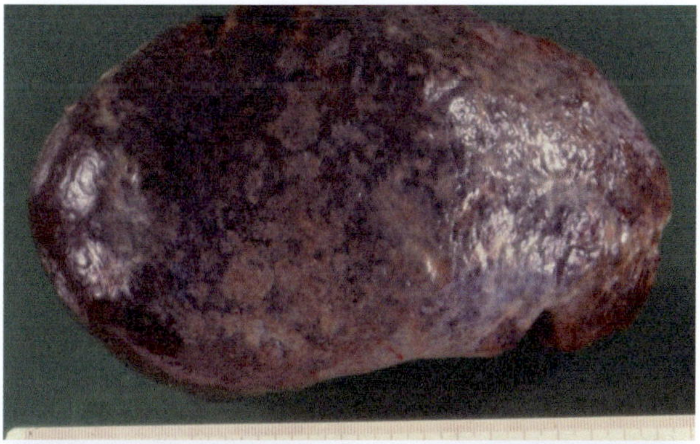

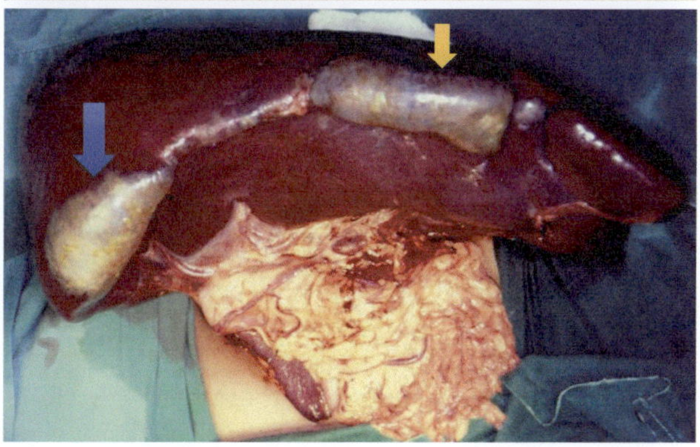

Figs. 5.47, 5.48, 5.49, and 5.50 Clinical photographs showing spleens of patients with SCA. Note the small and multiple infarcts. Note the variable extent and size of these infarcts

Figs. 5.47, 5.48, 5.49, and 5.50 (continued)

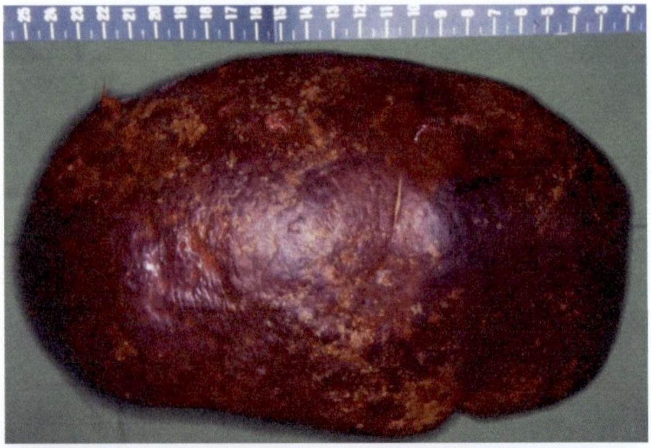

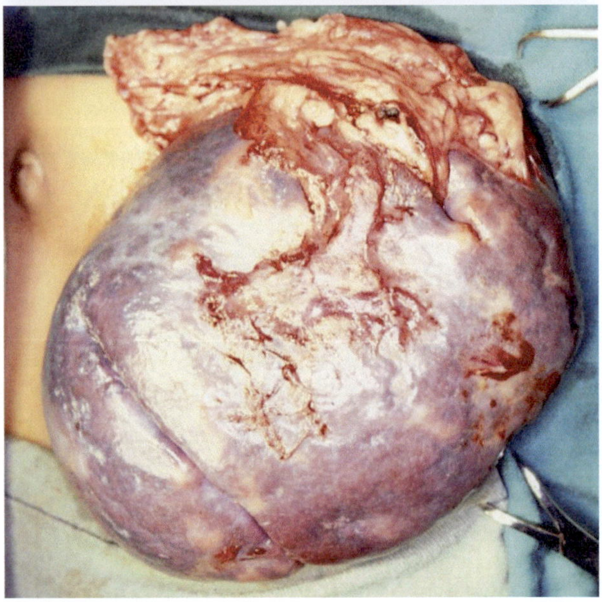

- Persistence of splenomegaly in these patients makes them liable to develop splenic complications including massive splenic infarctions (Figs. 5.51 and 5.52).
- Splenic infarctions secondary to vaso-occlusion are common in patients with SCA. They however occur early and usually are small, unnoticeable, and repetitive leading to progressive atrophy and ultimately to autosplenectomy.
- Massive splenic infarction is arbitrarily defined as infarction involving more than 50 % of the spleen size (Figs. 5.53, 5.54, 5.55, 5.56, and 5.57).

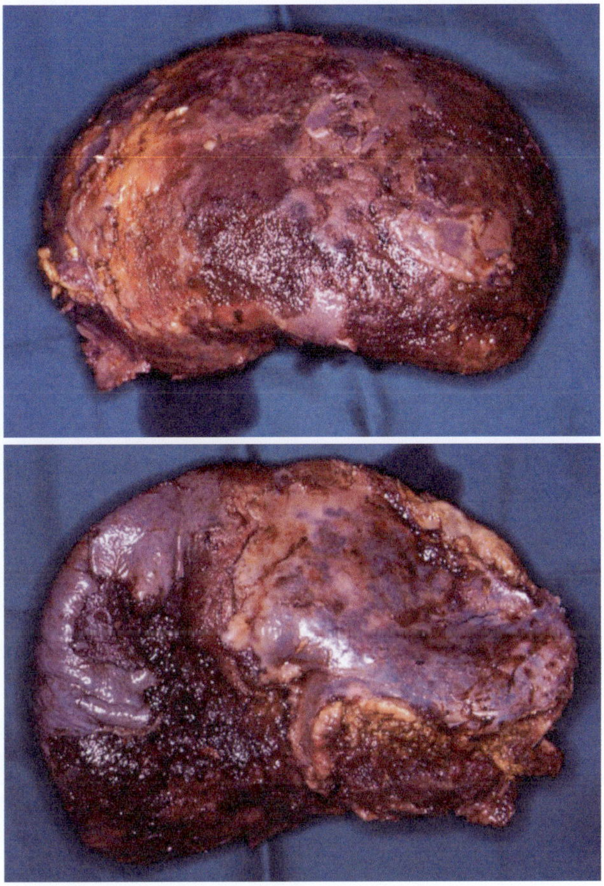

Figs. 5.51 and 5.52 Clinical photographs showing massive splenic infarction in a patient with SCA. Note the infarction involving almost the whole spleen

Figs. 5.53, 5.54, 5.55, 5.56, and 5.57 Clinical photographs showing spleens with massive splenic infarction. Note the variation in the size of the infarction involving more than half the size of the spleen or the whole spleen

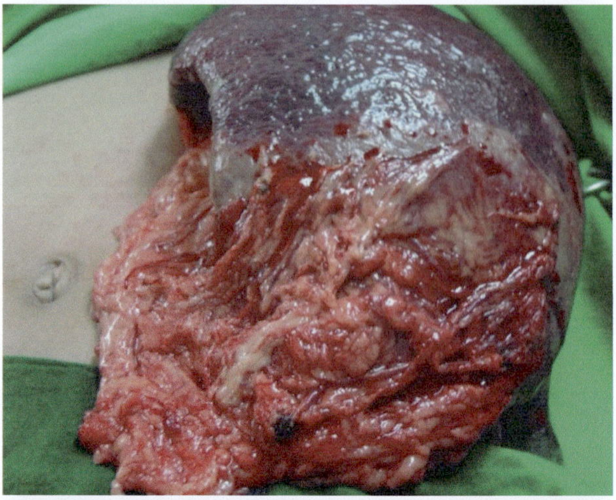

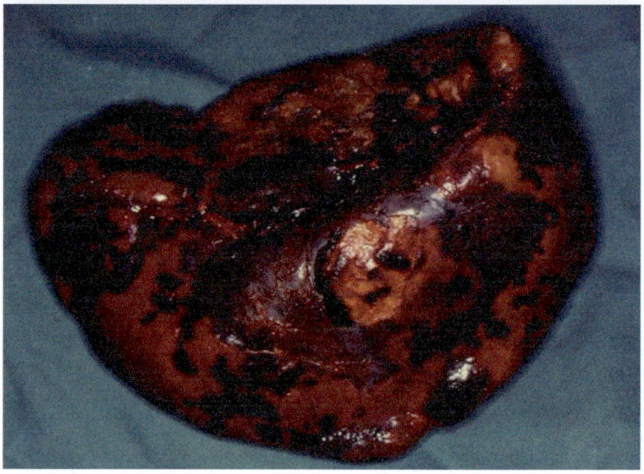

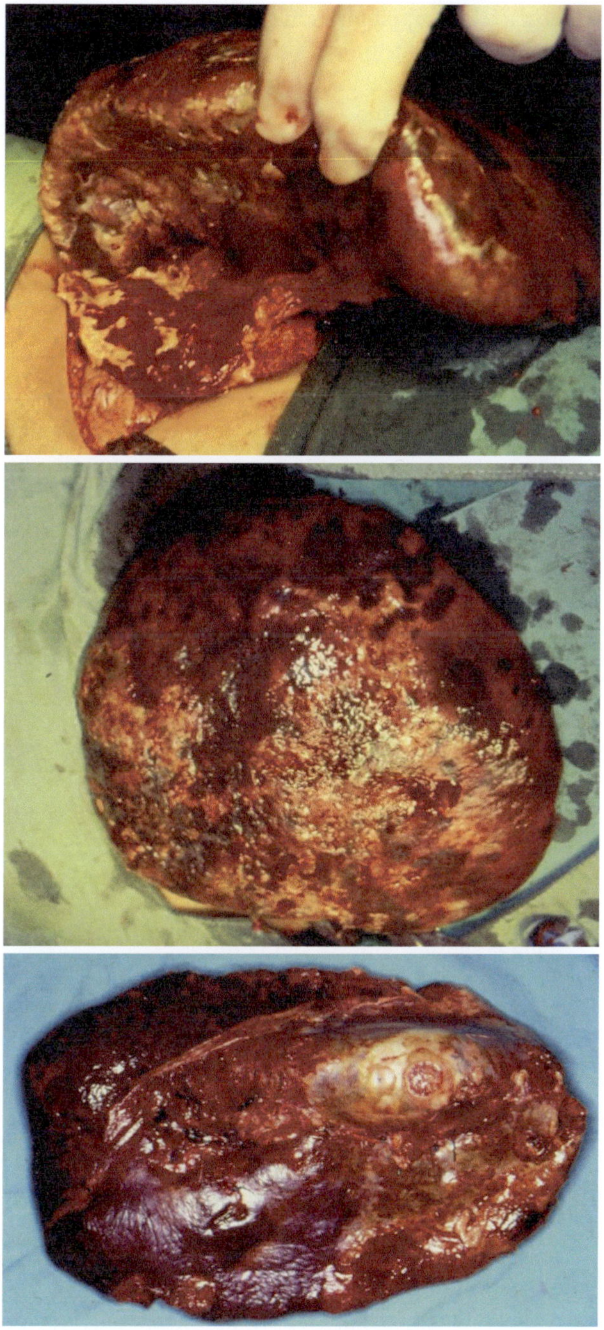

Figs. 5.53, 5.54, 5.55, 5.56, and 5.57 (continued)

- Massive splenic infarction (MSI) is a very rare condition.
- Massive splenic infarction of various etiologies including hematological and non-hematological causes has been published. These include:
  - Evans syndrome
  - Endocarditis
  - Polycythaemia vera
  - Paroxysmal nocturnal hemoglobinuria
  - Sickle cell hemoglobin C disease
  - Sickle cell-beta-thalassemia
  - Sickle cell trait
  - Hemoglobin SE
- These are seen particularly in association with stress or following air travel especially in an unpressurized aircrafts.
- While the majority of patients with sickle cell trait lead to normal, healthy lives, they may, however, still experience potentially life-threatening complications similar to sickle cell anemia under low oxygen tension. These include painful crisis, splenic infarction, and, rarely, sudden death. These adverse events usually occur under certain conditions including severe physical exertion, dehydration, high altitude, and scuba diving.
- In sickle cell trait, large splenic infarcts in the normal-sized spleen were reported following exposure to hypoxia during high-altitude flights in an unpressurized airplanes or during mountain climbing.
- Although splenic infarction has been reported to occur in patients with sickle cell trait at high altitude, there are also reports of splenic infarction not related to high-altitude exposure.
- Sleep apnea with attendant hypoxia was also implicated as a possible cause in some cases of splenic infarcts in patients with sickle cell trait without apparent precipitating factor.
- Massive splenic infarction in patients with sickle cell anemia (SCA) on the other hand is unique and extremely rare.
- The precipitating factor for massive splenic infarction in these patients is usually high-altitude-induced hypoxia typically in unpressurized airplanes but also has been reported to occur at mountain altitudes of 5000–7000 feet above sea level.
  - This promotes sickling by metabolic effects such as acidosis, hypoxia, and dehydration.
  - Other precipitating factors include septicemia, severe vaso-occlusive crisis, and acute chest syndrome.
  - The additional hypoxemia due to acute chest syndrome in these patients is presumed to contribute to the development of splenic infarction.
  - This may explain the occurrence of massive splenic infarction in patients with sickle cell anemia admitted to the hospital with other medical complications such as acute chest syndrome, severe vaso-occlusive crisis, and septicemia.

- Clinical features:
  - The presentation of massive splenic infarction is variable but the majority present with:
    - Sudden onset of severe left upper quadrant abdominal pain.
    - This may be associated with nausea, vomiting, fever, and chills.
  - These symptoms are nonspecific and may be confused with other causes of acute abdominal pain, and physicians caring for these patients should be aware of this.
  - Clinically, there is a tender enlarged spleen.
  - A history of recent travel to a high-altitude area is important.
  - This should hint to the possibility of splenic infarction, and with the availability of ultrasound examination, it is now possible to diagnose splenic infarction early and to follow the progress of this complication.

Massive Splenic Infarction

- Massive splenic infarction has been reported in patients with:
  - Sickle cell trait
  - Evans syndrome
  - Endocarditis
  - Polycythaemia vera
  - Paroxysmal nocturnal hemoglobinuria
  - Sickle cell hemoglobin C disease
  - Sickle cell-beta-thalassemia
  - Sickle cell trait
  - Hemoglobin SE
- Massive splenic infarction in these was associated with stress.
- Massive splenic infarction is rare in patients with sickle cell anemia.

  - Computerized tomography (CT) of the abdomen on the other hand is more valuable in demonstrating the site and extent of the infarct (Figs. 5.58, 5.59, 5.60, and 5.61).
  - The clinical presentation and radiological features of massive splenic infarction can resemble those with splenic abscess, and it is important to differentiate between the two as massive splenic infarction can be treated conservatively ultimately leading to autosplenectomy.
  - The management of such a complication is challenging both to the physicians and the surgeons, and a team work approach is most fruitful.
  - The majority of the patients are febrile, and in the presence of massive splenic infarct, the possibility of splenic abscess although rare must be excluded.

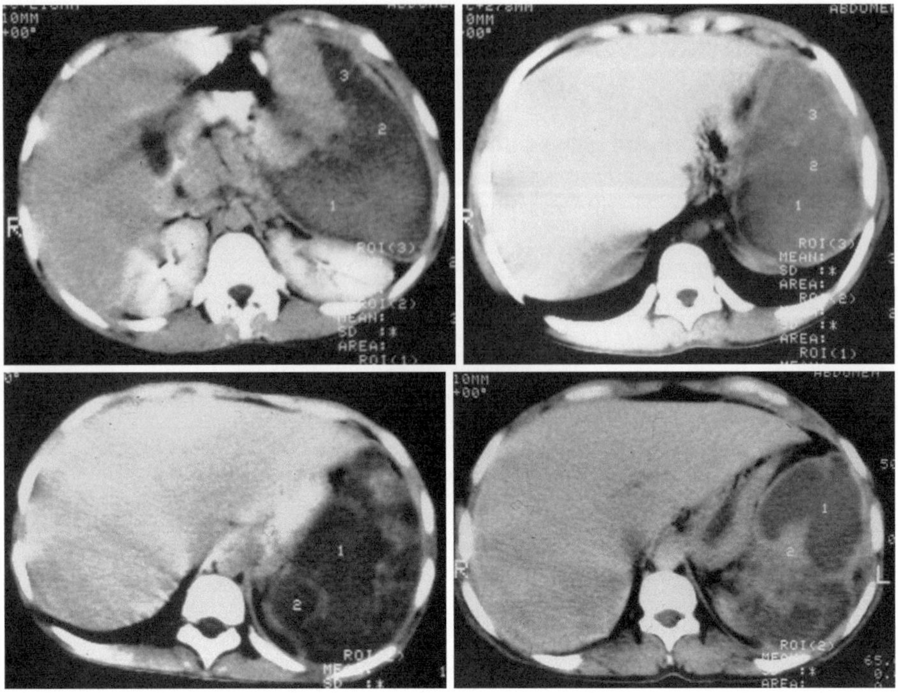

Figs. 5.58, 5.59, 5.60, and 5.61 Abdominal CT scans showing massive splenic infarction in patients with SCA. Note the variable extent of the infarction which involves more than half the spleen in some and almost the whole spleen in others

  - The two conditions and in doubtful cases can also be differentiated by percutaneous aspiration under ultrasound guidance.
  - These patients should be covered with antibiotics after obtaining the necessary cultures, and a conservative approach is now recommended in the management of these cases.
  - Surgery is reserved for cases where there is doubt about the possibility of splenic abscess or if there is persistent left upper quadrant abdominal pain.

- Diagnosis:
  - Abdominal ultrasound is the main noninvasive investigation.
  - Abdominal CT scan is more valuable.
  - It accurately outlines the site and size of splenic infarction and helps in differentiating this from other conditions, namely, splenic abscess (Fig. 5.62).
- Treatment:
  - The treatment of splenic infarction should be supportive and directed toward correcting any predisposing conditions.
  - Hydration with I.V. fluids.

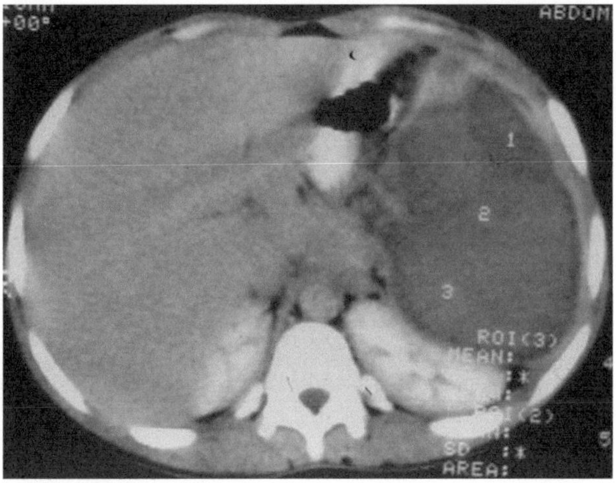

Fig. 5.62 Abdominal CT scan showing massive splenic infarction in a patient with sickle cell anemia. Note the extent of splenic infarction involving almost the whole spleen

- Adequate oxygenation.
- Blood transfusion where necessary.
- Analgesia.
- This however warrants close follow-up of these patients as they are liable to develop complications including:
  - Splenic rupture
  - Hemorrhage
  - Splenic abscess
  - Pseudocyst formation
- The role of splenectomy in patients with massive splenic infarction remains unclear. Most cases tend to be self-limiting ultimately leading to atrophy of the spleen.
- Splenectomy however is indicated for those with persistent abdominal pain or in the presence of complications such as hemorrhage, rupture, abscess, or persistent pseudocyst. Splenectomy is also indicated if there is difficulty differentiating splenic infarction from splenic abscess (Figs. 5.63, 5.64, and 5.65).

Massive Splenic Infarction: Treatment

- Conservative
- Splenectomy
  - Suspicion of superadded infection
  - Persistent left upper abdominal pain

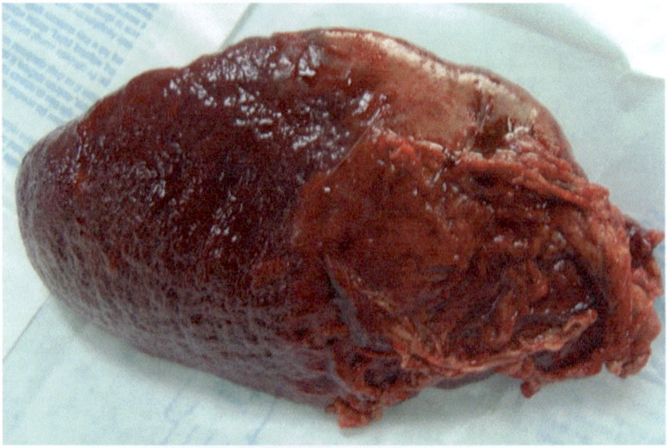

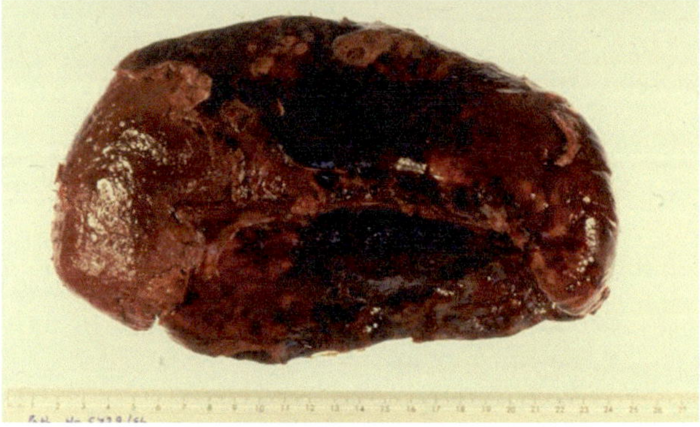

Figs. 5.63 and 5.64 Clinical photographs showing removed spleen with massive splenic infarcts. Note the extent of the infarct which is involving about 50 % of the size of the spleen in the first one and almost the whole spleen in the second one

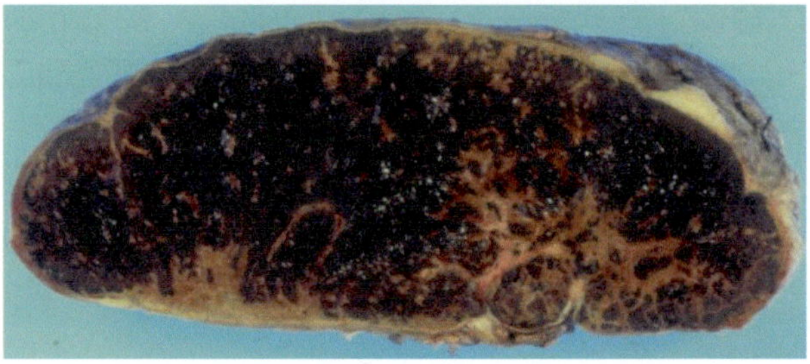

Fig. 5.65 A clinical photograph showing a cut section of a spleen showing massive splenic infarction

5.11 Partial Splenectomy

- Splenectomy is usually done through an open incision (upper midline or left upper transverse), but currently and with the recent advances in minimal invasive surgery, laparoscopic splenectomy is the preferred procedure.
- This is the preferred procedure in cases where the spleen is not too large and when splenectomy is elective.
- Total splenectomy should however be avoided whenever possible.
- This is to obviate the increased risk of post-splenectomy sepsis.

- While vaccination and antibiotics provide good protection against the risks of asplenia, this is not 100 % effective and not always available especially in poorer countries.
- Add to this the poor compliance of patients specially children in taking these antibiotics.
- To overcome this, partial splenectomy or partial splenic arterial embolization has been advocated (Figs. 5.66, 5.67, 5.68, 5.69, 5.70, and 5.71).

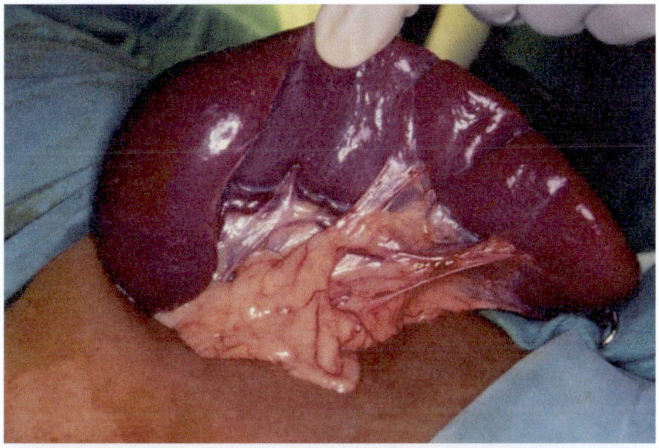

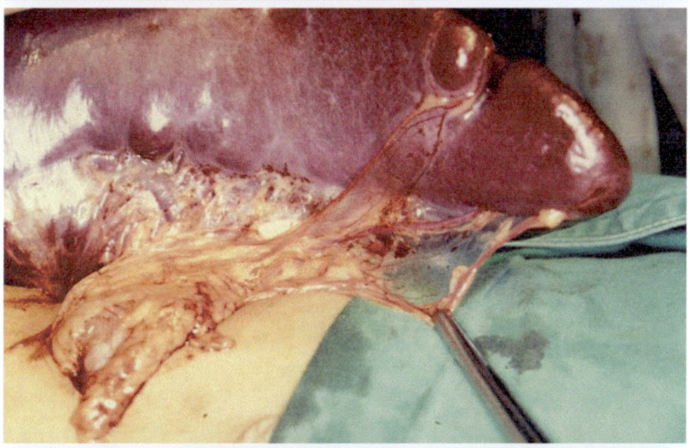

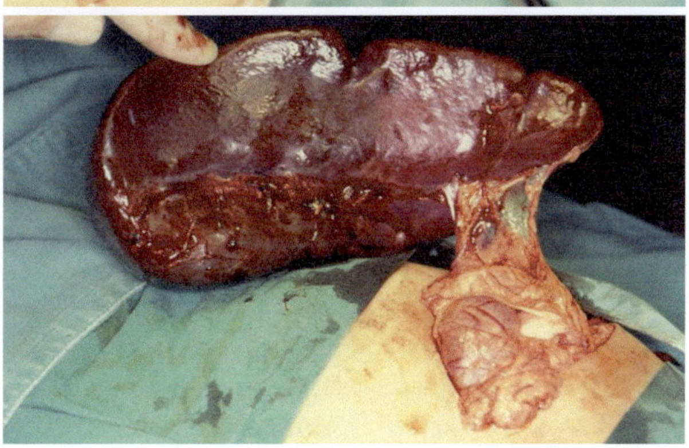

Figs. 5.66, 5.67, and 5.68 Clinical photographs showing enlarged spleen. Note also the vascular supply and distribution of vessels at the hilum. Note also preservation of the lower polar vessels for partial splenectomy

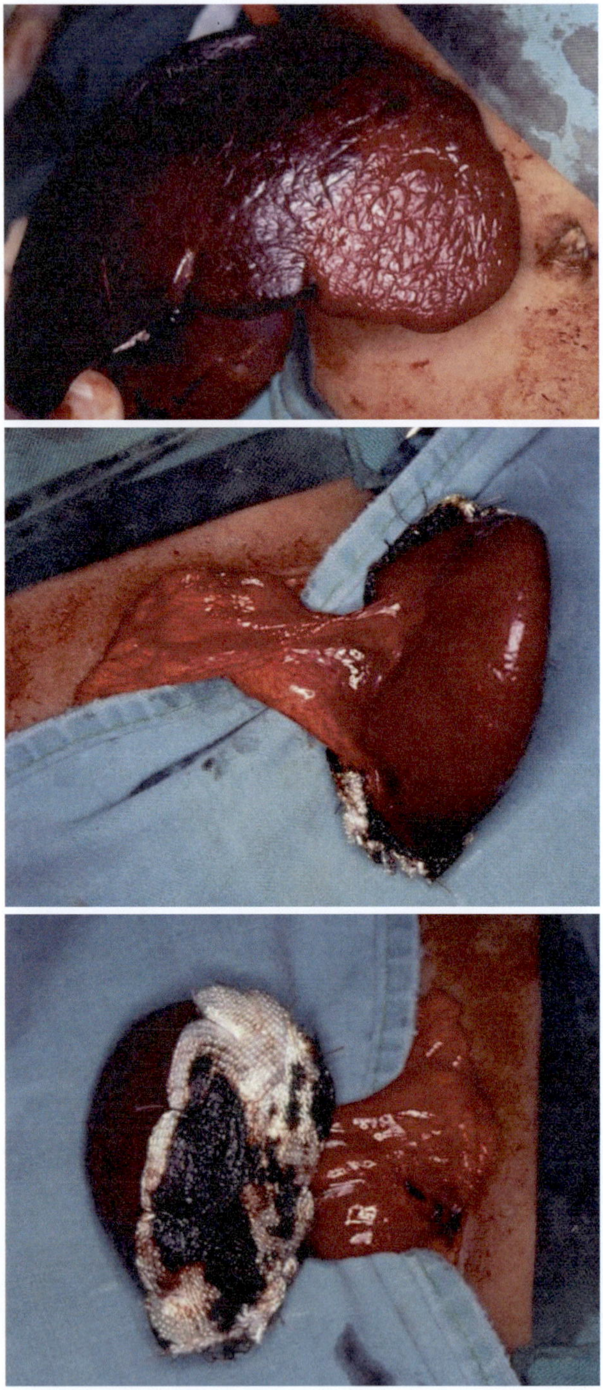

Figs. 5.69, 5.70, and 5.71 Clinical photographs showing partial splenectomy. Note the preservation of the lower pole of the spleen. Note also the Surgicel which is used for hemostasis of the cut surface of the spleen

- The spleen's protective functions can be maintained if a small part of the spleen can be left behind (up to 1/3 of the size of the normal spleen).
- Currently and where clinically appropriate, attempts are now made to perform either surgical subtotal (partial) splenectomy, or partial splenic embolization.
- Partial splenectomy is usually performed through an open technique, but recently, laparoscopic partial splenectomy was shown to be feasible and safe.
- As it may take some time for the preserved splenic tissue to provide full immunological protection, it is advisable to immunize these patients preoperatively and cover them with antibiotics.

5.12 Laparoscopic Splenectomy

- In the past, open splenectomy was the only option to treat splenic complications of children with SCD. Open splenectomy is done through an upper transverse of upper midline incision (Fig. 5.72).
- Large abdominal wounds are associated with more pain and may interfere with respiration. This may lead to immobility and increased risk of acute chest syndrome (Figs. 5.73, 5.74, 5.75 and 5.76).
- In 1991, Delaitre performed the first laparoscopic splenectomy, and since then it has become the procedure of choice to treat patients with hematological diseases requiring splenectomy.

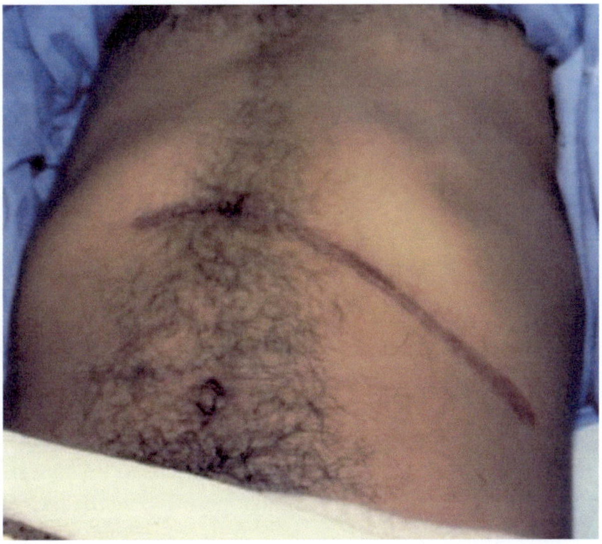

Fig. 5.72 A clinical photograph showing a large wound following open splenectomy for a patient with sickle cell anemia

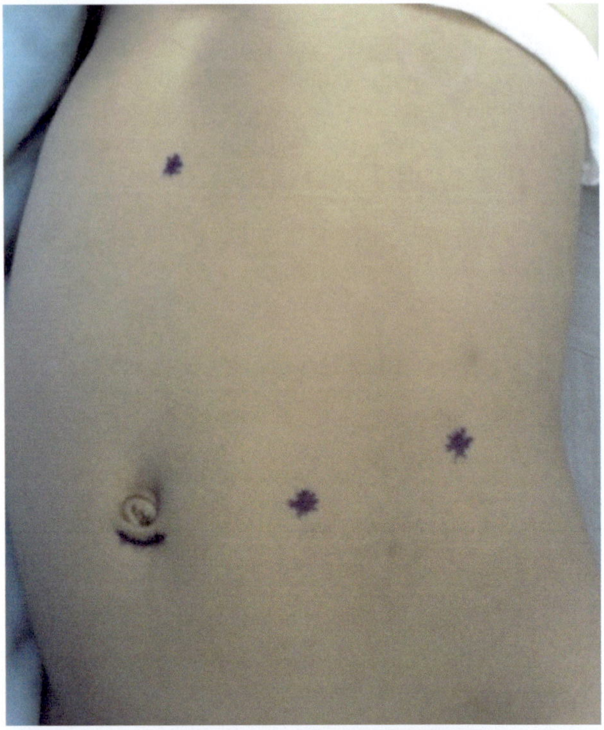

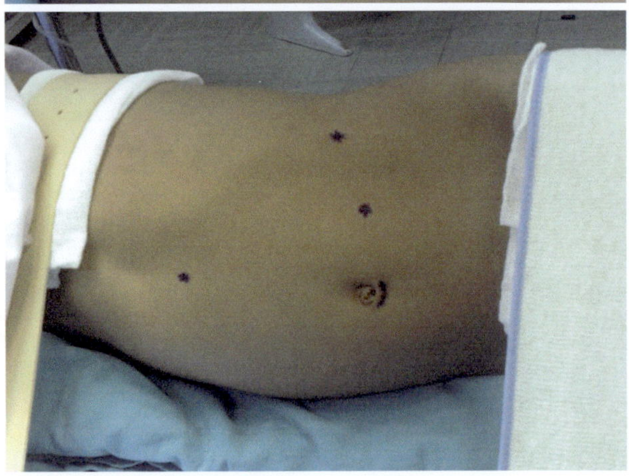

Figs. 5.73 and 5.74 Clinical photographs showing the sites of trocars used for laparoscopic splenectomy. These sites can be modified according to the size of the spleen and whether the position is supine or a lateral position

- Laparoscopic splenectomy was reported to be feasible and safe both in adults and children.
- Laparoscopic splenectomy should be the procedure of choice to treat patients with SCA-related splenic complications.
- Laparoscopic splenectomy was shown to be superior to open splenectomy with regard to hospital stay, postoperative recovery, complications, and cosmetic appearance.

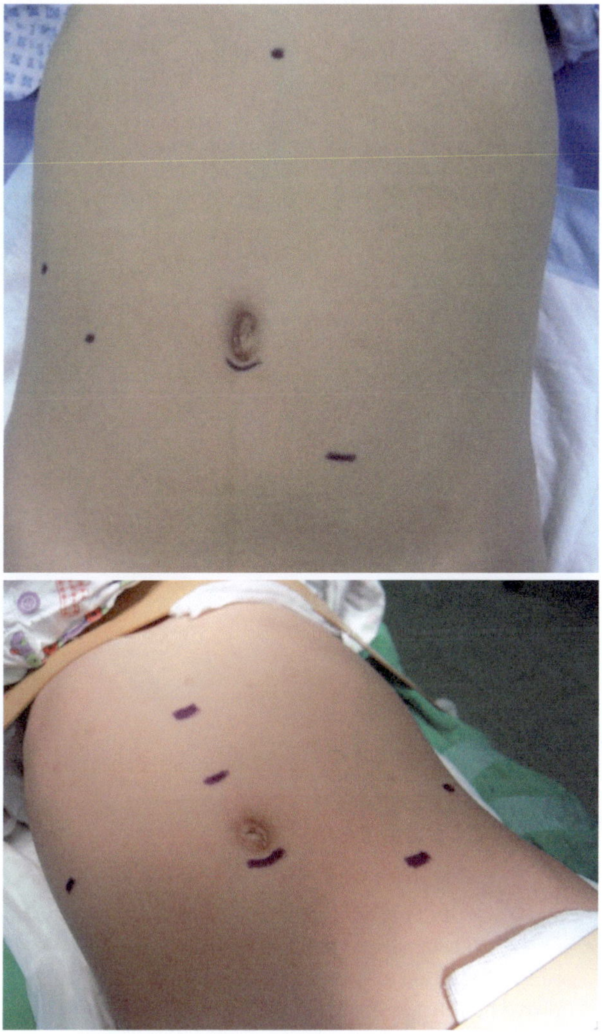

Figs. 5.75 and 5.76 Clinical photographs showing the sites of trocars used for laparoscopic splenectomy and cholecystectomy whether a supine or a lateral position is used. The number of ports can be modified depending on the size of the spleen

- Another common complication of SCA is cholelithiasis. The frequency of this is however variable, but it is known to increase with increasing age, and overall 70 % of patients with SCA develop gallstones.
- The treatment of symptomatic gallstones is well established, and currently laparoscopic cholecystectomy is the treatment of choice. The treatment of asymptomatic gallstones is still controversial.
- With good perioperative management, laparoscopic splenectomy is feasible and safe in children with SCA and can be done concomitantly with cholecystectomy. There is a definite learning curve where laparoscopic splenectomy and cholecystectomy take more operative time than the open technique. This is specially so for children with SCA who are known to have large spleens with severe adhesions.

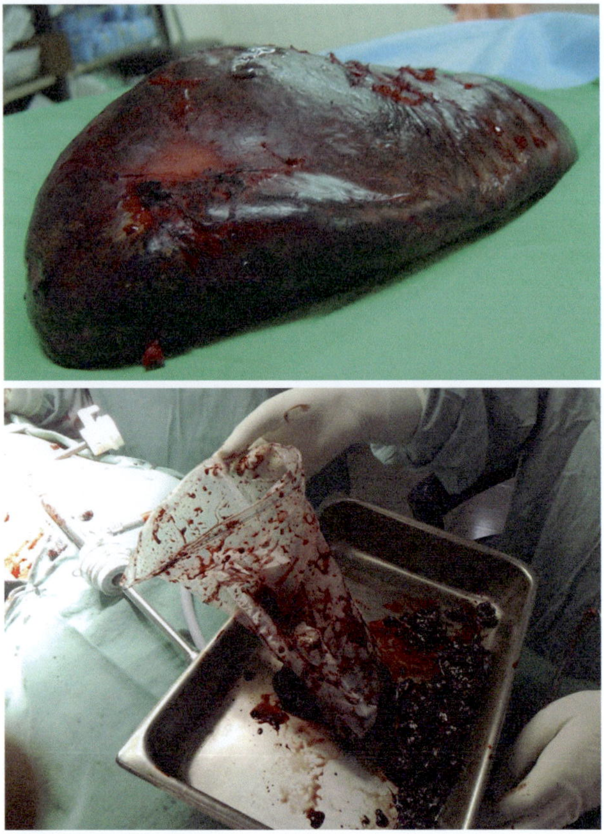

Figs. 5.77 and 5.78 Clinical intraoperative photographs showing an enlarged spleen that was removed intact via a large laparotomy wound and a large spleen that was remove laparoscopically, put into a retrieval bag, and removed in pieces via small trocar wounds

- Laparoscopic partial splenectomy is now feasible and safe in experienced hands.
- In the past, large spleens are removed through large laparotomy wounds, but currently these are removed laparoscopically through few small wounds. This may prove beneficial in reducing the frequency of postoperative acute chest syndrome (Figs. 5.77 and 5.78).

5.13 Perioperative Management of Children with SCA

- In the past and because of a perioperative mortality as high as 10 % and a postoperative morbidity up to 50 %, surgery was not advocated in patients with SCA except in symptomatic patients.
- This however is not the case nowadays as with better understanding of SCA and improved perioperative care, surgery is safer. This is also the case for children undergoing splenectomy and or cholecystectomy.
- In the past, post-splenectomy complications including acute chest syndrome which can be severe and life-threatening were common (Fig. 5.79).

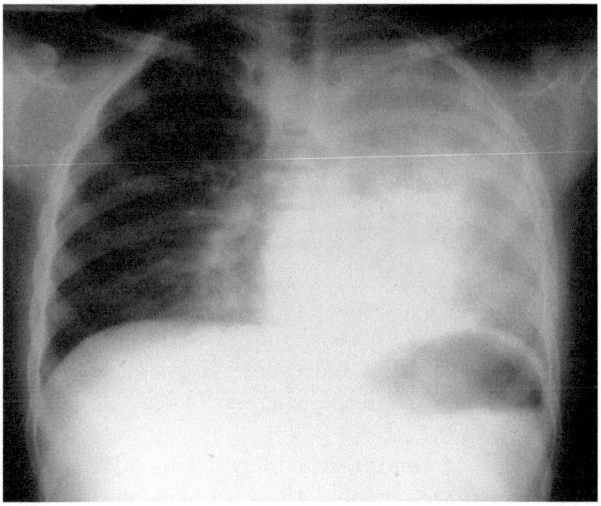

Fig. 5.79 A chest X-ray showing acute chest syndrome in a patient who had splenectomy

- To overcome this, a perioperative management protocol for all these patients should be adopted.
- The perioperative management protocol includes:
  1. Clinical evaluation.
  2. Preoperative hydration with intravenous fluids at a rate of 1.5 as their maintenance. This starts the night before surgery and continues postoperatively till they have adequate oral intake.
  3. All patients are immunized with pneumococcal, meningococcal, *H. influenzae* vaccines at least 10–14 days preoperatively. This is given postoperatively for those who require an emergency splenectomy.
  4. Preoperative blood transfusion to increase their hemoglobin to 10 g/dl with packed red blood cells and using this formula (weight in kg × (hemoglobin desired – actual hemoglobin) × 3) is advocated.
  5. At the time of surgery, avoid hypoxia, acidosis, hypothermia, and hypercarbia.
  6. Adequate analgesia postoperatively.
  7. Early mobilization and chest physiotherapy using incentive spirometry.

5.14 Overwhelming Post-splenectomy Infection (OPSI)

- There is growing concern about overwhelming post-splenectomy infection, which is certainly a hazard.
- The true incidence of OPSI, however, remains to be established, but it is greatest in children in whom splenectomy was performed in the first few years of life.
- OPSI is seen commonly within the first two years following splenectomy.

- *Streptococcus pneumoniae* is the commonest organism causing OPSI, followed by *Haemophilus influenzae* and *Neisseria meningitidis*.
- To obviate this, children undergoing splenectomy should be immunized with the following vaccines:
  - Pneumococcal
  - *H. influenzae*
  - Meningococcal
- These children should also be covered with penicillin prophylaxis either orally or intramuscularly for 2–3 years following splenectomy depending on the age at the time of splenectomy.
- The effectiveness of such prophylaxis in an era of increasing microbial resistance to antibiotics needs however to be evaluated.
- The parents should be educated to seek medical help at the earliest sign of an infection.
- A point of concern in children with SCA is their increased susceptibility to *Salmonella* infections. This should be evaluated further in terms of long-term antibiotic prophylaxis as well as the feasibility of finding a vaccine against *Salmonella*.

Further Reading

Al Jam'a A, Al Salem AH, Al Dabous I. Massive splenic infarction in Saudi patients with sickle cell anemia: a unique manifestation. Am J Hematol. 2002;69:205–9.

Al-Awamy BH, Niazi GA, El-Mouzan MI, et al. Relationship of haemoglobin F and alpha-thalassemia to severity of sickle cell anemia in the eastern province of Saudi Arabia. Ann Trop Pediatr. 1986;6:261–5.

Al-Salem AH. Indications and complications of splenectomy for children with sickle cell disease. J Pediatr Surg. 2006;41:1909–15.

Al-Salem AH. Splenic complications of sickle cell anemia and the role of splenectomy. ISRN Hematol. 2011;2011:864257.

Al-Salem AH. Massive splenic infarction in children with sickle cell anemia and the role of splenectomy. Pediatr Surg Int. 2013;29(3):281–5.

Al-Salem AH, Qaisaruddin S, Al Jam'a A, Al-Kalaf J, Al-Bashier AM. Splenic abscess and sickle cell disease. Am J Hematol. 1998;58:100–4.

Al-Wabari A, Parida L, Al-Salem AH. Laparoscopic splenectomy for children with hematological disorders: our initial experience with 45 cases. J Pediatr Surg Speci. 2008;2(3):18–20.

Al-Wabari A, Parida L, Al-Salem AH. Laparoscopic splenectomy and / or cholecystectomy for children with sickle cell disease. Pediatr Surg Int. 2009;25(5):417–21.

Bhattacharyya N, Ablin DS, kosloske AM. Stapled partial splenectomy for splenic abscess in a child. J Pediatr Surg. 1989;24:316–7.

Corcione F, Pirozzi F, Aragiusto G, Galante F, Sciuto A. Laparoscopic splenectomy: experience of a single center in a series of 300 cases. Surg Endosc. 2012;26:2870–6.

Elbashier AM, Al-Salem AH, Aljama A. Salmonella as a causative organism of various infections in patients with sickle cell disease. Ann Saudi Med. 2003;23:358–62.

Fernandes ET, Tavares PB, Gaarcette CBM. Conservative management of splenic abscess in children. J Pediatr Surg. 1992;27:1578–9.

Haricharan RN, Roberts JM, Morgan TL, et al. Splenectomy reduces packed red cell transfusion requirements in children with sickle cell disease. J Pediatr Surg. 2008;43(6):1052–6.

Lerner RM, Spataro RF. Splenic abscess: percutaneous drainage. Radiology. 1984;153:643–5.

Platt O, Brambilla DJ, Roses WF, et al. Mortality in sickle cell disease: life expectancy and risk factors for early death. N Engl J Med. 1994;330:1639–44.

Pugliese R, Sansonna F, Scandroglio I, et al. Laparoscopic splenectomy: a retrospective review of 75 cases. Int Surg. 2006;91:82–6.

Waghorn DJ. Overwhelming infection in asplenic patients: current best practice preventive measures are not being followed. J Clin Pathol. 2001;54(3):214–8.

Hepatobiliary Complications of Sickle Cell Anemia

6

6.1 Introduction

- SCA can affect any part of the body and poses diagnostic and therapeutic dilemmas to the treating physicians.
- The hepatobiliary system is one of the common organs to be affected either directly from the sicklening process or indirectly as a result of chronic hemolysis and multiple blood transfusions.
- This can manifest in several clinical conditions.

6.2 Cholelithiasis

- Cholelithiasis is one of the common complications of SCA (Figs. 6.1 and 6.2).
- These are usually pigment stones that result from chronic hemolysis leading to increased bilirubin production (Fig. 6.3).
- The frequency of cholelithiasis in patients with SCA is however variable depending on the age of the patients and the diagnostic method used.
- A frequency ranging from 5–55 % has been reported but an overall 70 % of patients with SCA will develop gallstones at one stage of their life.
- With better understanding of SCA, improved medical and surgical management of these patients and the development of new drugs such as hydroxyurea have contributed to a better survival and increased life expectancy of these patients.
- This will lead to an increased frequency of cholelithiasis in these patients as the frequency of gallstones in patients with SCA increases with age.
- An overall of 19.7 % frequency of gallstones was reported in children with SCA. This frequency increased from 8.7 % in those less than 10 years of age to 36 % in those 15–18 years of age.

A. Al-Salem, *Medical and Surgical Complications of Sickle Cell Anemia*,
DOI 10.1007/978-3-319-24762-5_6

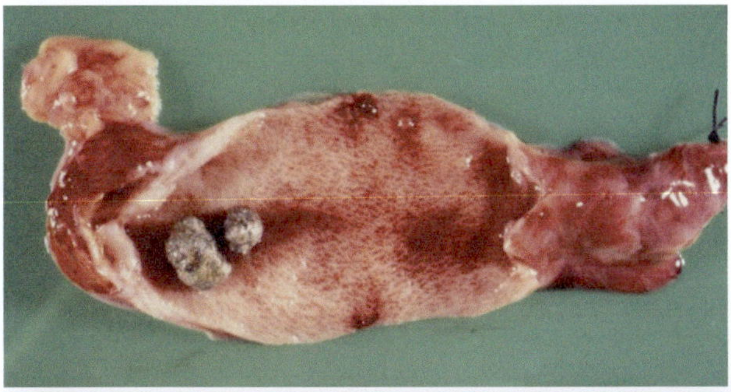

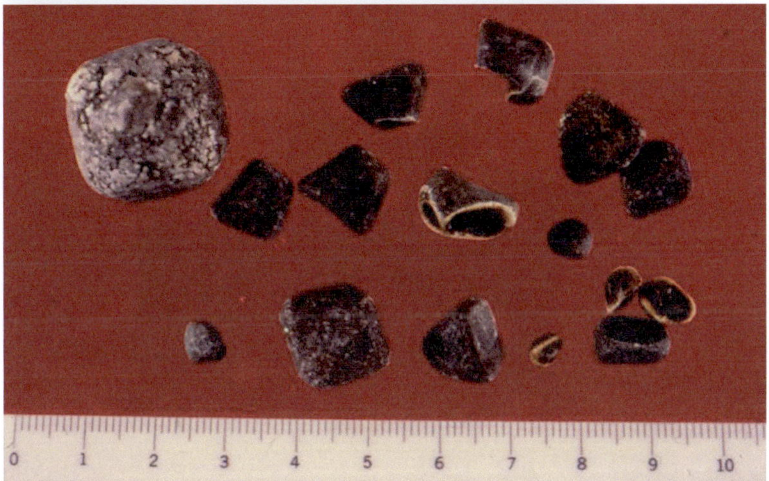

Figs. 6.1 and 6.2 Clinical photographs showing cholelithiasis

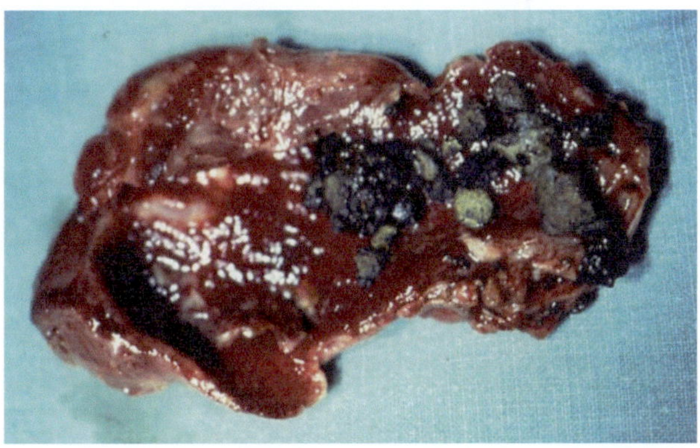

Fig. 6.3 A clinical photograph showing pigmented gallstones in a patient with SCA

6.3 Presentation

- The presentation of cholelithiasis in patients with SCA is variable.
- The classic presentation is that with biliary colic, right upper quadrant abdominal pain and discomfort, and dyspepsia or upper abdominal pain and discomfort.
- A small number of these patients present acutely with acute cholecystitis (Figs. 6.4 and 6.5).
- The recent liberal use of abdominal ultrasound as a diagnostic investigation resulted in the discovery of a large number of these patients with asymptomatic gallstones.

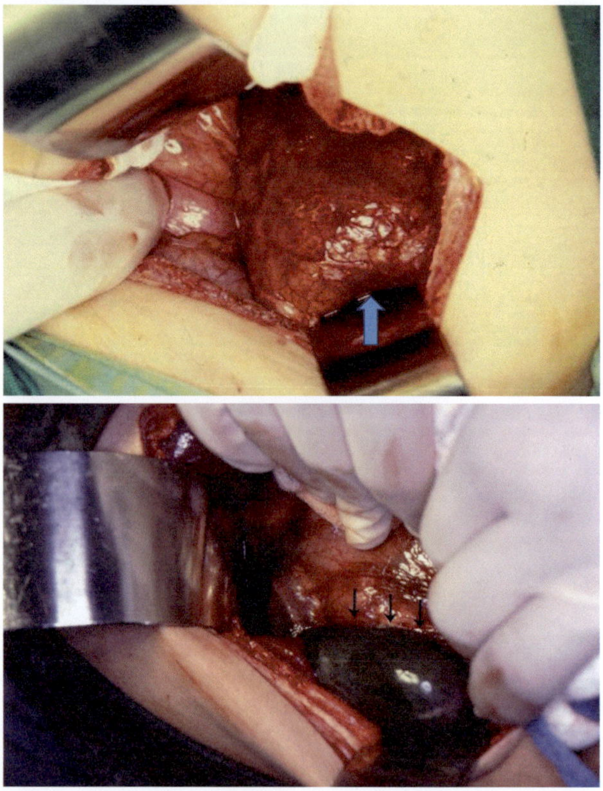

Figs. 6.4 and 6.5 A clinical intraoperative photograph showing acute cholecystitis and acute gangrenous cholecystitis in two patients with SCA

6.4 Diagnosis

- Abdominal ultrasound is the main diagnostic investigation to diagnose gallstones (Figs. 6.6 and 6.7).
- This is a simple, relatively cheap and noninvasive investigation which can accurately diagnose gallstones. Abdominal ultrasound can easily be repeated.
- The stones can be single or multiple (Fig. 6.8).
- Plain abdominal X-ray may also show these gallstones (Figs. 6.9 and 6.10).

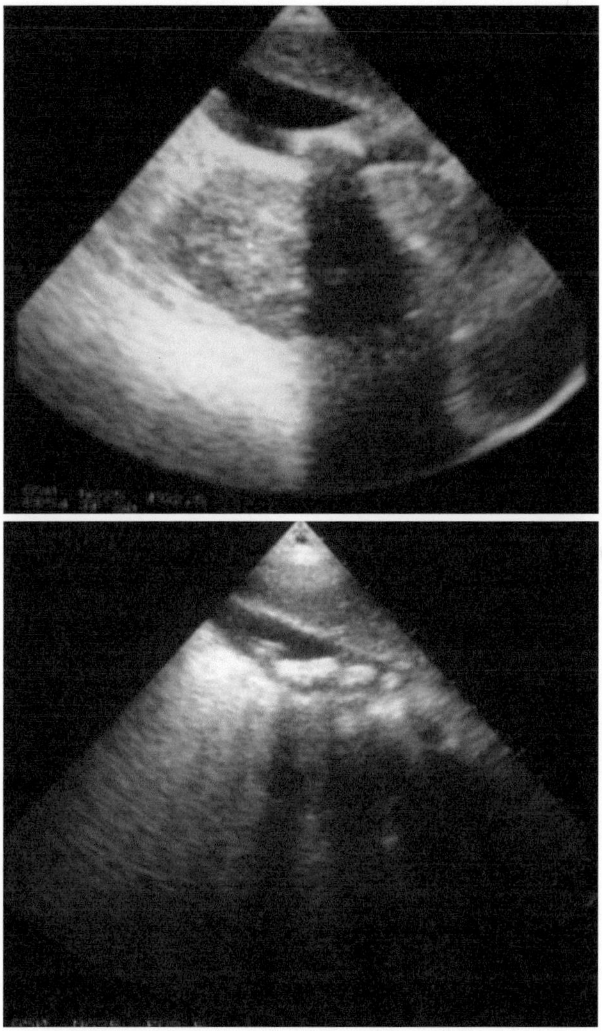

Figs. 6.6 and 6.7 Abdominal ultrasound showing gallstones in patients with SCA

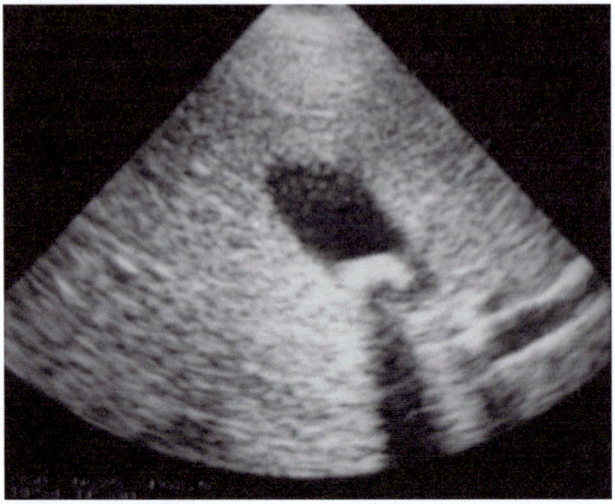

Fig. 6.8 Abdominal ultrasound showing a single gallstone in a patient with SCA

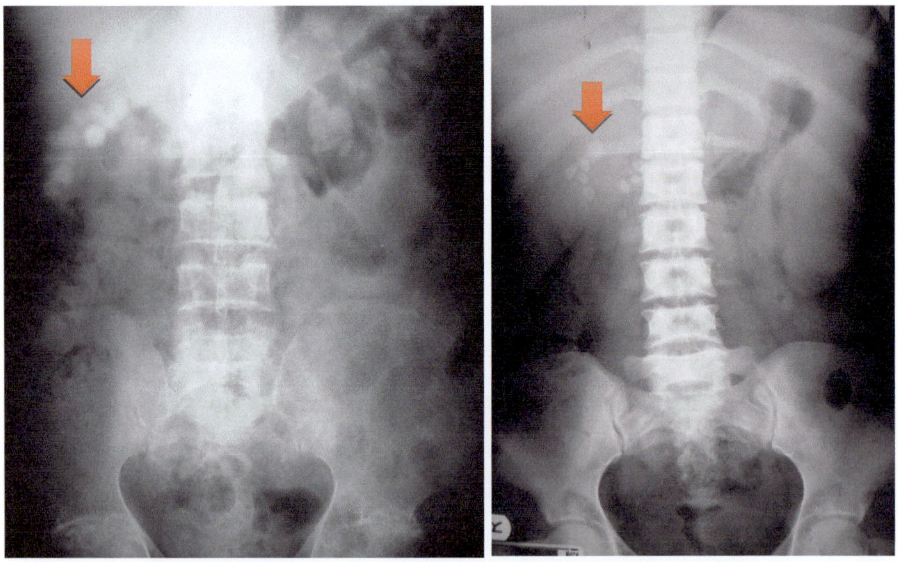

Figs. 6.9 and 6.10 Abdominal X-rays showing multiple gallstones

- Abdominal CT scan is rarely used to diagnose gallstones but can be used to diagnose gallstone-related complications such as common bile duct obstruction, live abscess, and pancreatitis.
- Endoscopic retrograde cholangiopancreatography (ERCP) is a valuable investigation to diagnose common bile duct stones and delineate the anatomy of the biliary system (Figs. 6.11 and 6.12).
- It is also valuable as a therapeutic modality to treat common bile duct stones.

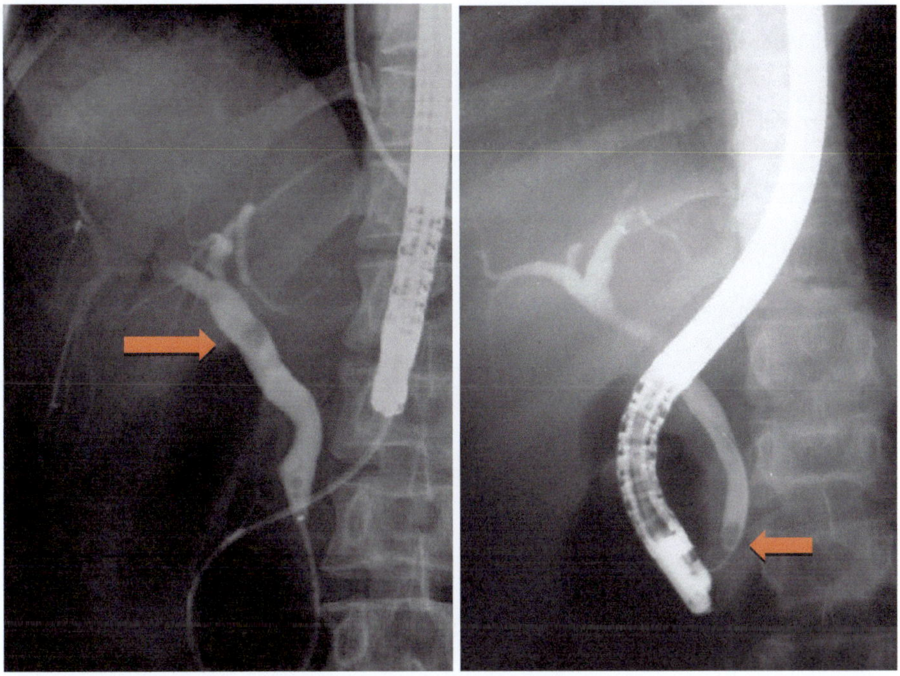

Figs. 6.11 and 6.12 ERCP showing common bile duct stones

6.5 Treatment

- The treatment of cholelithiasis in patients with SCA is cholecystectomy.
- In the era of minimal invasive surgery, laparoscopic cholecystectomy is now the procedure of choice. This is specially so for patients with SCA where it was shown to be feasible, beneficial, and safe.
- The fact that there is no large abdominal wound, laparoscopic cholecystectomy should be advantageous to patients with SCA. Not only is the hospital stay short and cosmetically better but the associated postoperative pain is much less. This makes their early mobilization much easier and will not interfere with their breathing which may prove beneficial in reducing the incidence of postoperative acute chest syndrome.
- The treatment of asymptomatic gallstones in patients with SCA is still controversial.
- In the past and because of a reported perioperative mortality rate as high as 10 % and a postoperative complication rate up to 50 %, surgery in patients with SCA was not advocated except in symptomatic patients.
- This however is not the case nowadays, as with better understanding of SCA and improved perioperative care, surgery is safer.
- Many surgeons now advocate cholecystectomy for asymptomatic gallstones in patients with SCA.

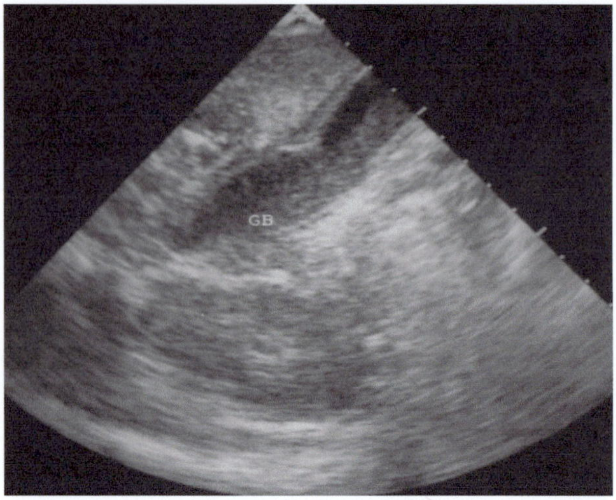

Fig. 6.13 An abdominal ultrasound showing acute cholecystitis with biliary sludge. Note the thickened wall of the gallbladder

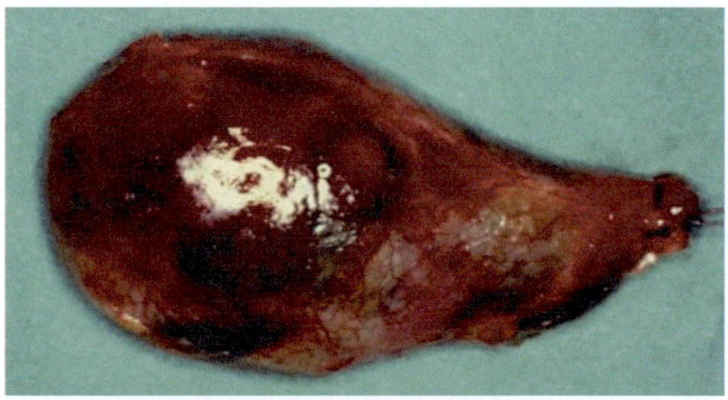

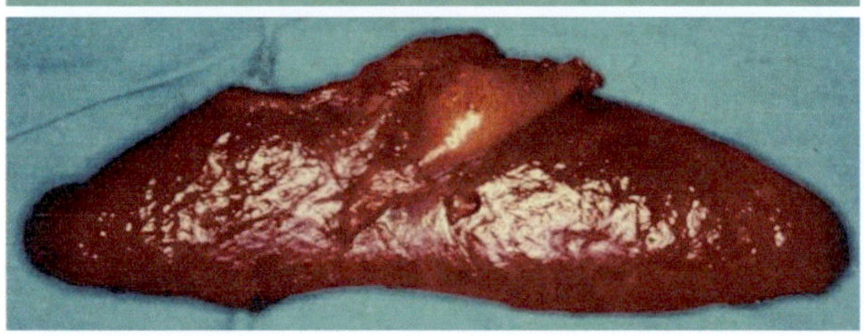

Figs. 6.14 and 6.15 Clinical photographs showing acute cholecystitis in already excised gallbladders

- The life expectancy of patients with SCA is known to be shorter than the general population and they usually die of SCA-related complications, but as a result of better understanding of SCA and its complications, the use of hydroxyurea, as well as improved medical and surgical care, SCA patients are now living longer. This makes them liable to develop gallstone-related complications including:
  - Biliary colic
  - Acute cholecystitis (Figs. 6.13, 6.14 and 6.15)
  - Choledocholithiasis (Fig. 6.16)

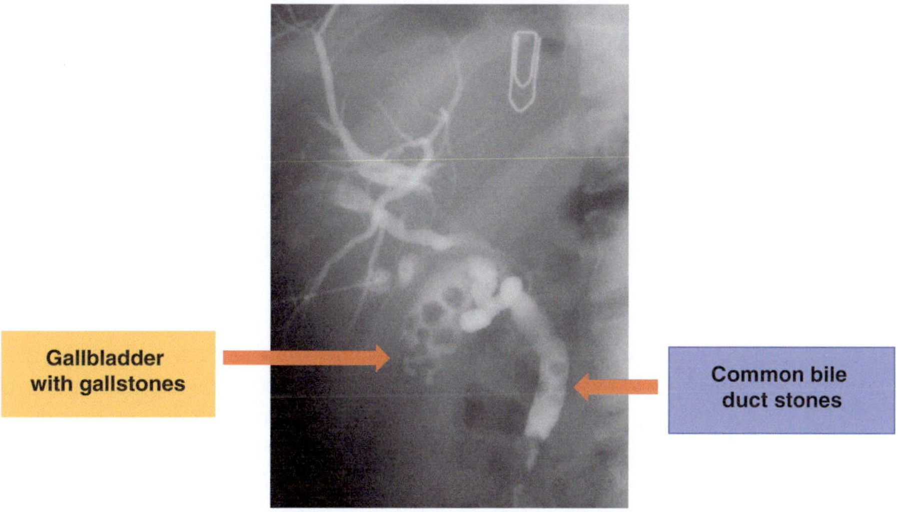

Fig. 6.16 Percutaneous transhepatic cholangiogram showing gallstones and common bile duct stones

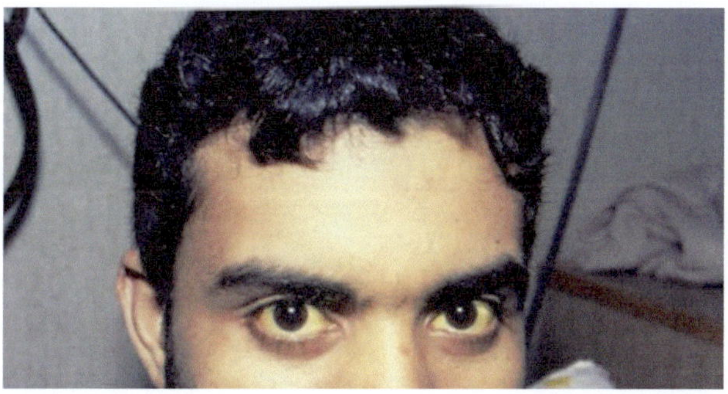

Fig. 6.17 A clinical photograph of a patient with SCA who presented with obstructive jaundice

  - Obstructive jaundice (Fig. 6.17)
  - Ascending cholangitis
  - Pancreatitis
- Operating on these patients on an emergency basis not fully prepared is definitely associated with a high morbidity and mortality (Fig. 6.2). It is much better to operate on these patients electively when they are well prepared.
- Add to this the fact that cholecystectomy should simplify the future management of abdominal crisis as the possibility of acute cholecystitis is eliminated.

Complications of Cholelithiasis

- Biliary colic and dyspepsia
- Acute and chronic cholecystitis
- Choledocholithiasis
- Obstructive jaundice
- Ascending cholangitis
- Acute pancreatitis

- It has been estimated that about 70 % of patients with SCA will develop gallstones at one stage of their life. This is a high frequency and a question that is being raised nowadays is whether this justifies incidental cholecystectomy for SCA patients who are having abdominal surgery electively for some other reason such as splenectomy or hiatal hernia repair. This is still controversial and most surgeons are not supportive of this.

6.6 Choledocholithiasis

- Another relatively common complication of SCA is the development of choledocholithiasis which is usually secondary to cholelithiasis but there are also primary choledocholithiasis (Figs. 6.18, 6.19, 6.20, 6.21, 6.22 and 6.23).
- In the general population with cholelithiasis, the incidence of common bile duct stones has been reported as 10–15 %. In patients with SCA, the frequency of common bile duct stones is 18–30 %.
- As a result of this high incidence of choledocholithiasis, routine intraoperative cholangiogram was advocated for those undergoing cholecystectomy (Fig. 6.24).
- In the era of laparoscopy and endoscopic retrograde cholangiopancreatography (ERCP), the question is whether laparoscopic cholangiography with or without common bile duct exploration is necessary in patients with SCA.
- Laparoscopic cholangiography will increase the operative time and makes it difficult to decide when CBD stones are diagnosed whether to convert the operation to open cholecystectomy or wait and do a post-laparoscopic cholecystectomy ERCP. Added to this is a 25 % false-positive rate that may lead to unnecessary CBD exploration or conversion to open cholecystectomy.
- Laparoscopic cholangiography and CBD exploration and extraction of CBD stones is feasible and safe in experienced hands.
- ERCP however is valuable both as a diagnostic and therapeutic procedure for SCA patients with choledocholithiasis both pre- and post-laparoscopic cholecystectomy. This sequential approach of endoscopic sphincterotomy and stone extraction followed by laparoscopic cholecystectomy is a safe and effective

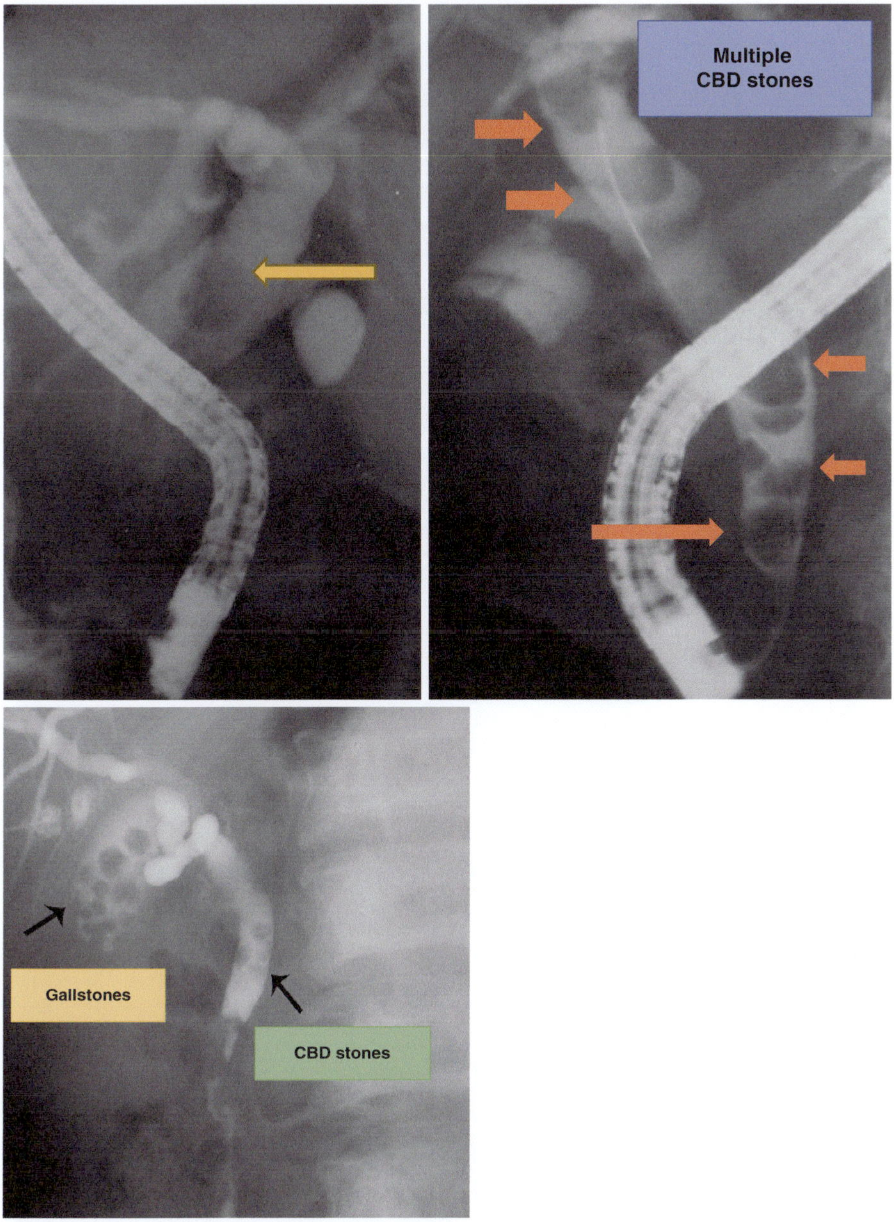

Figs. 6.18, 6.19, and 6.20 ERCP, percutaneous transhepatic cholangiogram (PTC) and ERCP showing single CBD stone, gallstones, and multiple CBD stones

Figs. 6.22 and 6.23 ERCP showing multiple gallstones without common bile duct stones and ERCP showing common bile duct stones complicated by a choledochoduodenal fistula. Note the air in the biliary tree

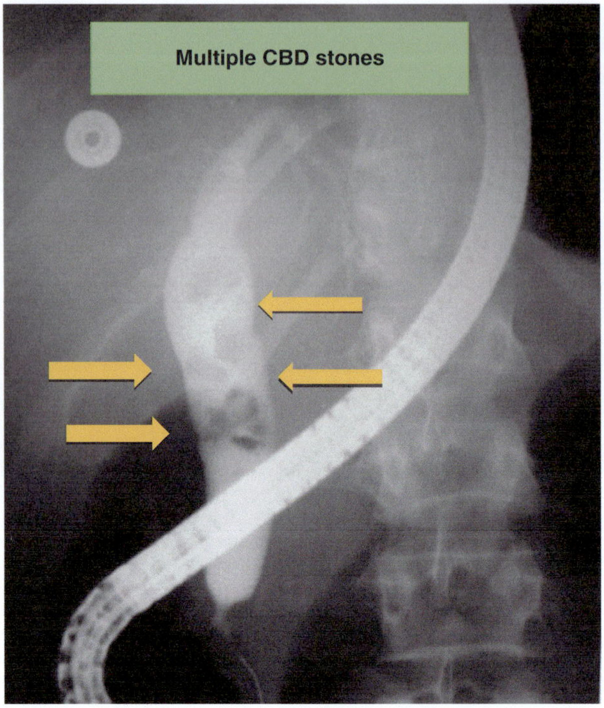

Fig. 6.21 ERCP showing multiple common bile duct stones

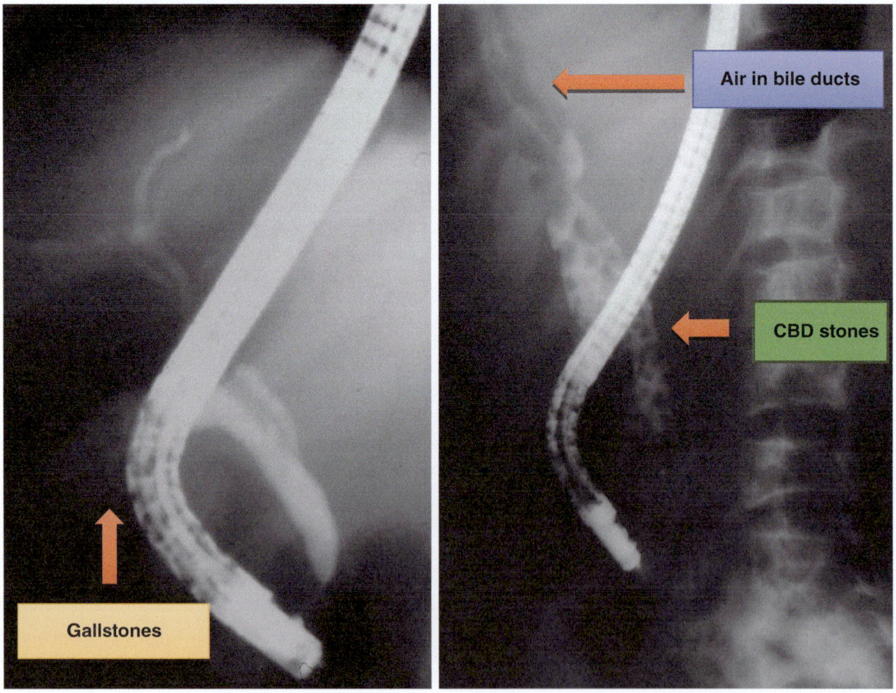

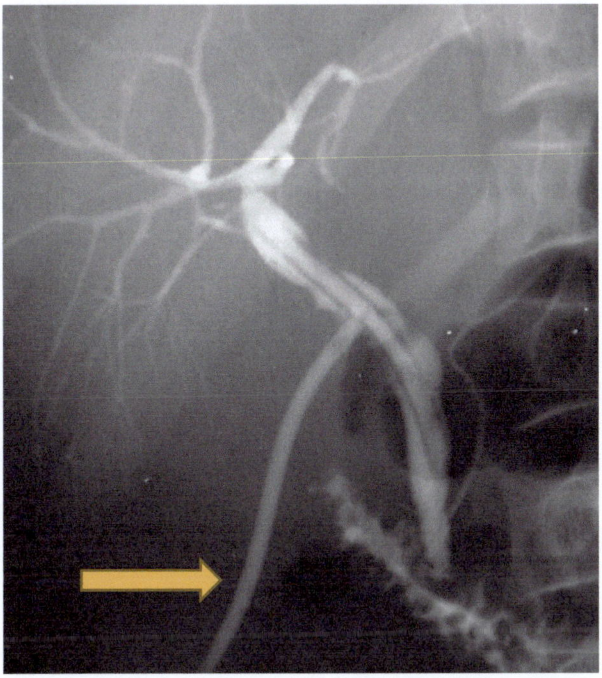

Fig. 6.24 T-tube cholangiogram following intraoperative cholangiogram and CBD exploration for CBD stones. Note the patent biliary ducts and T-tube for temporary drainage of common bile duct

approach for the management of SCA patients with cholelithiasis and choledocholithiasis (Figs. 6.25, 6.26, 6.27 and 6.28).

- The use of ERCP both pre- and post-laparoscopic cholecystectomy in experienced hands has markedly decreased common bile duct exploration (Figs. 6.29 and 6.30).
- ERCP can be used preoperatively in those with suspected common bile duct stones for both diagnosis and treatment.
- ERCP can be used to remove common bile duct stones followed by laparoscopic cholecystectomy.
- ERCP can also be used to diagnose and remove retained common bile duct stones following laparoscopic cholecystectomy.

6.7 Biliary Sludge

- This is one of the common and interesting complications of SCA.
- Biliary sludge, which is a sequel of chronic hemolysis, is a mixture of calcium bilirubinate and cholesterol crystals within viscous bile that contains a high concentration of mucus and proteins.

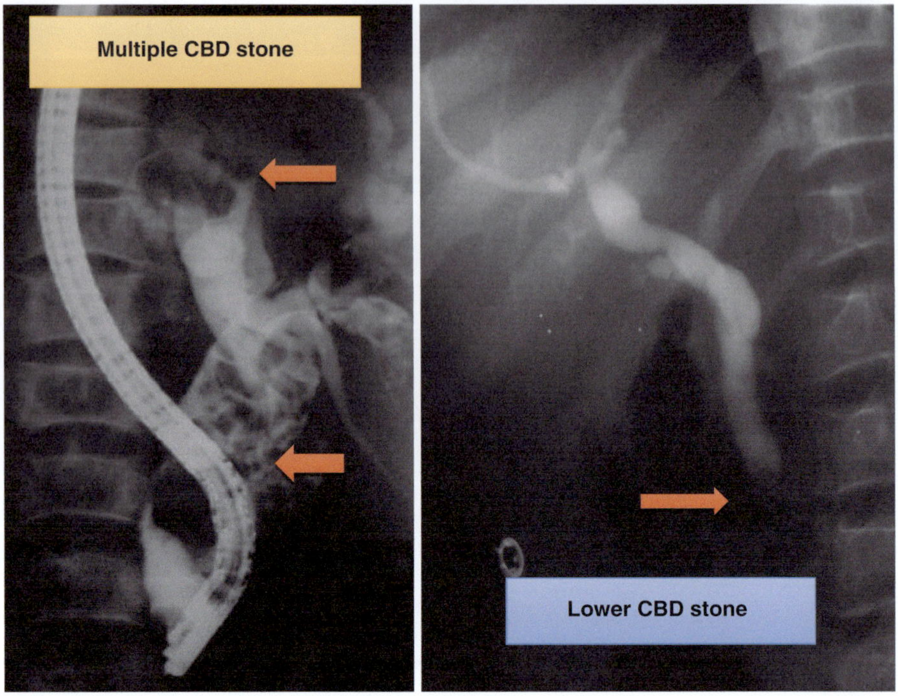

Figs. 6.25 and 6.26 ERCP showing multiple bile duct stones in the first one and a single CBD stone following laparoscopic cholecystectomy in the second one

- It can be seen in the gallbladder or sometimes in the bile ducts (Figs. 6.31, 6.32, 6.33, 6.34, 6.35, and 6.36).
- On ultrasound, it characteristically produces a low-amplitude echo pattern, intraluminal layers in the dependent part of the gallbladder.
- The exact incidence of biliary sludge in patients with SCA is not known.
- A frequency of as high as 16.4 % of biliary sludge was reported in children with SCA (Fig. 6.37).
- What is the significance of biliary sludge?
- It was shown that a large number of patients with biliary sludge (65.7 %) developed gallstones on follow-up.
- Biliary sludge is usually asymptomatic discovered incidentally on abdominal ultrasound. Sometimes biliary sludge can be symptomatic causing biliary colic and biliary dyspepsia.
- Management of patients with biliary sludge:
  - Patients with biliary sludge should be followed-up, and those who develop gallstones undergo elective laparoscopic cholecystectomy.
  - Symptomatic patients with biliary sludge should be offered laparoscopic cholecystectomy to relieve them from their symptoms (Figs. 6.38 and 6.39).

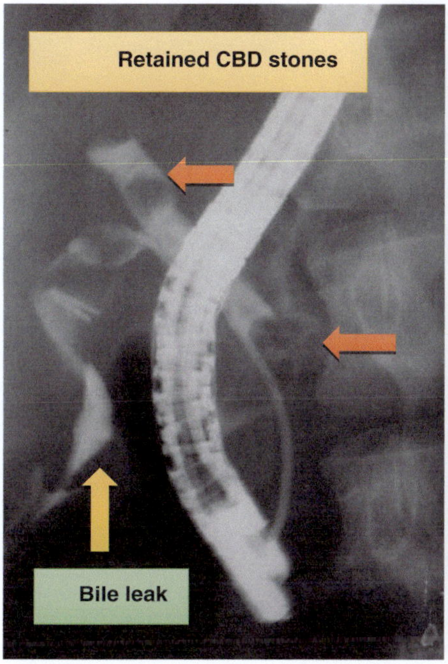

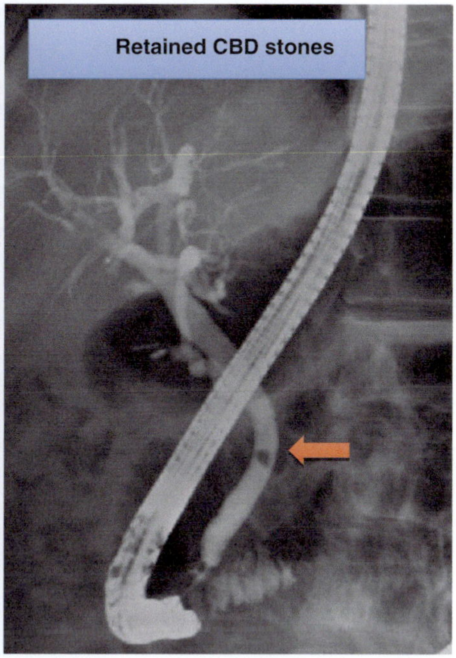

Figs. 6.27 and 6.28 ERCP showing retained common bile duct stones following laparoscopic cholecystectomy. Note the retained CBD stones which caused bile leak

- A question that still needs an answer is: since the majority of patients with biliary sludge will develop gallstones, is it advisable to offer these patients whether symptomatic or not elective laparoscopic cholecystectomy?
- There are those who advocate conservative treatment and follow-up of patients with biliary sludge and offer them laparoscopic cholecystectomy when they develop gallstones while others and based on the high rate of development of cholelithiasis in these patients advocate elective laparoscopic cholecystectomy. This will obviate the subsequent risk of developing biliary sludge and cholelithiasis-related complications.

6.8 Sickle Cell Cholangiopathy

- This is an interesting but still not well-established complication of SCA.
- It is seen in patients who present with cholestatic jaundice and on ultrasound and ERCP are found to have bile duct dilatation without an obstructive cause (Figs. 6.40 and 6.41).

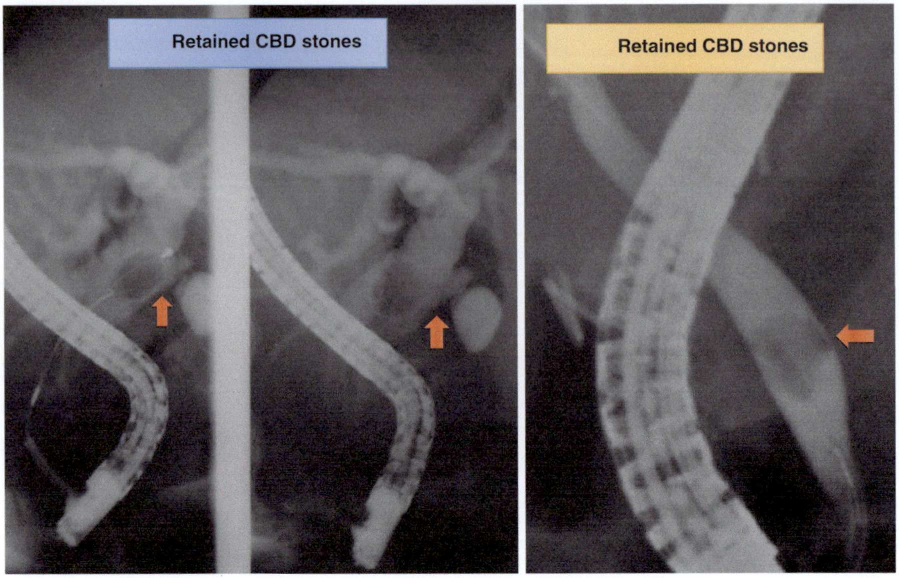

Figs. 6.29 and 6.30 ERCP showing CBD stone being removed in the first one and a retained CBD stone following laparoscopic cholecystectomy

- Sickle cell cholangiopathy is not rare but the exact incidence is not known.
- A frequency as high as 25 % of sickle cell cholangiopathy was found in SCA patients who present with cholestatic jaundice. They have bile duct dilatation without an obstructive cause when evaluated by ERCP.
- Etiology:
  - The reason for this bile duct dilation is not exactly known and none of these patients had previously cholelithiasis or choledocholithiasis.
  - This is a form of cholangiopathy that is a consequence of sickling in the end arteries of the biliary arterial tree leading to hypoxia and dilatation of the biliary system.
  - The bile ducts are supplied via the hepatic arteries and ischemic bile duct injury may occur when these vessels are injured or occluded.
  - This ultimately will result in ischemia of the bile ducts and the effect depends on the extent and velocity of the occlusive process.
  - In patients with SCA, the occlusion which is usually not complete is of the peribiliary vascular plexus and is a result of sickling within these vascular channels.
  - This ultimately will lead to hypoxia of the bile ducts leading to their dilatation rather than ischemia and stricture formation.

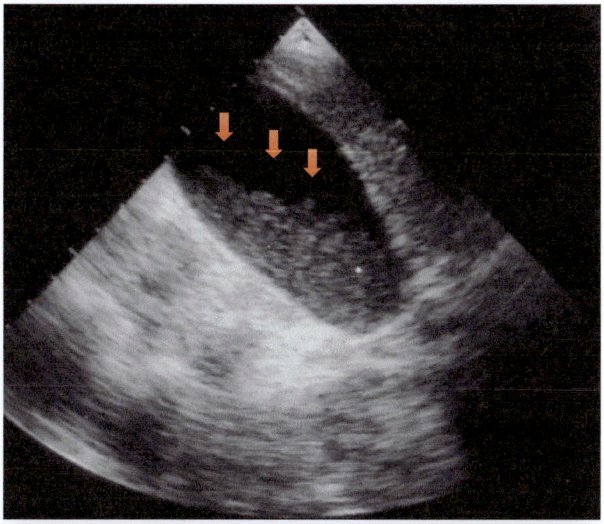

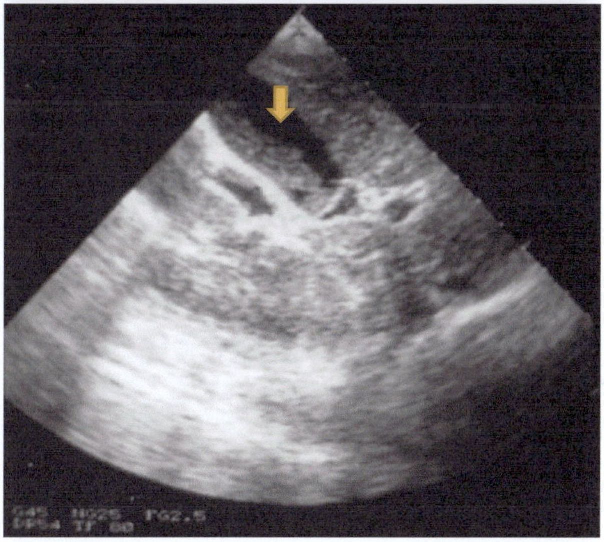

Figs. 6.31, 6.32, 6.33, 6.34, 6.35, and 6.36 Abdominal ultrasound and ERCP showing biliary sludge in the gallbladder and CBD

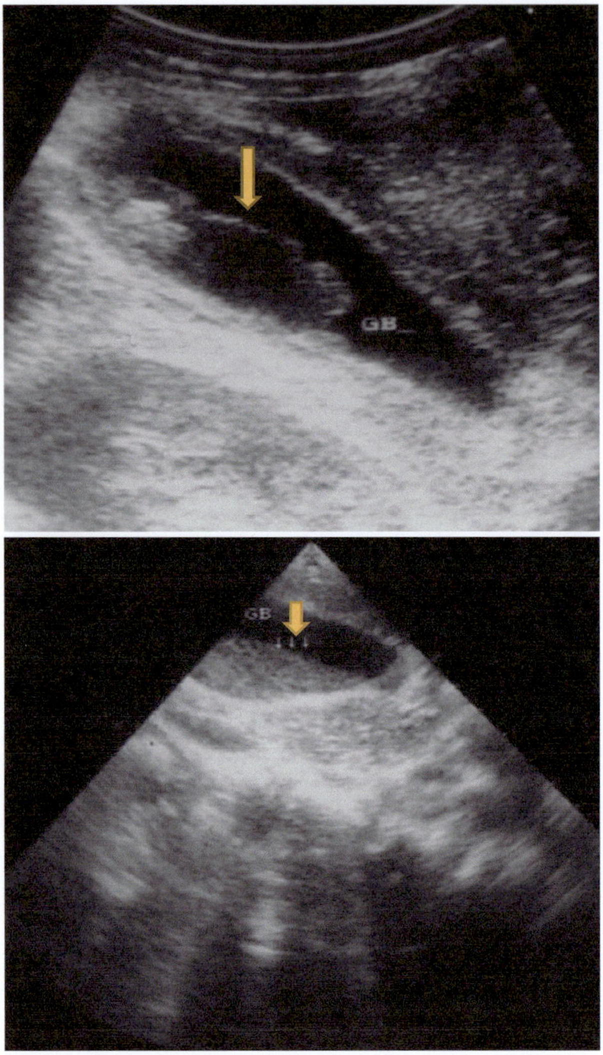

Figs. 6.31, 6.32, 6.33, 6.34, 6.35, and 6.36 (continued)

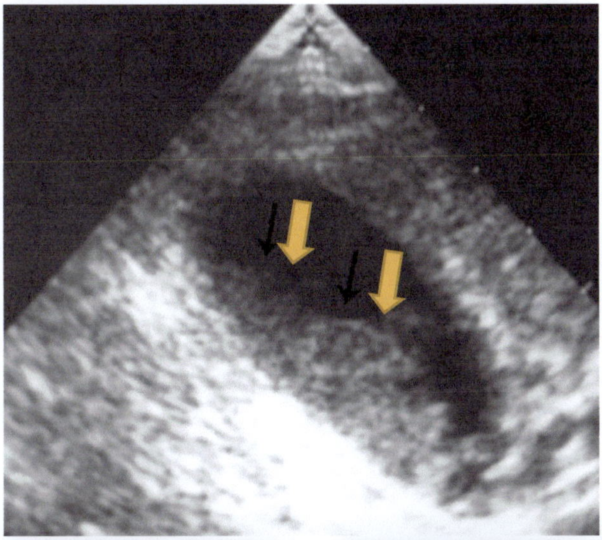

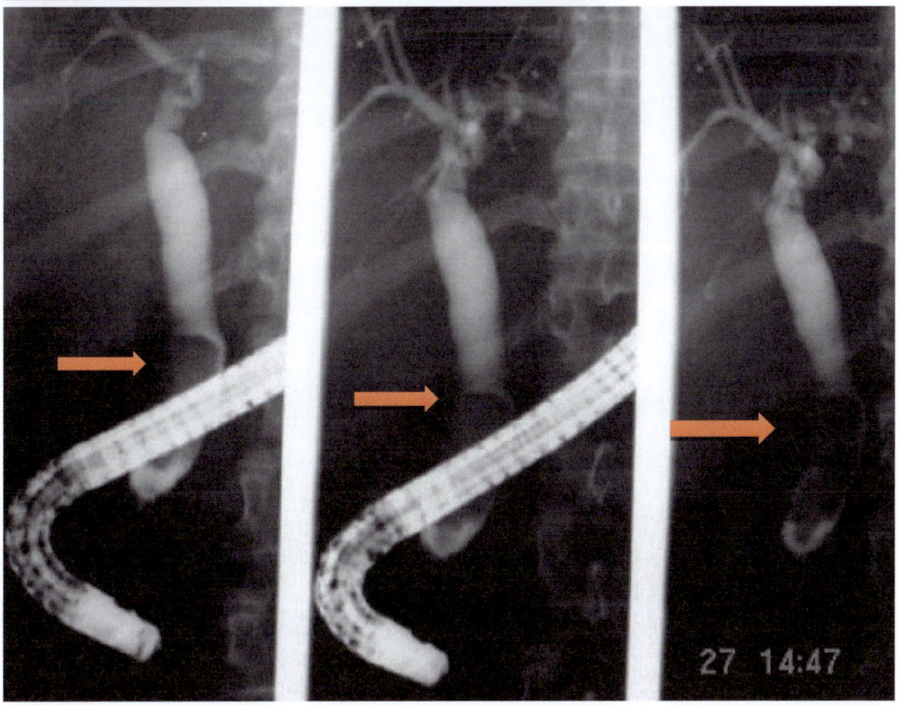

Figs. 6.31, 6.32, 6.33, 6.34, 6.35, and 6.36 (continued)

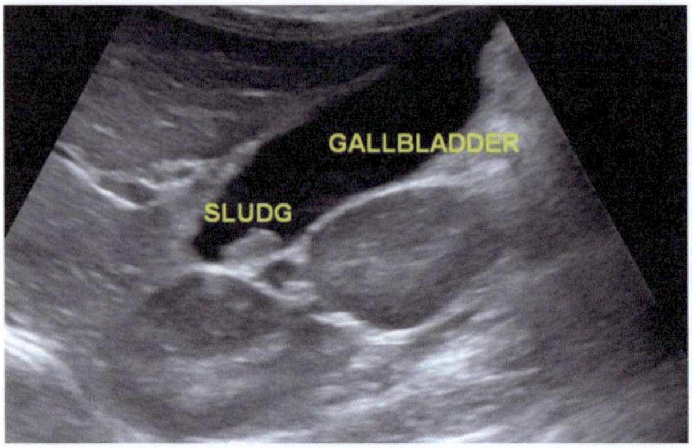

Fig. 6.37 Abdominal ultrasound showing biliary sludge in a child with sickle cell anemia

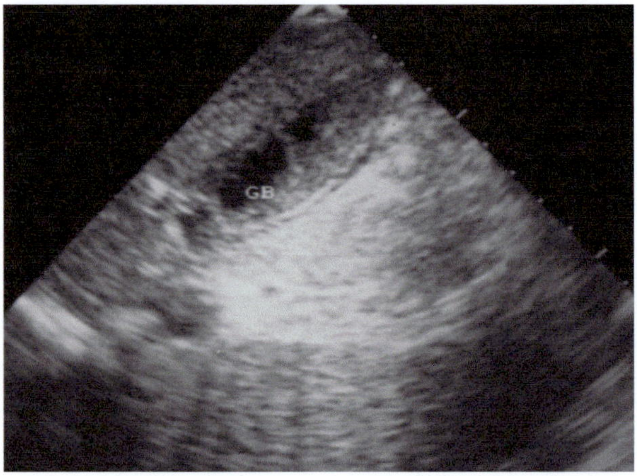

Fig. 6.38 Abdominal ultrasound showing biliary sludge and evidence of acute cholecystitis

- This is called SCA cholangiopathy and the extent of this is also variable (Figs. 6.42 and 6.43).
- There are patients with bile ducts dilatation limited to the common bile duct, but there are also those with dilatation involving both extra- and intrahepatic bile ducts.

- Documenting this is of great importance as these patients need to be followed up regularly for the possibility of developing bile duct stones.
- The dilated bile ducts lead to stasis of bile with the possibility of subsequent development of biliary sludge and bile duct stones.
- Taking in consideration the high frequency of biliary sludge and the possibility of bile duct stone formation in these patients, ERCP and endoscopic

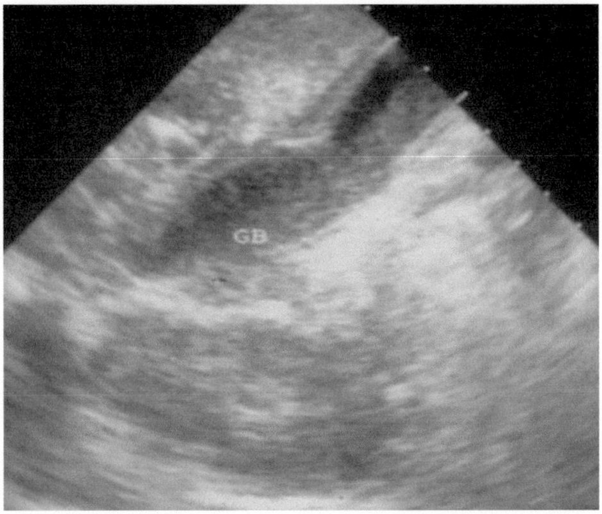

Fig. 6.39 Abdominal ultrasound showing biliary sludge and evidence of acute cholecystitis

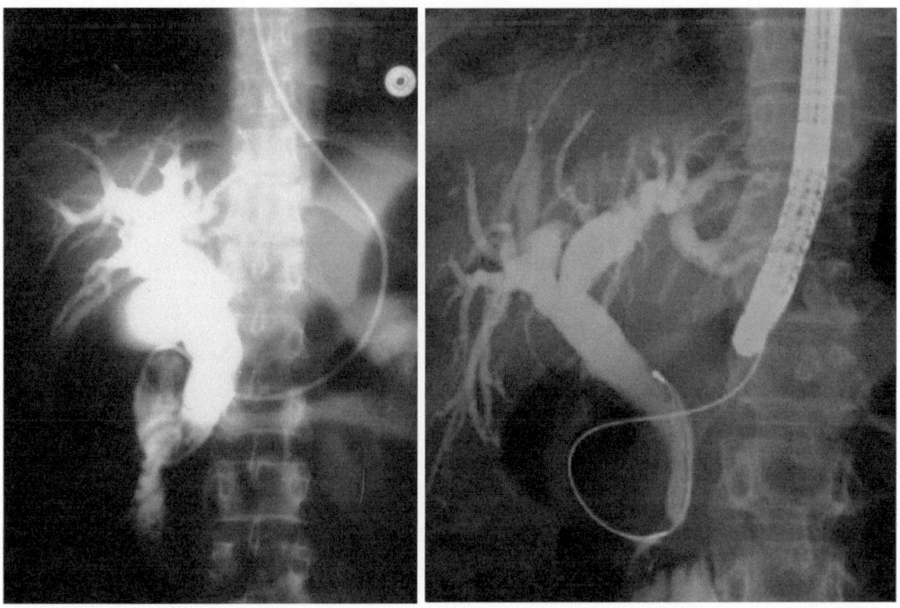

Figs. 6.40 and 6.41 ERCP showing dilated biliary ducts without an obstructive cause. Note the extent of the dilatation involving the whole biliary ducts

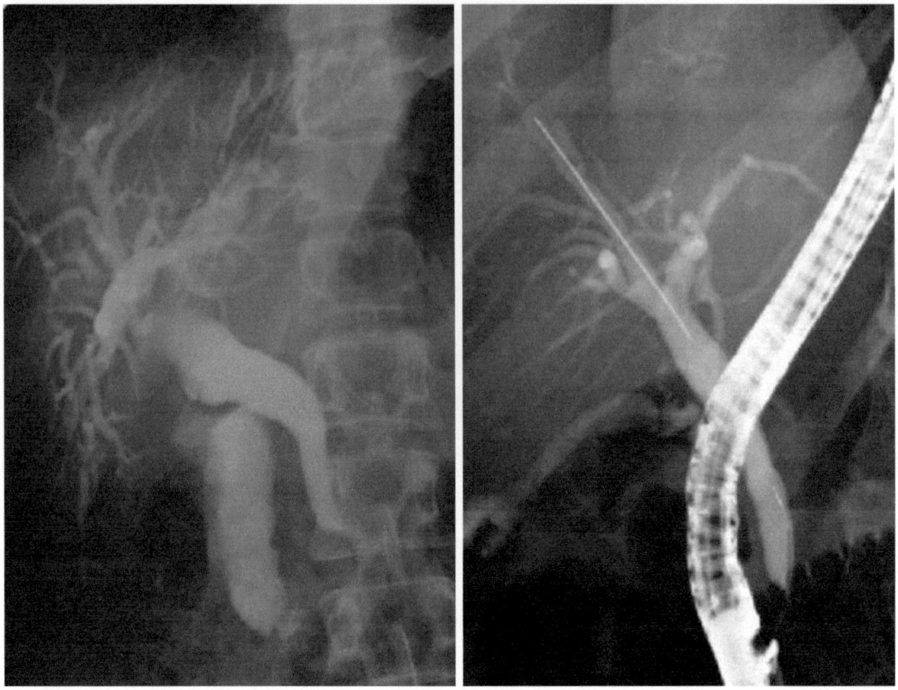

Figs. 6.42 and 6.43 ERCP showing dilated bile ducts without an obstructive cause. The dilatation is limited to the CBD and hepatic ducts

sphincterotomy may be beneficial as these may obviate the future development of bile duct stones.

- Sphincterotomy may allow free drainage of bile from the bile ducts to the duodenum, avoiding bile stasis in the bile ducts.

6.9 Pancreatitis

- Primary or idiopathic pancreatitis is not a common complication of SCA.
- Commonly, pancreatitis is seen in patients with cholelithiasis and/or choledocholithiasis as a result of common bile duct obstruction but there are reports of pancreatitis in patients with SCA without cholelithiasis.

- In these patients, pancreatitis may be due to microvascular occlusion and ischemic injury to the pancreas.
- Acute pancreatitis should be considered in the differential diagnosis of abdominal pain in patients with SCA.
- There are also reports of pancreatitis in SCA patients following ERCP. These are usually mild and transient and procedure-related complications.
- It is also important to observe and follow-up these patients as SCA patients may also develop pancreatic pseudocyst (Figs. 6.44, 6.45, and 6.46).
- The treatment of pancreatitis is usually conservative with:
  - Intravenous hydration.
  - Antibiotics.
  - Analgesia.
  - Laparoscopic cholecystectomy is advocated in those with gallstone-related pancreatitis. This should be done electively once their condition becomes stable to avoid further attacks.

6.10 Sickle Cell Hepatopathy

- One of the common manifestations of SCA is jaundice which can be caused by a variety of hepatobiliary diseases including cholestatic jaundice (Fig. 6.47).
- There are however certain causes of cholestatic jaundice that are SCA related. One of these is intrahepatic sickling of RBC. This can lead to cholestasis and a clinical picture that may resemble extrahepatic bile duct obstruction which causes diagnostic and therapeutic dilemmas.
- Intrahepatic sickling produces a constellation of signs and symptoms, and although they are divided into distinct clinical syndromes, there is however overlap between them and the overall effect is called sickle cell hepatopathy.
- Early recognition of these syndromes, diagnosis, and prompt treatment are important to achieve a favorable outcome.
- The aim should be early diagnosis and treatment to prevent irreversible liver injury, and every mean possible including the laboratory findings, radiological investigations, and liver biopsy should be utilized to establish the diagnosis.

6.11 Acute Sickle Cell Hepatic Crisis

- The exact etiology of acute hepatic crisis is not known.
- It is thought to result from stagnation of sickled red blood cells within the liver sinusoids.
- This will result in a decrease in circulation through the hepatic sinusoids.
- The clinical presentation of acute liver cell hepatic crisis is variable depending on the severity but the majority present with:

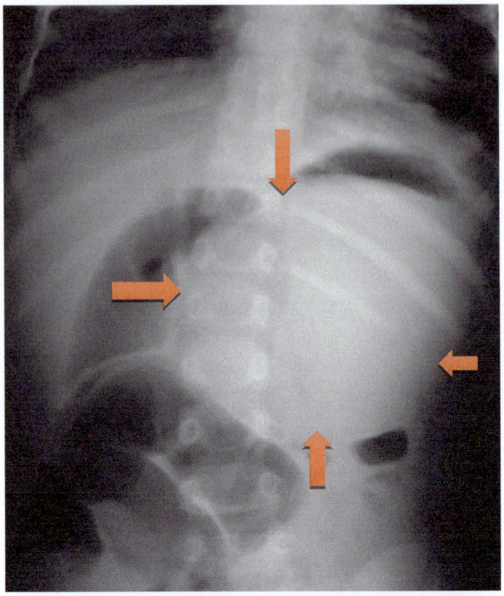

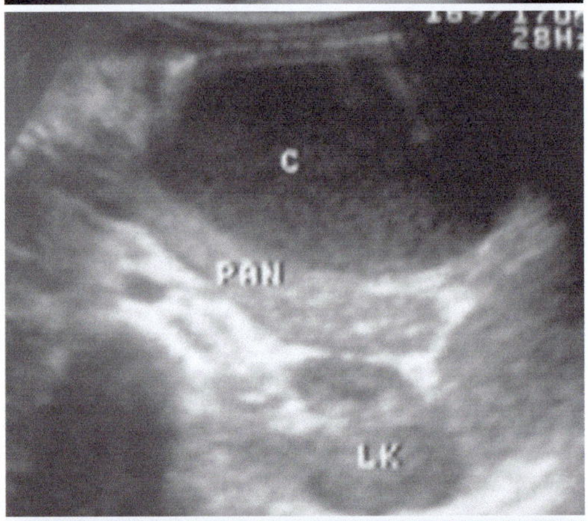

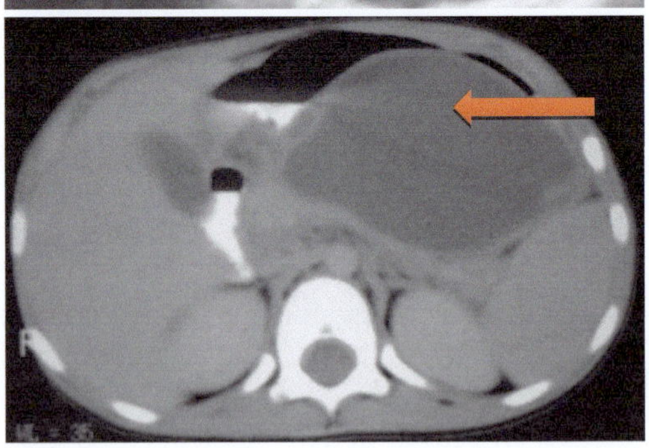

Figs. 6.44, 6.45, and 6.46 Abdominal radiograph, abdominal ultrasound, and CT scan showing pancreatic pseudocyst following an attack of acute pancreatitis. Note the soft tissue density pushing the intestine and stomach representing a pancreatic pseudocyst

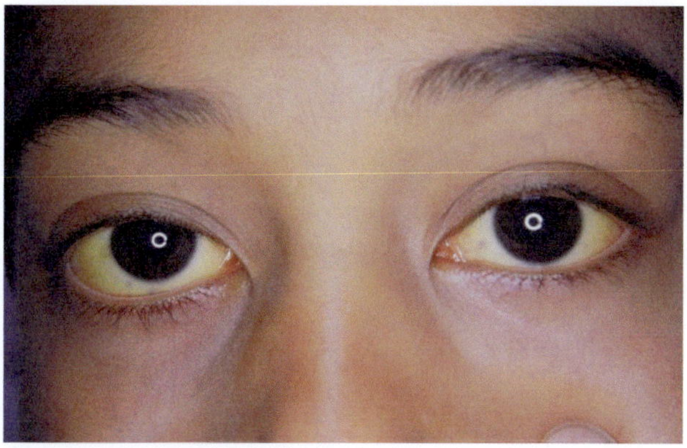

Fig. 6.47 A clinical photograph showing a child with sickle cell anemia and jaundice

- Right upper quadrant abdominal pain.
- Low-grade fever.
- Vomiting.
- This is usually associated with leukocytosis and mild to moderated elevations of the liver enzymes and bilirubin levels.
- The increase in bilirubin is that of the conjugated part.

• The treatment is conservative and supportive as it is self-limiting and it usually resolves spontaneously.
• In severe cases, simple or partial exchange blood transfusion may be necessary.
• An extremely rare complication of acute severe hepatic crisis that must be kept in mind is hepatic infarction. This is usually seen as a characteristic wedge-shaped, peripherally located hypodense lesion on CT scan.

6.12 Hepatic Sequestration Crisis

• Sequestration of red blood cells is a common complication of SCA.
• This is commonly seen in the spleen and to a lesser extent in the lungs.
• Acute splenic sequestration crisis is considered the second most common cause of death after infection during the first 5 years of life in children with SCA.
• Hepatic sequestration crisis is not common and it is caused by obstruction of the blood flow from the liver sinusoids by the sickled red blood cells leading to compression of the bile ducts.
• This will lead to pooling of blood within the liver leading to acute hepatic enlargement (Fig. 6.48).
• It is also associated with a rapid drop in hemoglobin and hematocrit levels and an increase in the reticulocyte count and bilirubin level.
• This differentiates it from acute hepatic crisis.

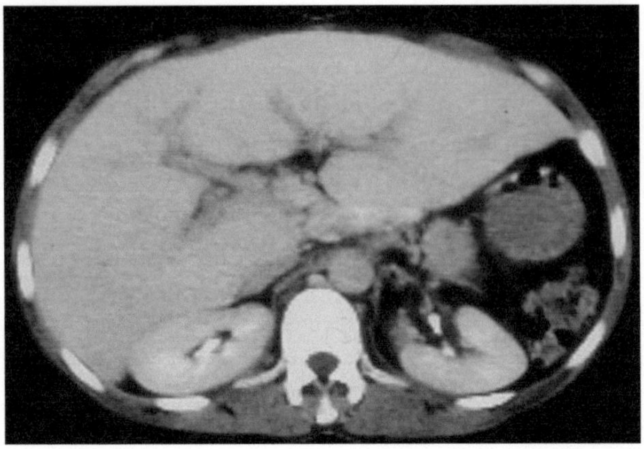

Fig. 6.48 Abdominal CT scan showing liver sequestration in a patient with SCA

- The liver enzymes are only mildly elevated and the hyperbilirubinemia is that of the conjugated fraction.
- Once diagnosed and treated with hydration and blood transfusion, it behaves like acute splenic sequestration with regression of the hepatic size and increase in hemoglobin level.
- Recurrence is common and a chronic hepatic sequestration form was also described.

6.13 Acute Sickle Cell Intrahepatic Cholestasis

- Acute sickle cell intrahepatic cholestasis is a rare but a serious and sometimes fatal complication of SCA.
- It is a distinct clinical entity but some consider it a severe form of sickle cell hepatic crisis.
- It results from sever obstruction of the liver sinusoids leading to stasis, hypoxia, and intracanalicular cholestasis secondary to ballooning of the hepatocytes.
- Clinically, it resembles acute hepatic crisis but the main differentiating points are the associated:
  - Extreme hyperbilirubinemia
  - Coagulopathy
  - Acute hepatic failure
- Early recognition of this potentially fatal complication is crucial as ultimately it will lead to liver failure, encephalopathy, and renal impairment.
- Early diagnosis and intensive supportive care including exchange blood transfusion, fresh frozen plasma, platelet transfusion, and plasmapheresis may reverse the process of intrahepatic sickling and cholestasis resulting in a favorable outcome.
- A variant of chronic intrahepatic cholestasis was also described.
- This is a mild benign condition characterized by prolonged hyperbilirubinemia in the absence of right upper guardant abdominal pain and evidence of hemolysis.

- Once it is recognized, it can be successfully treated with a regular exchange blood transfusion program with or without hydroxyurea.
- A similar condition of benign hyperbilirubinemia was also described in children with SCA.

6.14 Hepatitis B and C

- SCA is a chronic illness characterized by periods of remissions and exacerbations which are called crisis.
- One of these is hemolytic crisis.
- Although there is a chronic hemolysis in patients with SCA, they can also have an acute hemolytic crisis. This will lead to acute anemia which will require blood transfusion.
- Frequent blood transfusion is also required for other complications of SCA such as:
  - Acute splenic sequestration crisis
  - Acute hepatic sequestration crisis
  - Acute chest syndrome
  - Priapism
  - Central nervous system crisis
- Add to this the need for blood transfusion as part of their preoperative preparation for major surgery.
- This makes them liable to develop blood transfusion-related complications including iron overload, alloimmunization, and hepatitis B and C (Fig. 6.49).

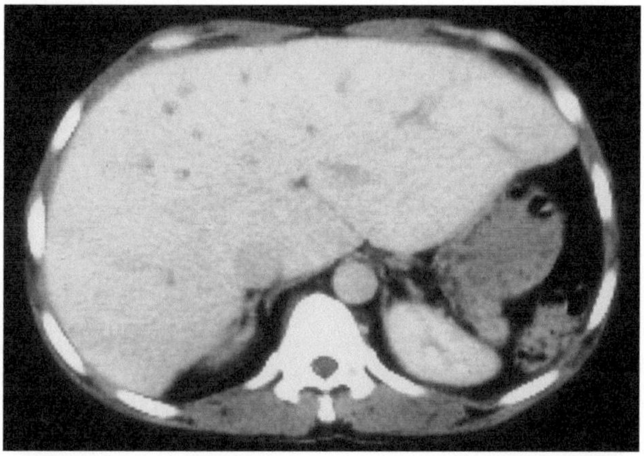

Fig. 6.49 Abdominal CT scan showing the liver with iron overload in a patient with SCA receiving multiple blood transfusions

- Hepatic iron overload is a serious complication of chronic blood transfusion therapy in patients with SCA.
- The degree of liver iron overload is clearly associated with the number of previous blood transfusions. This will lead to liver fibrosis and, eventually, liver cirrhosis.
- There is also a definite increase in the prevalence of hepatitis B and C infections among patients with SCA.
- The prevalence of chronic hepatic B in patients with SCA is reported to be low, less than 3.3 %, but in parts of the world where hepatitis B is more prevalent, the rate is much higher.
- One important contributing factor for this is the availability of vaccination against hepatitis B. Hence early vaccination against HBV would probably be the only effective way of controlling HBV infection in these patients.
- This is in contrast to hepatitis C where so far no vaccination against it is available.
- Preventive measures such as blood screening for anti-HCV before transfusion and stringent infection control measures are crucial steps to be implemented for the control of spread of HCV among these patients.
- The frequency of hepatitis C is much higher in those with SCA but this is variable.
- In patients with SCA, the prevalence of HCV antibody is directly related to the number of blood transfusions.
- It was found that patients who received more than ten blood transfusions had a 26.4–30.3 % prevalence of anti-HCV antibodies, in comparison to 8.6–10.7 % in those who received less than ten blood transfusions.
- Patients with chronic hepatitis C if left untreated are susceptible for liver damage, liver cirrhosis, hepatocellular carcinoma, and live failure.
- Add to this the fact that the combination of iron overload and chronic hepatitis C can lead to more rapidly progressive liver disease.
- In the past there was no well-proven treatment for chronic hepatitis C, but the recent progress has made treatment and cure of chronic hepatitis C possible.
- Patients with SCA and chronic hepatitis C for many years were considered to be unsuitable for such treatment.
- One reason for this is that ribavirin may induce hemolysis which can further aggravate their already existing anemia. This is not the case nowadays and patients with SCA and chronic hepatitis C can be treated with pegylated interferon and ribavirin.
- The treatment is safe and effective and the response rate is comparable to those patients without SCA.
- Recently, new and safe drugs are being used to treat patients with hepatitis B and C.

Further Reading

Ahmed S, Siddiqui AK, Siddiqui RK, Kimpo M, Russo L, Mattana J. Acute pancreatitis during sickle cell vaso-occlusive painful crisis. Am J Hematol. 2003;73(3):190–3.

Ahmed M, Dick M, Mieli-Vergani G, Harrison P, Karani J, Dhawan A. Ischaemic cholangiopathy and sickle cell disease. Eur J Pediatr. 2006;165(2):112–3.

Al-Salem AH, Nourallah H. Sequential endoscopic laparoscopic management of cholelithiasis and choledocholithiasis in children who have sickle cell disease. J Pediatr Surg. 1997;32:1432–5.

Al-Salem AH, Qaisaruddin S. The significance of biliary sludge in children with sickle cell disease. Pediatr Surg Int. 1998;13:14–6.

Al-Salem AH, Nanglia R, Kolar K, Qaisaruddin S, Al-Dabbous I, Al-Jam'a A. Cholecystectomy in children with sickle cell disease. Perioperative management. Pediatr Surg Int. 1995;10:472–4.

Al-Salem AH, Qaisaruddin S, Al-Dabbous I, et al. Cholelithiasis in children with sickle cell disease. Pediatr Surg Int. 1996;11:471–3.

Ancel D, Amiot X, Chaslin-Ferbus D, Hagege I, Garioud A, Girot R, Pol S, Grange JD. Treatment of chronic hepatitis C in sickle cell disease and thalassaemic patients with interferon and ribavirin. Eur J Gastroenterol Hepatol. 2009;21(7):726–9.

Banerjee S, Owen C, Chopra S. Sickle cell hepatopathy. Hepatology. 2001;33(5):1021–8.

Curro G, Meo A, Ippolito D, Pusiol A, Cucinotta E. Asymptomatic cholelithiasis in children with sickle cell disease: early or delayed cholecystectomy? Ann Surg. 2007;245(1):126–9.

DeVault KR, Friedman LS, Westerberg S, Martin P, Hosein B, Ballas SK. Hepatitis C in sickle cell anemia. J Clin Gastroenterol. 1994;18(3):206–9.

Harmatz P, Butensky E, Quirolo K, et al. Severity of iron overload in patients with sickle cell disease receiving chronic red blood cell transfusion therapy. Blood. 2000;96:76–9.

Hassan M, Hasan H, Giday S, et al. Hepatitis C virus in sickle cell disease. J Natl Med Assoc. 2003;95:939–42.

Hatton CS, Bunch C, Weatherall DJ. Hepatic sequestration in sickle cell anaemia. Br Med J. 1985;290:744–5.

Issa H, Al-Haddad A, Al-Salem A. Sickle cell cholangiopathy: an endoscopic retrograde cholangiopancreatography evaluation. World J Gastroenterol. 2009;15(42):5316–20.

O'Callaghan A, O'Brien SG, Ninkovic M, Butcher GP, Foster CS, Walters JRF, et al. Chronic intrahepatic cholestasis in sickle cell disease requiring exchange transfusion. Gut. 1995a; 37:144–7.

O'Callaghan A, O'Brien SG, Ninkovic M, et al. Chronic intrahepatic cholestasis in sickle cell disease requiring exchange transfusion. Gut. 1995b;37:44–147.

Platt O, Brambilla DJ, Roses WF, et al. Mortality in sickle cell disease: life expectancy and risk factors for early death. N Engl J Med. 1994;330:1639–44.

Shao SH, Orringer EP. Sickle cell intrahepatic cholestasis: approach to a difficult problem. Am J Gastroenterol. 1995;90:2048–50.

Streinberg MH, Barton F, Castro O, Pegelow CH, Ballas SK, Kutlar A, et al. Effect of hydroxyurea on mortality and morbidity in adult sickle cell anemia: risks and benefits up to 9 years of treatment. JAMA. 2003;289:1645–51.

Swaim MW, Agarwal S, Rosse WF. Successful treatment of hepatitis C in sickle-cell disease. Ann Intern Med. 2000;133:750–1.

Tagge EP, Othersen Jr HB, Jackson SM, et al. Impact of laparoscopic cholecystectomy on the management of cholelithiasis in children with sickle cell disease. J Pediatr Surg. 1994;29: 209–13.

The Acute Chest Syndrome in Sickle Cell Anemia

7

7.1 Introduction

- Acute chest syndrome (ACS) is defined as a new infiltrate on chest X-ray that is associated with one or more of the following symptoms:
  - Fever
  - Cough
  - Dyspnea
  - Hypoxia
  - Productive cough
- The ACS is a common complication of sickle cell anemia and a cause of morbidity and mortality in these patients (Fig. 7.1).
- The acute chest syndrome is considered the leading cause of death and hospitalization among patients with sickle cell anemia.
- Acute chest syndrome is the second most common cause of hospitalization, second to vaso-occlusive crisis for patients with SCA.
- It is considered the most common cause of death, with one-fourth of SCA-related deaths due to ACS.
- The extent and severity of ACS is variable:
  - It can affect one segment of the lung.
  - Or it can extend to affect the whole lobe of the lung.
  - Sometimes, ACS can affect the whole lung.
  - Or it can be bilateral (Figs. 7.2, 7.3, and 7.4).
- ACS is seen in patients with:
  - Sickle cell anemia (Hb SS).
  - Hb SC.
  - Sickle-beta-thalassemia.
  - The incidence is higher in patients with sickle cell anemia.
- The exact incidence of acute chest syndrome is not known but an estimated incidence of 10,500/100,000 patients/year was reported.

A. Al-Salem, *Medical and Surgical Complications of Sickle Cell Anemia*,
DOI 10.1007/978-3-319-24762-5_7

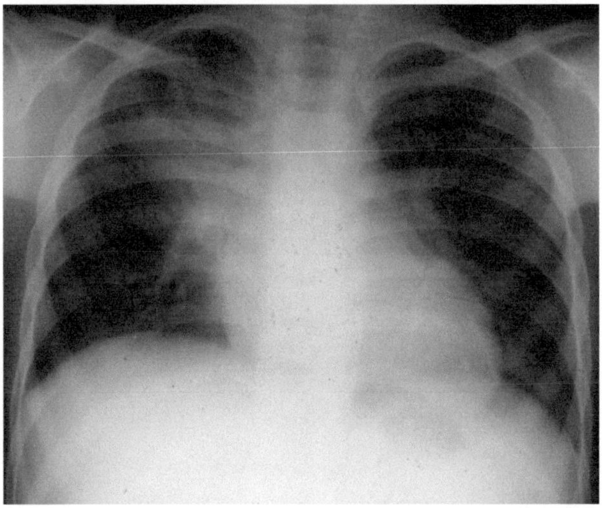

Fig. 7.1 Chest X-ray showing a mild attack of acute chest syndrome in a child with sickle cell anemia

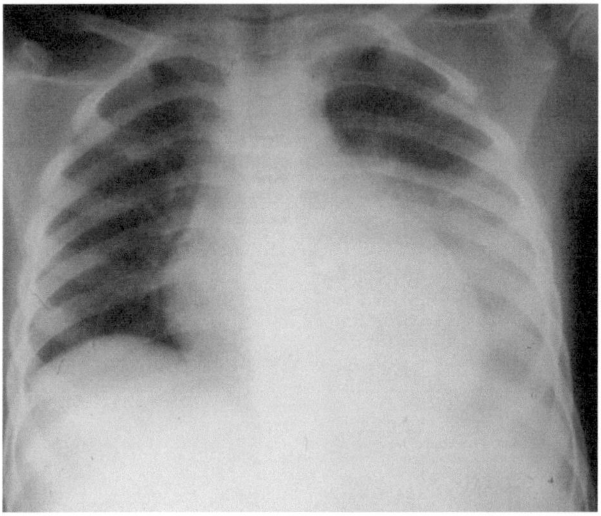

Fig. 7.2 Chest X-ray showing ACS affecting the left lower lobe of the lung and part of the left upper lobe

- An estimated incidence of 25.3 per 100 patient-years was also reported among children with sickle cell anemia.
- ACS occurs most often as a single episode, but there are certain patients who suffer multiple episodes.
- The mortality is higher in those who have more than one episode of ACS.

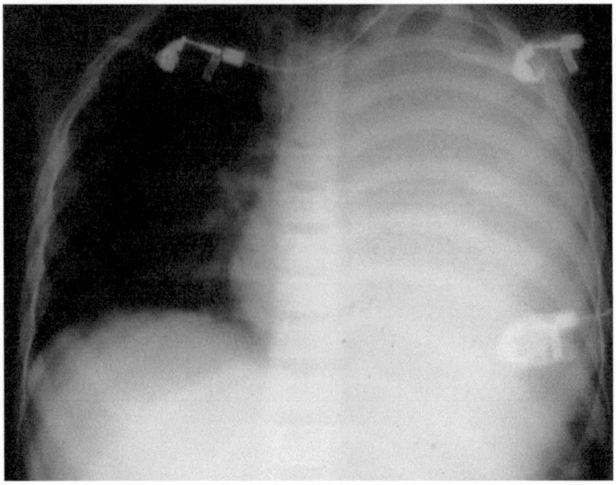

Fig. 7.3 Chest X-ray showing ACS affecting the whole left lung

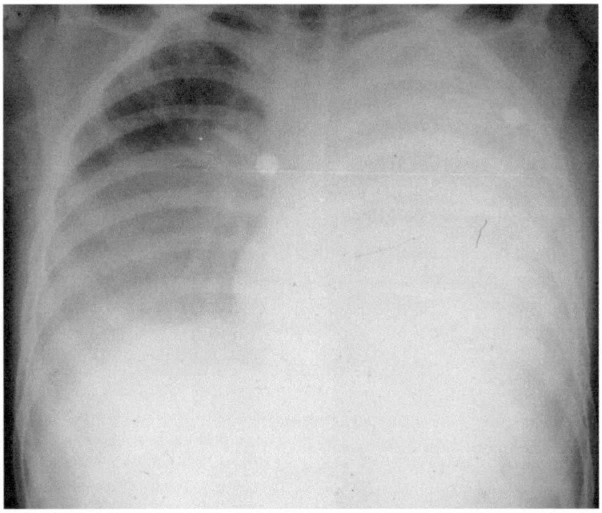

Fig. 7.4 Chest X-ray showing bilateral ACS involving the left lung and part of the right lung

- Recurrent episodes of ACS are known to be associated with an increased risk of chronic lung disease.
- Acute chest syndrome is seen commonly in children 2–4 years of age.
- The incidence of ACS gradually declines with age.
- The incidence of ACS is inversely proportional to the level of fetal hemoglobin and the degree of anemia and directly proportional to the steady state white blood cell count.

- It is believed that high Hb F level exerts a protective effect on those less than 2 years of age and also in older patients with high HbF levels.
- ACS is a common complication in children with SCA and considered the most common cause of death, with one-fourth of SCA-related deaths due to ACS.
- ACS can develop:
  - Following an attack of vaso-occlusive crisis
  - Secondary to hypoxia following postoperative atelectasis
  - Secondary to bronchospasm due to an attack of bronchial asthma
- ACS is more likely to occur in children with a history of bronchial asthma.

7.2 Etiology

- The cause of ACS remains largely unknown and it is believed to be multifactorial.
- Both infectious and noninfectious causes have been described.
- In about 40 % of cases, a specific cause of ACS can be determined.
- Infection is considered the most common cause (30 %). This is followed by pulmonary infarction (15 %) and fat embolism (10 %).
- The list of causes of ACS includes the following:
  - Pulmonary infarction
  - Intrapulmonary sickling
  - Fat embolism
  - Fibrin embolism
  - Hypoventilation secondary to ribs or sternum infarction
  - Hypoventilation secondary to narcotics
  - Pulmonary edema secondary to narcotics or fluid overload
  - Postoperative hypoventilation secondary to atelectasis
  - Postoperative bronchospasm
  - Bronchospasm secondary to an attack of bronchial asthma
  - Infections (bacterial, viral, fungal, protozoa)
  - Foreign body aspiration
- In about 45 % of ACS, no definite cause could be identified.
- The relative frequency of the other causes of ACS is as follows:
  - Pulmonary infarction (15–16 %)
  - Fat embolism (9–10 %)
  - Chlamydophila pneumonia (6–7 %)
  - Mycoplasma pneumonia (6–7 %)
  - Viral infection (respiratory syncytial virus, parvovirus, rhinovirus) (5–6 %)
  - Mixed infections (4–5 %)
- Infection is considered the most common cause of ACS in children below 9 years of age (35 %). This is in contrast to children older than 9 years of age where infection is the cause of ACS in 22 %. In adults, infection is the cause of ACS in 26 %.

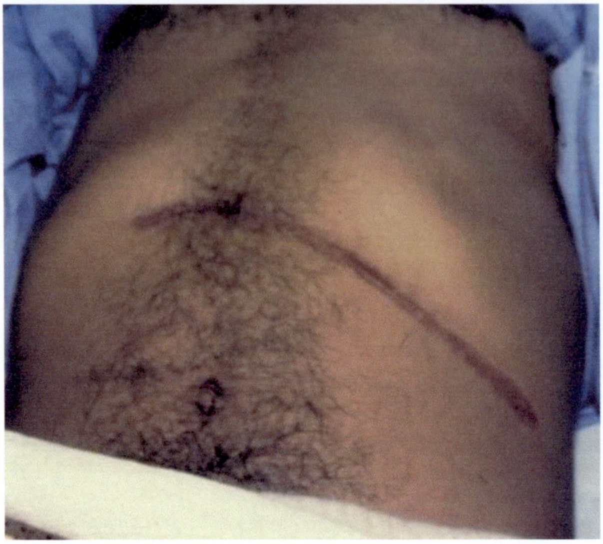

Fig. 7.5 Clinical photograph showing a patient with a large abdominal scar following splenectomy and cholecystectomy

- The relative frequency of infectious agents as a cause of ACS is as follows:
  - Chlamydia (30 %)
  - Mycoplasma (20 %)
  - Respiratory syncytial virus (10 %)
  - *Staphylococcus aureus* (4 %)
  - *Streptococcus pneumoniae* (3 %)
- It is estimated that about 50 % of all patients who develop ACS were initially admitted to the hospital with vaso-occlusive crises. This is especially so in those with vaso-occlusive crisis affecting the spine, ribs, and abdomen. This is attributed to several factors:
  - Vaso-occlusive crisis leads to pain, hypoventilation, hypoxemia, and development of atelectasis.
  - Add to this the respiratory depressive effect of opioids used to treat the vaso-occlusive crisis.
  - Both factors lead to low oxygenation which increases sickling of red blood cells.
- Pulmonary infarction is a well-known cause of ACS in patients with SCA. This results from:
  - Vaso-occlusive crisis
  - Intrapulmonary sickling
  - Pulmonary embolus
- Postoperative ACS (Figs. 7.5, 7.6, 7.7, and 7.8):
  - This is a well-known and serious complication in patients with SCA.

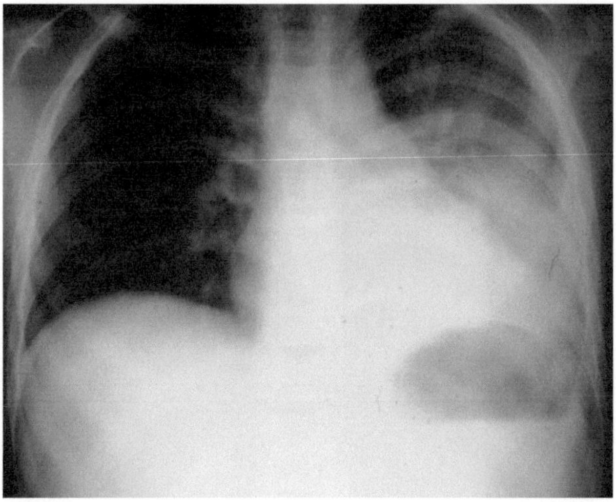

Fig. 7.6 Chest X-ray showing ACS involving the left lower lobe in a child with sickle cell anemia who had splenectomy

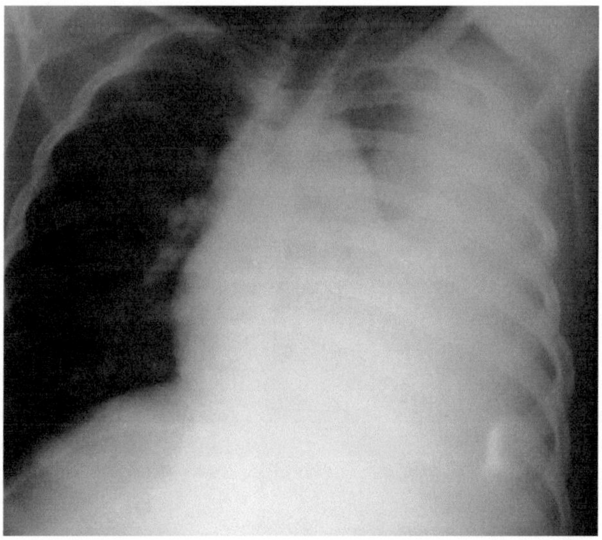

Fig. 7.7 Chest X-ray showing extensive ACS involving the whole left lung in a postoperative patient with sickle cell anemia

- This is seen especially following abdominal surgeries with large wounds that interfere with breathing secondary to the associated pain.
- The recent advancement of minimal invasive surgery may play a role in reducing the incidence of postoperative ACS. Other factors that may decrease the incidence of postoperative ACS include:
  - Proper preoperative evaluation.
  - Proper perioperative hydration.

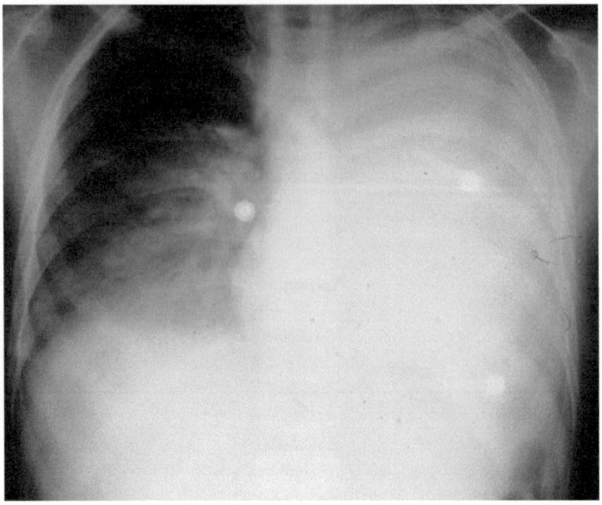

Fig. 7.8 Chest X-ray showing bilateral ACS in a postoperative patient with SCA

    - Preoperative blood transfusion when necessary to increase their Hb to around 10 g/dl for major surgeries.
    - Close intraoperative monitoring and every effort should be made to avoid hypoxemia, hypothermia, acidosis, and hypercarbia.
    - Early mobilization and chest physiotherapy including incentive spirometry.
  - Postoperative ACS may develop as a result of:
    - Postoperative deep vein thrombosis with pulmonary embolism
    - Postoperative atelectasis
    - Postoperative chest infection
- Asthmatic patients with SCA appear to be at increased risk for ACS.
- It has been estimated that patients with SCA who were diagnosed with asthma were two to four times more likely to develop ACS and recurrent episodes of ACS than those without asthma.

7.3 Investigations and Diagnosis

- The diagnosis of ACS in a patient with SCA is made clinically and it is based on the following criteria:
  - A new pulmonary infiltrate detected by chest radiograph involving at least one complete lung segment that is not consistent with the appearance of atelectasis
  - One or more of the following signs or symptoms:
    - Chest pain
    - Temperature >38.5 °C

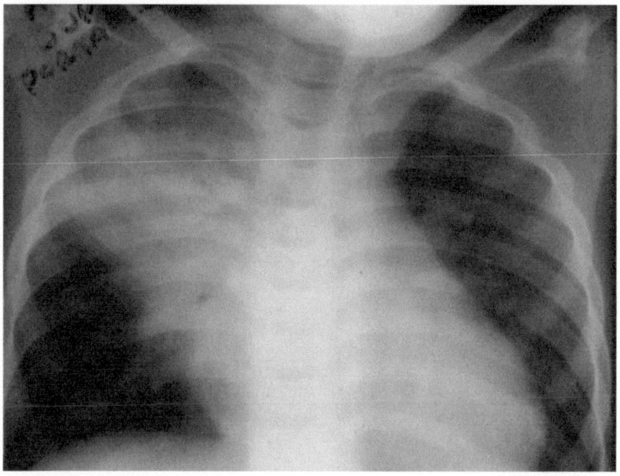

Fig. 7.9 Chest X-ray showing a pulmonary infiltrate in a patient with ACS

  - Tachypnea, wheezing, cough, or the appearance of increased work of breathing
  - Hypoxemia
- Chest radiographs (Figs. 7.9, 7.10, 7.11, and 7.12):
  - The pulmonary infiltrate in ACS may involve one segment of the lung or extend to involve one lobe or sometimes the whole lung.
  - ACS may in severe cases affect both lungs.
  - It is important to diagnose ACS early to avoid subsequent morbidity and mortality.
  - An early chest X-ray should be part of the investigations of all patients with SCA who have fever, chest pain, or respiratory symptoms and those admitted with severe vaso-occlusive crisis, particularly with chest or rib pain.
  - The chest radiograph should be repeated within 24–48 h after admission in those with an initial normal chest X-ray and also to detect progression of the ACS in those already diagnosed to have ACS.
  - Complete blood count (CBC), platelet count, reticulocyte count, and differential WBC count
- Blood grouping and cross-matching for possible packed RBC transfusion or exchange blood transfusion
- Blood, urine, stool, and sputum cultures when clinically indicated
- Arterial blood gas analysis
- Liver function tests
- Electrolytes, BUN and creatinine
- Blood, urine, stool and sputum cultures when clinically indicated
- Arterial blood gas analysis
- Liver function tests
- Electrolytes, BUN, and creatinine

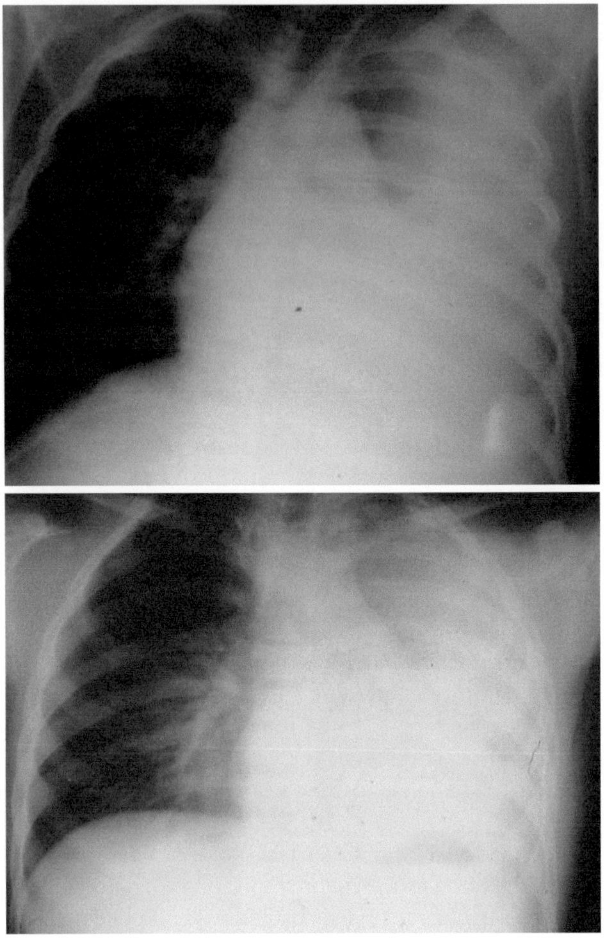

Figs. 7.10 and 7.11 Chest X-ray showing severe ACS involving the whole left lung

7.4 Complications of ACS

- There is a strong relation between ACS and the occurrence of neurologic complications. These include:
  - A reversible posterior leukoencephalopathy syndrome
  - A silent cerebral infarct
  - Acute necrotizing encephalitis
- Respiratory failure requiring mechanical ventilation occurs in about 10 % of ACS cases.
- Deep veins thrombosis.
- Pulmonary embolism.

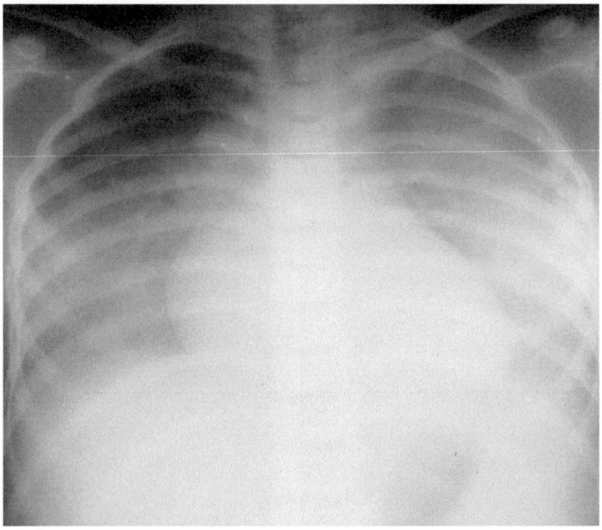

Fig. 7.12 Chest X-ray showing bilateral ACS in a child with sickle cell anemia

- Pulmonary infarction.
- Pulmonary hypertension is an increasingly recognized complication of SCA.
- Chronic lung disease.
- ACS is one of the causes of mortality in patients with SCA.

7.5 Management

- The clinical severity of ACS is variable ranging from a clinically mild to a severe progressive condition.
- The clinical course of ACS is not only variable but also unpredictable and because of this even the clinically mild cases of ACS should be admitted to the hospital for close monitoring (Figs. 7.13, 7.14, 7.15, 7.16, 7.17, 7.18, 7.19, and 7.20).
- The management of SCA patients with ACS is challenging, and these patients should be admitted to the hospital for close observation and monitoring. Only those with very mild ACS can be admitted to the ward but all other cases should be admitted to the intensive care unit.
- Intravenous fluid hydration. Overhydration or rapid hydration should be avoided as this may complicate the clinical picture and lead to pulmonary edema or heart failure.
- Adequate analgesia is given especially to those with associated vaso-occlusive crisis.
  - This is to prevent hypoventilation and atelectasis.
  - It is also important to avoid using strong opioids unless necessary, and if these are used, it is important to avoid using high doses.

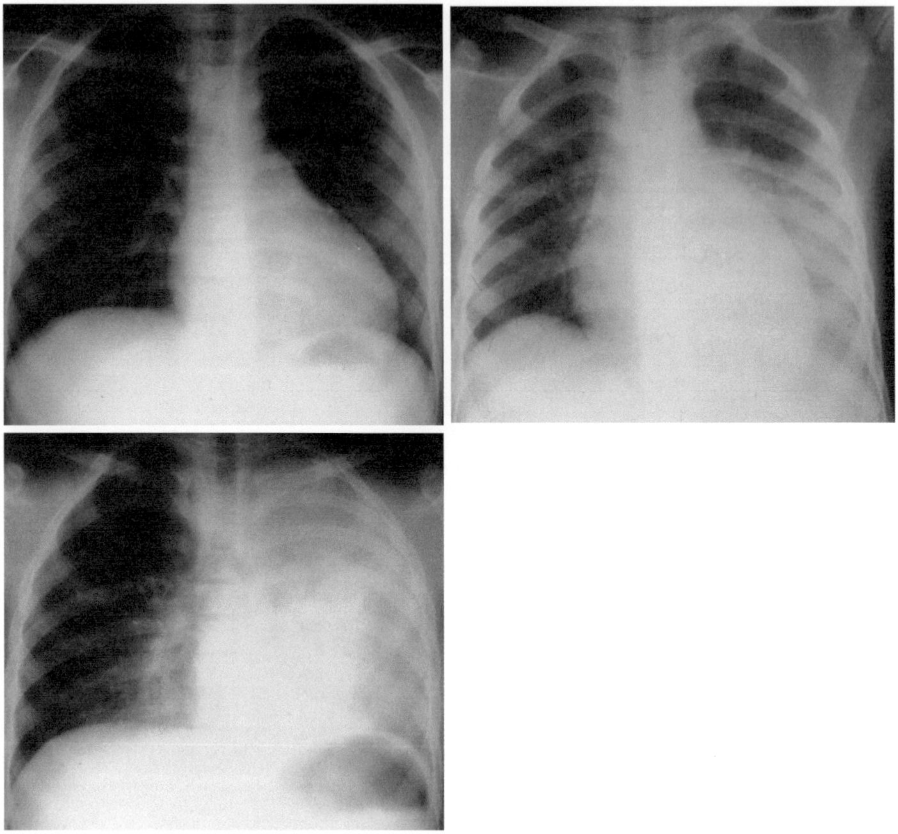

Figs. 7.13, 7.14 and 7.15 Chest X-rays showing progression of acute chest syndrome. The acute chest syndrome started as a mild attack involving part of the left lower lobe but progressed to involve the whole left lower lobe and finally it involved the whole left lung

   - A high dose of morphine or other opioids is known to cause respiratory depression and hypoventilation which subsequently can lead to atelectasis.
   - This in turn may lead to ventilation-perfusion mismatch and intrapulmonary sickling, which can complicate the clinical picture further and worsen or lead to progression of the ACS.
- Febrile patients should be treated with antipyretic (acetaminophen or paracetamol).
- Antibiotics:
   - Patients with ACS should be covered with broad-spectrum antibiotics.
   - The antibiotic coverage is empirical initially and should include a third-generation cephalosporin (e.g., cefotaxime or ceftriaxone) for bacterial coverage and a macrolide (e.g., azithromycin or erythromycin) for coverage of atypical organisms (e.g., mycoplasma and chlamydia).

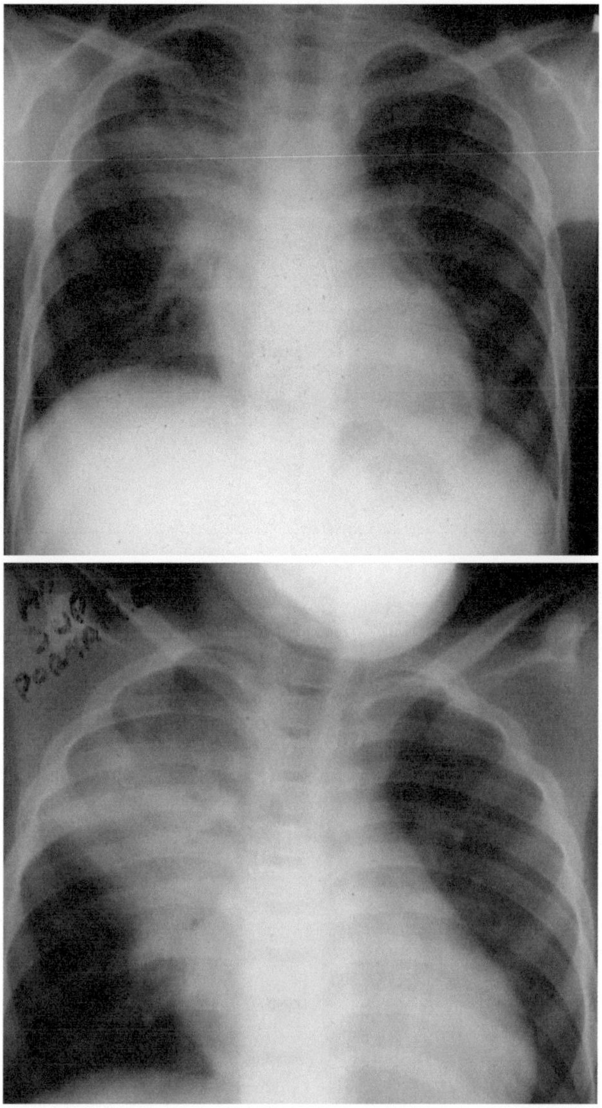

Figs. 7.16 and 7.17 Chest X-rays showing acute chest syndrome in a patient with sickle cell anemia that was mild to start with but progressed to involve the whole right upper lobe

- Clindamycin may be used instead of cephalosporin if the patient is allergic to cephalosporin.
- Vancomycin can be used in those with progressive disease and to cover methicillin-resistant *Staphylococcus aureus* (MRSA).

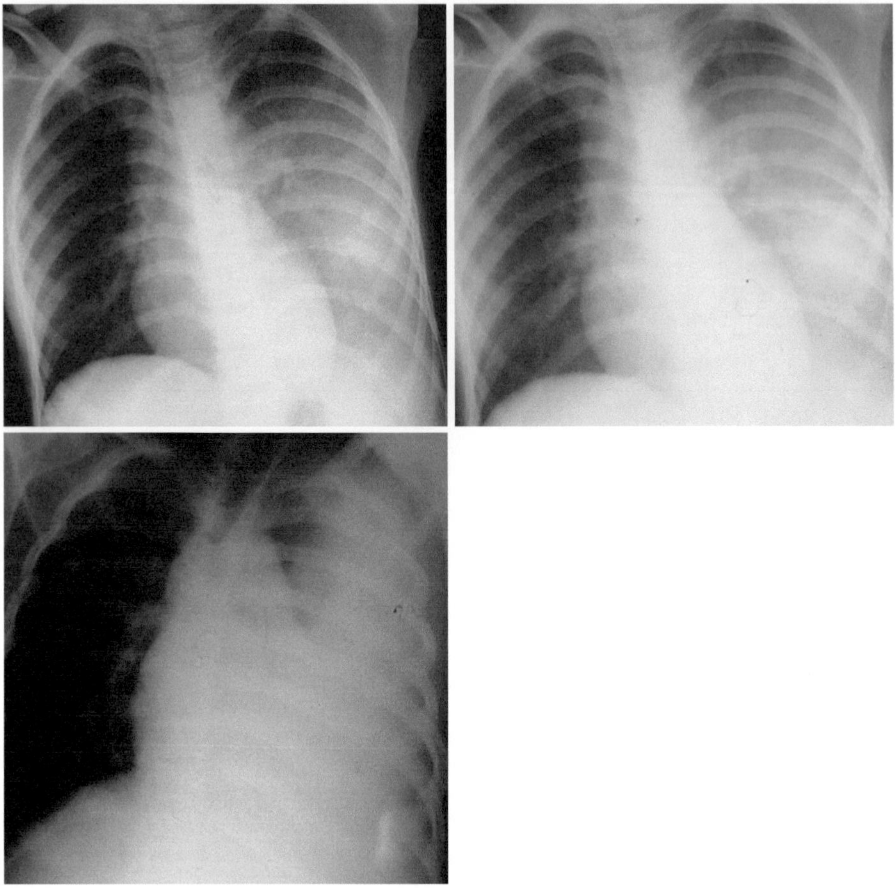

Figs. 7.18, 7.19, and 7.20 Chest X-rays showing progression of acute chest syndrome. It started in the left lower lobe and part of the left upper lobe but progressed to involve the whole left lung

- Respiratory support:
  - Patients with ACS require close monitoring as they can deteriorate rapidly.
  - It is important to maintain proper arterial oxygenation. Oxygen supplementation should be provided to maintain arterial oxygen saturation ≥ 92 %.
  - An incentive spirometer is used to prevent atelectasis.
  - For patients with rising oxygen requirements, it is important to assist these patients initially using noninvasive ventilation using:
    - Nasal mask continuous positive airway pressure (CPAP)
    - Positive airway pressure (BPAP)

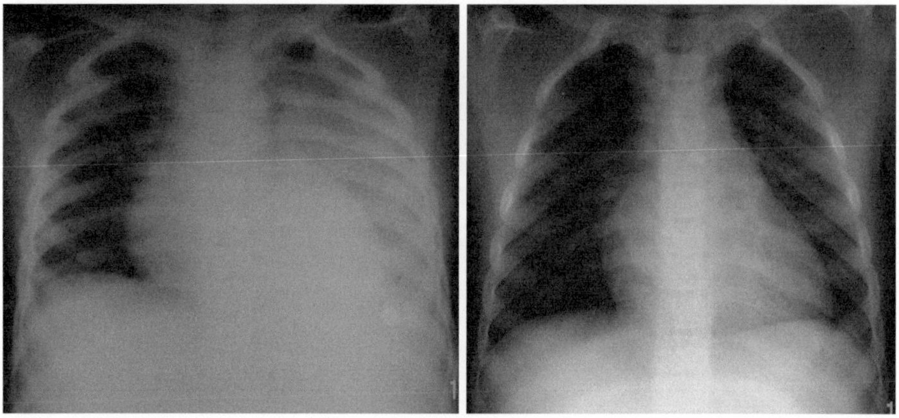

Figs. 7.21 and 7.22 Chest X-rays showing ACS before and after treatment including exchange blood transfusion. Note the disappearance of the lung infiltrate after treatment

  - For patients with respiratory failure, conventional or high-frequency oscillatory mechanical ventilation can be used.
  - For patients who fail to respond to mechanical ventilation, extra corporeal membrane oxygenation (ECMO) has been used successfully.
- In patients with a history of bronchial asthma, inhaled bronchodilators should be used.
- It has been suggested that bronchodilators should also be considered even if the patient does not have a prior history of bronchial asthma.
- The role of corticosteroids in the treatment of ACS remains unclear. A short-term course of corticosteroids may be used, but these should be tapered to reduce the risk of rebound vaso-occlusive crisis.
- Inhaled nitric oxide, a selective pulmonary vasodilator, can be used to treat these patients. The role of nitric oxide in treating ACS is however not well established.
  - Nitric oxide improves ventilation/perfusion mismatch and decrease pulmonary hypertension.
  - Nitric oxide also increases the oxygen affinity of HbS, thus potentially decreasing sickling of red blood cells.
- Bronchoscopy with bronchoalveolar lavage can be used as a diagnostic and therapeutic modality but should be reserved for patients with severe or progressive infiltrates. It provides both diagnostic and therapeutic benefits.
- Blood transfusion (Figs. 7.21, 7.22, 7.23, 7.24, 7.25, and 7.26):
  - The role of blood transfusion in the management of patients with SCA and ACS is now well established as it improves oxygenation.

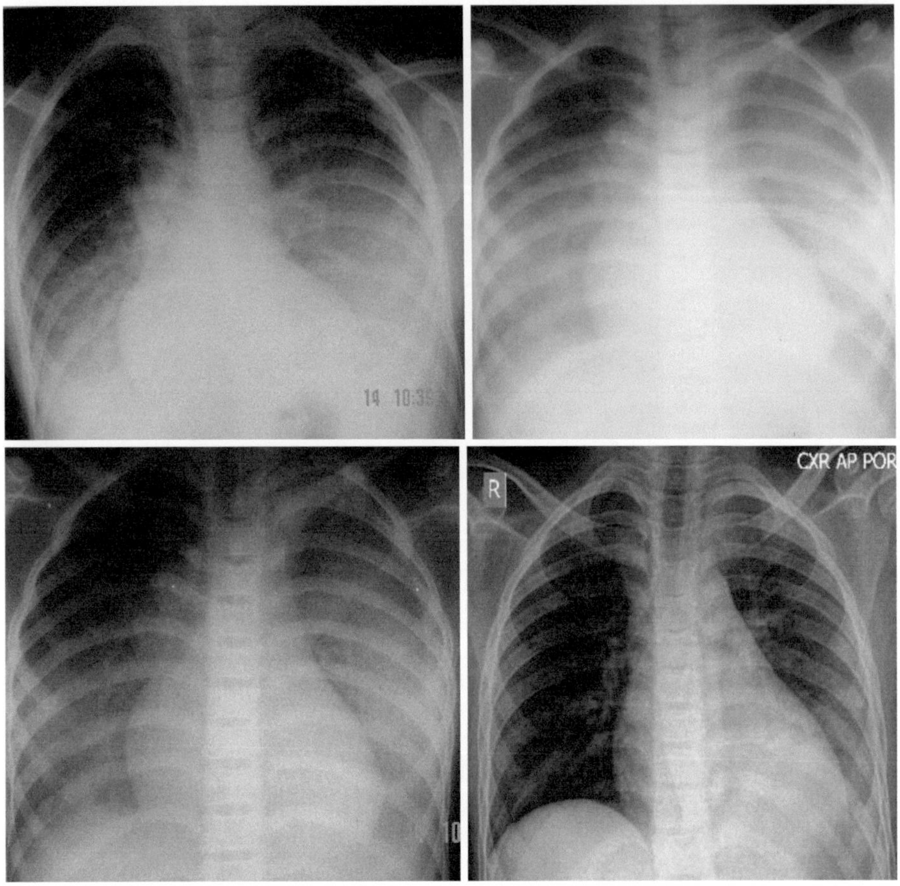

Figs. 7.23, 7.24, 7.25, and 7.26 Serial chest X-rays of patients with severe bilateral acute chest syndrome that responded to treatment including exchange blood transfusion

- This is based on several clinical series but there are no randomized controlled trials comparing transfusion therapy to standard supportive management without blood transfusion.
- Simple packed red blood cell transfusion and also exchange transfusions were used with similar results.
- The goal of simple transfusion is to increase the hematocrit to 30 % or the hemoglobin to 11 g/dL.
- The goal of partial exchange blood transfusion is to decrease the level of Hgb S to <30 % of the total hemoglobin concentration, while not exceeding an Hgb level of >10 g/dL.

- Partial exchange blood transfusion or erythrocytapheresis should be used in patients with ACS for the following indications:
  - Progression of ACS despite simple packed RBCs transfusion
  - Severe hypoxemia
  - Extensive ACS with multi-lobar involvement
  - Previous history of severe ACS or cardiopulmonary disease
  - Arterial oxygen saturation (SaO_2) persistently <80 % despite aggressive ventilatory support
  - Serial decline in SaO_2
  - Unstable and/or worsening vital signs
  - Persistent respiratory rate greater than 30/min
- Blood transfusion whether simple or exchange carries risks that are particularly relevant to patient with SCA. These include:
  - Transmission of viral infections including hepatitis B and C and HIV
  - Alloimmunization
  - Acute blood hyperviscosity
  - Iron overload

- Hydroxyurea:
  - Hydroxyurea is beneficial in preventing ACS.
  - It has been shown to decrease the frequency of ACS.
  - Hydroxyurea reduces the incidence of ACS by 40 % in adult patients with SCA.
  - In children with SCA, there was a threefold reduction of ACS in those who received hydroxyurea when compared to those who did not receive hydroxyurea.
- Hematopoietic cell transplantation:
  - This should be considered for patients who have experienced multiple ACS attacks.
  - And who have an HLA-matched sibling donor.
  - This has > 80 % success rate.
- Long-term management of patients with ACS:
  - This is directed toward preventing recurrence of ACS and its complications.
  - It includes:
    - Prophylactic antibiotics to decrease the risk of infection
    - Immunization
    - Proper management of asthma in patients with SCA
    - Treatment with hydroxyurea
    - Red blood transfusion therapy
    - Hematopoietic cell transplantation

Further Reading

Boyd JH, Macklin EA, Strunk RC, DeBaun MR. Asthma is associated with acute chest syndrome and pain in children with sickle cell anemia. Blood. 2006;108:2923.

Castro O, Brambilla DJ, Thorington B, et al. The acute chest syndrome in sickle cell disease: incidence and risk factors. The cooperative study of sickle cell disease. Blood. 1994;84:643.

Charache S, Terrin ML, Moore RD, et al. Effect of hydroxyurea on the frequency of painful crises in sickle cell anemia. Investigators of the multicenter study of hydroxyurea in sickle cell anemia. N Engl J Med. 1995;332:1317.
Crabtree EA, Mariscalco MM, Hesselgrave J, et al. Improving care for children with sickle cell disease/acute chest syndrome. Pediatrics. 2011;127, e480.
Dean D, Neumayr L, Kelly DM, et al. Chlamydia pneumoniae and acute chest syndrome in patients with sickle cell disease. J Pediatr Hematol Oncol. 2003;25:46.
Emre U, Miller ST, Gutierez M, et al. Effect of transfusion in acute chest syndrome of sickle cell disease. J Pediatr. 1995;127:901.
Hankins JS, Ware RE, Rogers ZR, et al. Long-term hydroxyurea therapy for infants with sickle cell anemia: the HUSOFT extension study. Blood. 2005a;106:2269.
Hankins J, Jeng M, Harris S, et al. Chronic transfusion therapy for children with sickle cell disease and recurrent acute chest syndrome. J Pediatr Hematol Oncol. 2005b;27:158.
Hyder O, Yaster M, Bateman BT, Firth PG. Surgical procedures and outcomes among children with sickle cell disease. Anesth Analg. 2013;117:1192.
Miller ST, Wright E, Abboud M, et al. Impact of chronic transfusion on incidence of pain and acute chest syndrome during the Stroke Prevention Trial (STOP) in sickle-cell anemia. J Pediatr. 2001;139:785.
Pelidis MA, Kato GJ, Resar LM, et al. Successful treatment of life-threatening acute chest syndrome of sickle cell disease with venovenous extracorporeal membrane oxygenation. J Pediatr Hematol Oncol. 1997;19:459.
Platt OS. The acute chest syndrome of sickle cell disease. N Engl J Med. 2000;342:1904.
Setty BN, Stuart MJ, Dampier C, et al. Hypoxaemia in sickle cell disease: biomarker modulation and relevance to pathophysiology. Lancet. 2003;362:1450.
Sobota A, Graham DA, Heeney MM, Neufeld EJ. Corticosteroids for acute chest syndrome in children with sickle cell disease: variation in use and association with length of stay and readmission. Am J Hematol. 2010;85:24.
Sullivan KJ, Goodwin SR, Evangelist J, et al. Nitric oxide successfully used to treat acute chest syndrome of sickle cell disease in a young adolescent. Crit Care Med. 1999;27:2563.
Velasquez MP, Mariscalco MM, Goldstein SL, Airewele GE. Erythrocytapheresis in children with sickle cell disease and acute chest syndrome. Pediatr Blood Cancer. 2009;53:1060.
Vichinsky EP, Styles LA, Colangelo LH, et al. Acute chest syndrome in sickle cell disease: clinical presentation and course. Cooperative study of sickle cell disease. Blood. 1997;89:1787.
Vichinsky EP, Neumayr LD, Earles AN, et al. Causes and outcomes of the acute chest syndrome in sickle cell disease. National acute chest syndrome study group. N Engl J Med. 2000;342:1855.
Wales PW, Carver E, Crawford MW, Kim PC. Acute chest syndrome after abdominal surgery in children with sickle cell disease: is a laparoscopic approach better? J Pediatr Surg. 2001;36:718.

Musculoskeletal Manifestations of Sickle Cell Anemia

8

8.1 Introduction

- One of the common manifestations of sickle cell anemia is vaso-occlusive crises which affect virtually all patients with sickle cell anemia.
- This starts early, often beginning in late infancy and characterized by recurrent attacks that continue throughout life.
- The majority of these attacks are self-limiting with full recovery and no further complications.
- This however is not the case always, and sometimes these attacks can be complicated by joint effusion or bone infarction (avascular necrosis).
- The presence of infarcted or necrotic bone in these patients makes them susceptible to develop osteomyelitis. This is predisposed to by the increased susceptibility of these patients to infections as a result of hyposplenism and impaired complement activity.

8.2 Acute Vaso-occlusive Crisis

- Sickle cell anemia is characterized by periods of remissions and exacerbations. These periods of exacerbations are called crisis.
- Bone and joint vaso-occlusive crisis is the most common manifestations of sickle cell anemia and a major cause of frequent emergency room visits and hospitalization.
- It is also called painful crisis.
- This commonly occurs in the bone marrow or epiphyses of the bones leading to bone marrow infarction.
- This can affect any part of the skeleton, but there is a predilection for the long bones.

A. Al-Salem, *Medical and Surgical Complications of Sickle Cell Anemia*,
DOI 10.1007/978-3-319-24762-5_8

- Pain caused by vaso-occlusive crisis may occur as often as every week, or these patients may go without any attacks for several months or sometimes years.
- As a result of these repeated attacks, many patients with SCA develop long-term consequences including avascular necrosis of the femoral heads, avascular necrosis of the humoral head, or collapsed vertebral bodies.
- The frequency and severity of these vaso-occlusive crises are variable. It has been suggested that concomitant alpha thalassemia trait and higher hemoglobin S levels in patients with sickle cell anemia appear to be associated with more frequent attacks of vaso-occlusive crisis, while high HbF levels appear to have a protective effect with less frequent and milder attacks.
- Vaso-occlusive crisis can affect any bony structure in the body but typically occurs in the long bones. The commonest sites are:
  - The tibia/fibula (25–30 %)
  - The femur (20–25 %)
  - The radius, ulna, and humorous (20–38 %)
- Pathogenesis:
  - The exact pathogenesis of vaso-occlusive crisis is not known and several factors may be involved.
  - In the bone marrow, there is slow progression of red blood cells through the bone marrow sinusoids and capillary beds. This together with the relatively hypoxic tissue environment increases the risk for RBCs sickling.
  - As a result, there will be activation and adhesion of leukocytes, platelets, and endothelial cells as well as hemoglobin S-containing erythrocytes leading to microvascular occlusion, impaired blood flow, regional hypoxia, and ischemia.
  - The inflammatory response to ischemia and infarction leads to pain in the affected area and surrounding tissues.
- Clinical features:
  - The clinical presentation of a vaso-occlusive crisis is variable in terms of severity and duration.
  - The usual presentation includes:
    - Pain along one of the bony parts of the skeleton.
    - The pain is usually deep seated and sometimes very severe excruciating making the patient scream and cry for help (Fig. 8.1).
    - The pain may be localized to one or more areas of the skeleton.
    - Others may have only mild pain that does not interfere with their daily normal activity.
    - The pain may be associated with localized swelling, erythema, and tenderness.
    - The pain may be associated with a low-grade fever and the affected area is warm.
  - These attacks are usually self-limiting and most patients recover with no further complications.

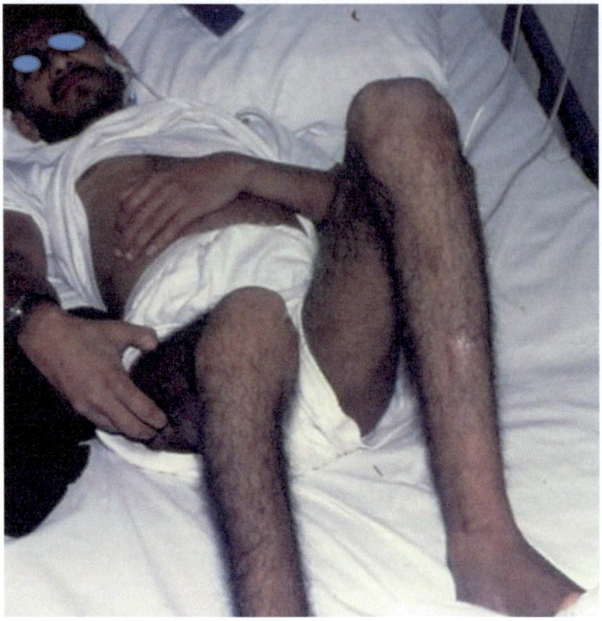

Fig. 8.1 A clinical photograph showing a patient with sickle cell anemia during a severe attack of vaso-occlusive crisis. Note the facial expressions indicating severe pain

  - When these attacks affect the epiphyses of the bones, there may be an associated effusion of the adjacent joint.
  - It is important to differentiate this from septic arthritis.
  - Affection and infarction of the vertebral bone marrow lead to collapse of the vertebrae with a typical "fish mouth" appearance.
- Diagnosis and investigations:
  - The diagnosis of a painful vaso-occlusive crisis is predominantly a clinical one.
  - The laboratory investigations during an acute vaso-occlusive crisis are usually normal apart from a mild leukocytosis.
  - It is important to differentiate acute vaso-occlusive crisis from osteomyelitis.
  - Febrile patients (38 °C) should have a complete blood count, ESR, C-reactive proteins, and blood cultures to evaluate for the possibility of osteomyelitis.
  - Plain radiographs initially are usually normal and do not show abnormalities, but subsequently and as a result of necrosis and remodeling, they may show areas of ill-defined translucency followed by arc-like subchondral and intramedullary lucent areas and patchy sclerosis and increased density and deformities in the vertebra of the spine.

- The most useful investigation is a radioisotope bone scan using a combination of ^{99m}technecium (Tc)-labeled sulfur colloid and ^{99M}Tc-diphosphonate which reliably detect areas of infarction. The bone scans with technetium-99 m methylene diphosphonate may show increased uptake, whereas a bone scan with technetium sulfur colloid often shows decreased or absent uptake in the affected area. The bone scan is however unreliable in distinguishing infarction from osteomyelitis.
- Magnetic resonance imaging (MRI) is a very sensitive imaging technique for detecting bone and bone marrow infarction, but the changes seen are often difficult to distinguish from those seen in osteomyelitis.
- MRI should be reserved for investigating those patients whose symptoms fail to settle with conventional management and/or where there is a high suspicion of osteomyelitis.

• Treatment:
  - Simple and mild attacks of vaso-occlusive crisis can be treated at home, and patients with SCA should be educated how to do this.
  - This includes:
    • Pain control using acetaminophen, ibuprofen, or acetaminophen with codeine depending on the severity of pain
    • Bed rest
    • Oral hydration fluids
    • Warm pads
  - Moderate and sever attacks require treatment in the hospital emergency room and sometimes hospitalization.
  - Pain control is the main issue in this regard which should be prompt, and pain medications should never be withheld from these patients.
  - These patients should be treated in centers specialized in sickle cell anemia. To avoid delay in treating these patients in emergency rooms, there are specialized dedicated centers with experienced nurses who can provide immediate care for these patients.
  - The treatment of moderate and severe attacks includes:
    • Hydration with oral or intravenous fluids.
    • Warm pads to the affected area or areas.
    • Analgesia and anti-inflammatory medications.
    • Severe attacks may necessitate the use of continuous infusion or regularly scheduled opioid dosing and patient-controlled analgesia.
    • It is also important to use these opioids carefully as an overdose may lead to respiratory depression.
    • Oxygen supplementation has no role in patients with a normal oxygen saturation or whose oxygen saturation is at that individual's baseline.
    • Packed RBC transfusion is given only to those with associated symptomatic anemia.
    • Hydroxyurea was shown to reduce the frequency of vaso-occlusive crisis, and it is used in children and adults with severe or recurrent vaso-occlusive crisis.

8.3 Osteomyelitis and Septic Arthritis

- Patients with sickle cell anemia are known to be susceptible to infections at various sites.
- This is predisposed to by hyposplenism and impaired complement activity.
- In the presence of infarcted or necrotic bone and bacteremia, these areas can be infected causing osteomyelitis and septic arthritis.
- Patients with sickle cell anemia have an increased incidence of septic arthritis and osteomyelitis as compared to the general population.
- The association between osteonecrosis and septic arthritis is well documented, but there are reports of septic arthritis without well-documented osteonecrosis.
- In general, osteomyelitis occurs in 18 %, while septic arthritis occurs in 7 % of patients with sickle cell anemia (Figs. 8.2 and 8.3).

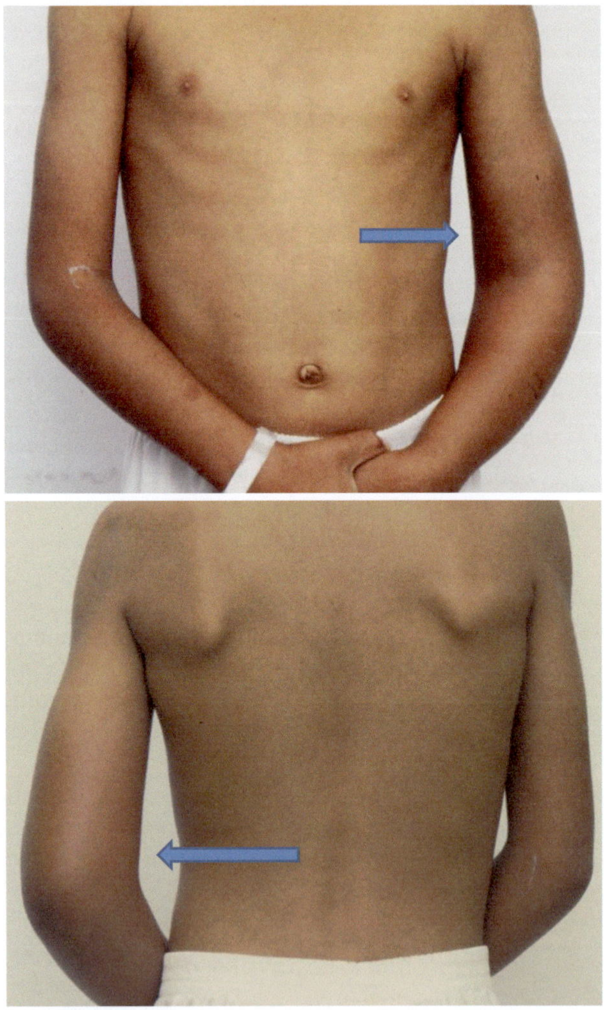

Figs. 8.2 and 8.3 Clinical photographs showing septic arthritis of the elbow. Note the swelling and redness of the elbow joint

- Osteomyelitis most commonly affects the diaphysis of long bones.
- There is an increased incidence of Salmonella osteomyelitis in patients with sickle cell anemia, where it is believed to be the most common pathogen causing osteomyelitis and septic arthritis followed by *S. aureus*.
- Early diagnosis of osteomyelitis and septic arthritis is important to avoid chronicity and irreversible joint damage.
- It is also important to be cautious as vaso-occlusive crisis affecting the bones or close to the articular surfaces may lead to a similar clinical picture to osteomyelitis and septic arthritis.
- Clinical features:
  - Osteomyelitis usually presents with:
    - Pain at the site of infection.
    - Swelling.
    - Tenderness over the affected area.
    - Erythema and redness.
    - Most patients also have fever.
    - Sometimes there is an associated joint effusion if the infection is close to a joint.
    - Difficulty in walking in those with osteomyelitis affecting the lower limb.
  - These signs and symptoms are similar to those found in vaso-occlusive crises, making the distinction between a painful crisis and osteomyelitis extremely difficult.
  - The most common sites of osteomyelitis are:
    - The femur
    - The tibia
    - The humerus
  - Osteomyelitis may not be suspected until the signs and symptoms of a typical painful crisis have failed to resolve after 1–2 weeks of standard therapy.
  - Patients with septic arthritis usually present with:
    - Pain at the site of involved joint and adjacent bones
    - Fever
    - An associated effusion in the affected joint
  - Septic arthritis can affect any joint but there is a predilection for large joints and lower extremities.
  - The distribution of septic arthritis is as follows:
    - The hip joint (40 %)
    - The knee joint (25 %)
    - The elbow joint (20 %)
    - The shoulder joint (10 %)
    - The ankle joint (0.5 %)
  - The diagnosis of septic arthritis must be made early to avoid subsequent joint destruction (Fig. 8.4).
  - Joint fluids should be aspirated for bacteriological evaluations and the antibiotics used should be adjusted accordingly.
  - The microorganisms causing septic arthritis are generally the same as in osteomyelitis.

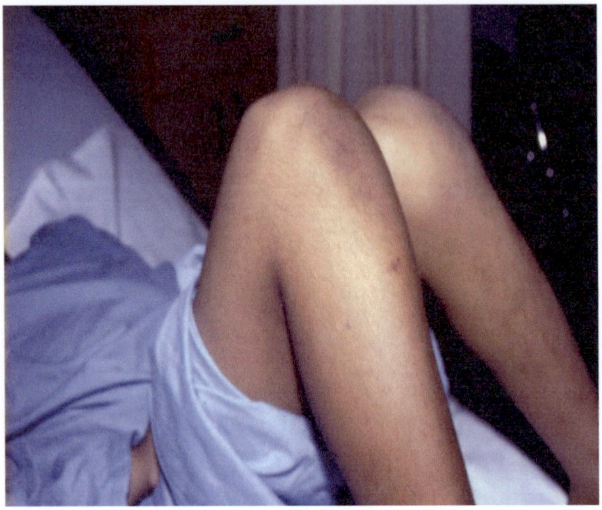

Fig. 8.4 A clinical photograph showing septic arthritis of the knee joint

- *Salmonella* sp. are the most common organisms causing septic arthritis in patients with sickle cell anemia.
- Other organisms reported include:
  - *Klebsiella pneumoniae*
  - *Staphylococcus aureus*
  - *Pneumococcus* sp.

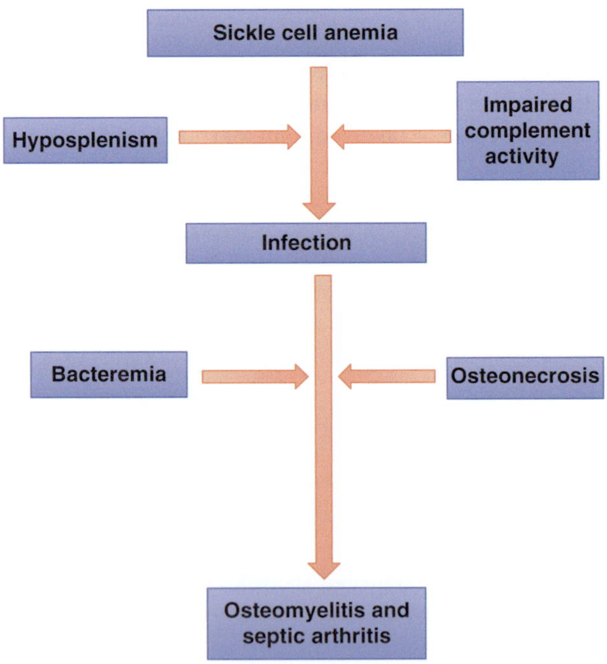

- Causative organisms:
  - Osteomyelitis in patients with sickle cell anemia is different than that in normal adults in terms of causative organisms.
  - The most common cause of osteomyelitis in sickle cell anemia is *Salmonella* (*Salmonella typhimurium*, *Salmonella enteritidis*, *Salmonella choleraesuis*, and *Salmonella paratyphi B*), followed by *Staphylococcus aureus* and Gram-negative enteric bacilli.
  - This is important when considering antibiotic coverage initially before the results of cultures.

Causes of Osteomyelitis and Septic Arthritis Patients with Sickle Cell Anemia

1. *Salmonella typhimurium*
2. *Salmonella enteritidis*
3. *Salmonella choleraesuis*
4. *Salmonella paratyphi B*
5. *Staphylococcus aureus*
6. *Haemophilus influenzae*
7. *Escherichia coli*
8. *Pneumococcus* sp.

- Diagnosis:
  - The diagnosis of SCA patients with suspected osteomyelitis and/or septic arthritis is challenging.
  - Plain radiographs, bone scan, and MRI are helpful in the diagnosis of osteomyelitis and or septic arthritis.
  - Plain radiographs may be normal initially, or the initial changes, namely, periostitis and osteopenia, are nonspecific and also can be seen in vaso-occlusive crisis, and therefore, they are of limited value (Figs. 8.5, 8.6, 8.7, and 8.8).
  - Subsequent follow-up radiographs may show lucent areas, sclerosis, and bone destruction (Figs. 8.9 and 8.10).
  - These changes may take 7–10 days to appear.
  - Ultrasonography is a simple, noninvasive, and valuable investigation for the diagnosis of osteomyelitis which shows the extraosseous pathology in acute osteomyelitis and may show periosteal elevation.
  - These changes are not specific and can also be seen in vaso-occlusive crises.
  - It has been reported that a fluid depth (>4 mm) detected during ultrasound evaluation is highly suggestive of osteomyelitis.

The Distribution of Septic Arthritis

- The hip joint (40 %)
- The knee joint (25 %)
- The elbow joint (20 %)
- The shoulder joint (10 %)

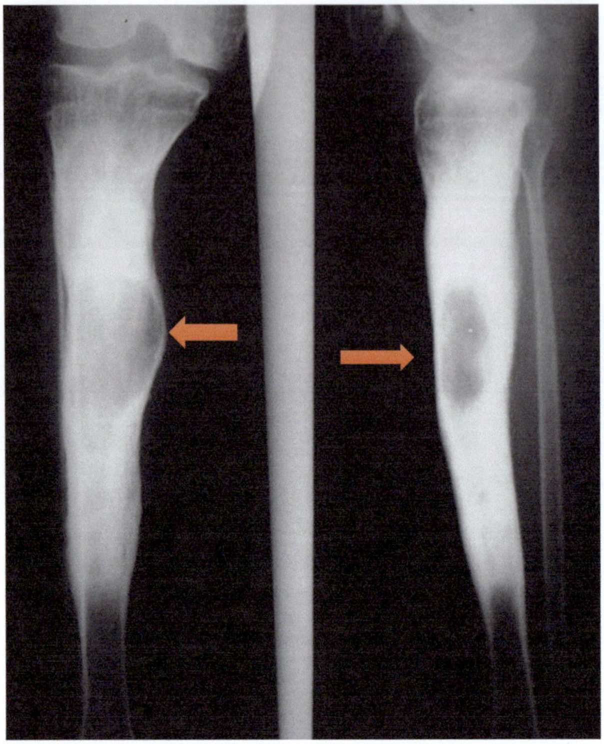

Fig. 8.5 Plain X-ray showing chronic osteomyelitis. Note the radiolucent area

- A bone biopsy or aspiration may be necessary to establish the diagnosis.
- A radioisotope bone scan is reliable but not 100 % accurate in distinguishing osteomyelitis from vaso-occlusive crisis.
- A combination of ^{99m}Tc-sulfur colloid and ^{99M}Tc-diphosphonate or ^{99M}Tc with gallium improves the diagnostic accuracy, as marrow uptake tends to be normal in osteomyelitis, while it is usually increased in vaso-occlusive crisis.
- Radiolabeled leukocyte scans are also used to differentiate osteomyelitis from vaso-occlusive crisis.
- MRI is increasingly being used to help diagnose osteomyelitis, but even this is not 100 % specific differentiating osteomyelitis from vaso-occlusive crisis.
- Blood cultures are often sterile when taken, as it is a common practice to treat patients with vaso-occlusive crises with broad-spectrum antibiotics upon admission, especially if they are febrile.
- CBC will show elevated WBCs and ESR and CRP will also be elevated.
- Joint effusion should be aspirated for bacteriological evaluation.

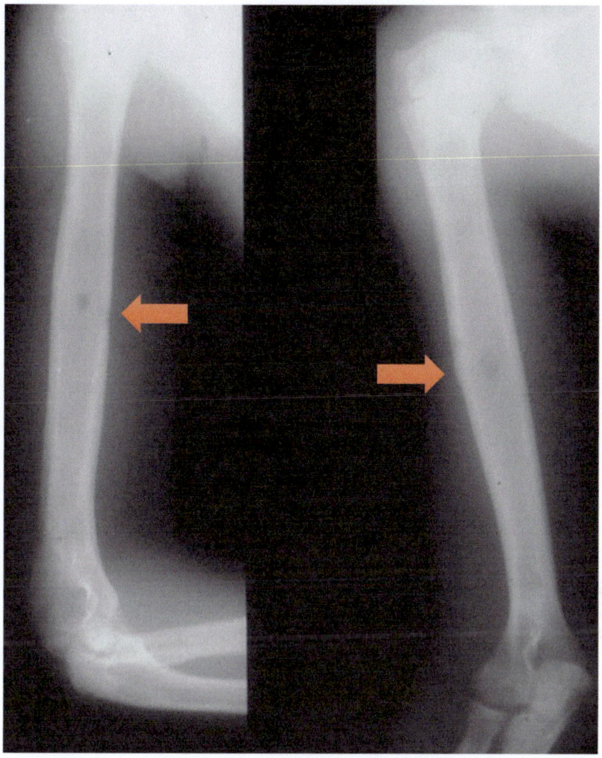

Fig. 8.6 Plain X-ray showing chronic osteomyelitis

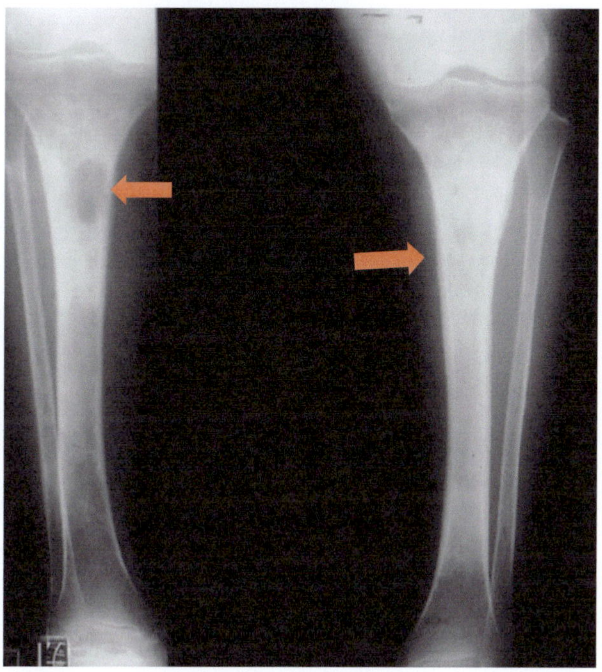

Fig. 8.7 Plain X-ray showing chronic osteomyelitis

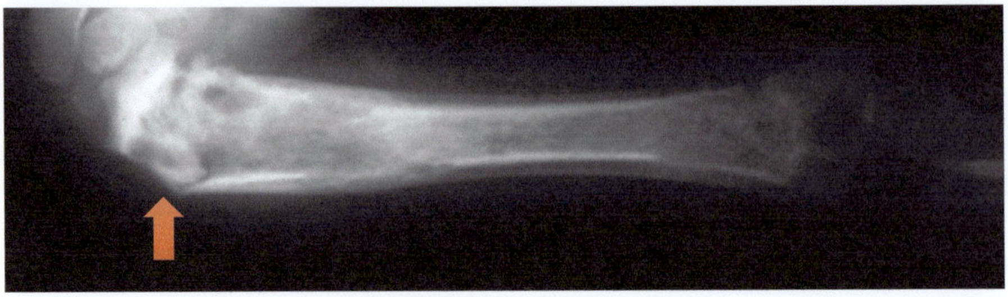

Fig. 8.8 Plain X-ray showing chronic osteomyelitis. Note the bony changes as well as the pathological fracture

- Treatment of osteomyelitis and septic arthritis in sickle cell anemia:
  - These patients should be treated with a prolonged course of intravenous antibiotics.
  - It is important to choose the antibiotics that are appropriate to the causative organisms.
  - The antibiotic treatment of a confirmed case of osteomyelitis should continue for at least 6 weeks. The empirical antibiotic treatment must be directed against *Salmonella* and *S. aureus*.
  - A third-generation cephalosporin such as ceftriaxone is used initially to cover Salmonella infections.
  - Ciprofloxacin is a useful alternative for older children with *Salmonella* osteomyelitis.
  - Other organisms such as *Staphylococcus* should also be covered by empirical antibiotic therapy.
  - Radiological evidence of accumulation of fluid at the site of infection should be drained.
  - However, there is no firm consensus regarding when to drill or drain, and these invasive procedures tend to be reserved for those who are not responding to antibiotic therapy or those who have localized encapsulated septic collections (Fig. 8.11).
  - In those with septic arthritis, early diagnosis, antibiotics, and evacuation of the collection are important for good functional outcome.
  - Drainage is preferred, if possible by arthroscopy.
  - Arthrotomy and drainage should be reserved for cases with a thick discharge which is difficult to evacuate via aspiration.
  - Early diagnosis, careful evacuation of the joint collection, and antibiotic therapy with immobilization are the keys to good functional outcome.

8.4 Avascular Necrosis

- Chronic skeletal problems are common in patients with sickle cell anemia.
- These include:
  - Avascular necrosis
  - Vertebral collapse

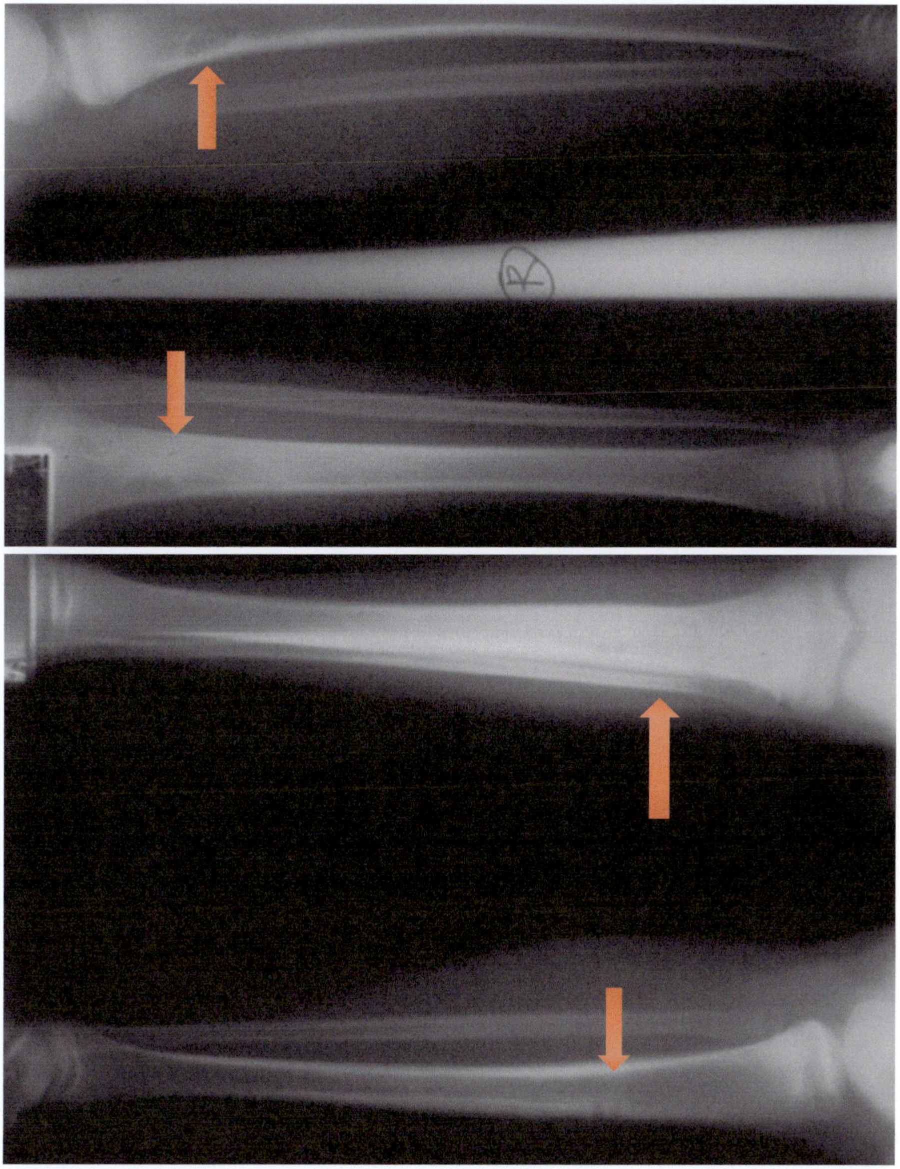

Figs. 8.9 and 8.10 Plain X-rays showing chronic osteomyelitis in a patient with sickle cell anemia. Note the lucent areas and increased sclerosis

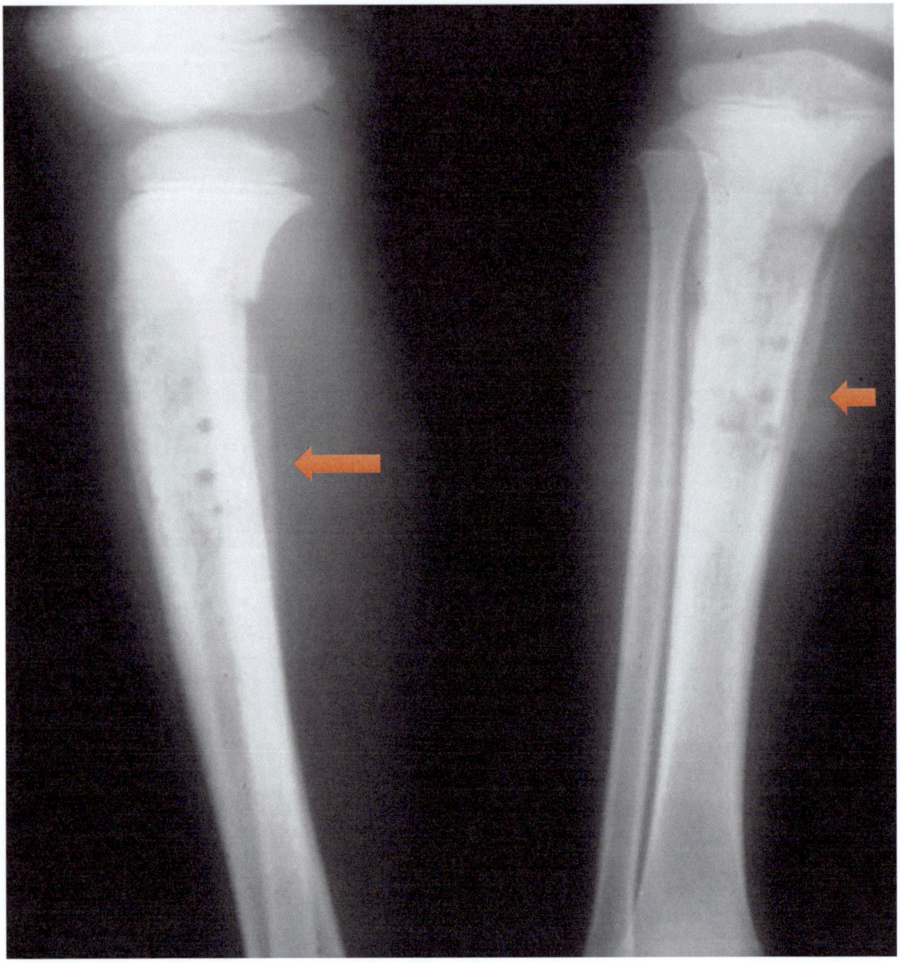

Fig. 8.11 An X-ray showing chronic osteomyelitis. Note also the effects of drilling

  - Chronic arthritis
  - Osteoporosis secondary to hyperplasia of the bone marrow
  - Growth retardation
- Avascular necrosis occurs when vaso-occlusion results in the infarction of the articular surfaces and heads of the long bones (Figs. 8.12, 8.13, 8.14, 8.15 and 8.16).
- Avascular necrosis is a well-known complication of sickle cell anemia.
- The true prevalence of avascular necrosis in sickle cell anemia is difficult to estimate because there patients are with asymptomatic avascular necrosis.
- It has been estimated that about 10 % of patients with sickle cell anemia will have avascular necrosis of one or more joints. Many think this an underestimation and the true frequency is higher.

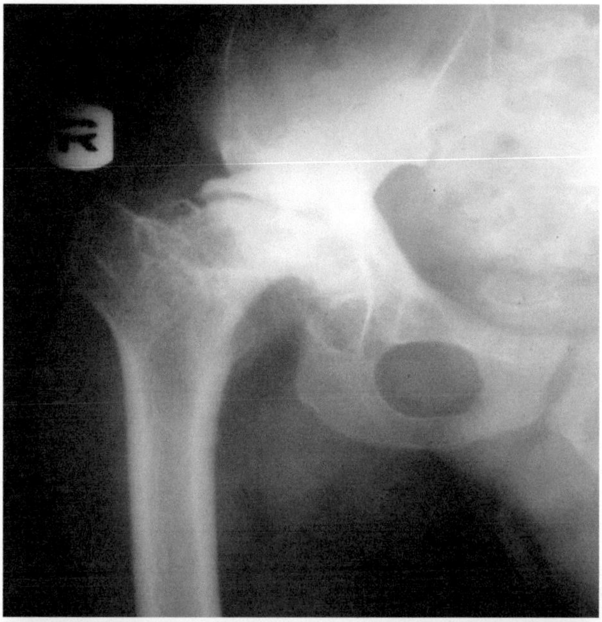

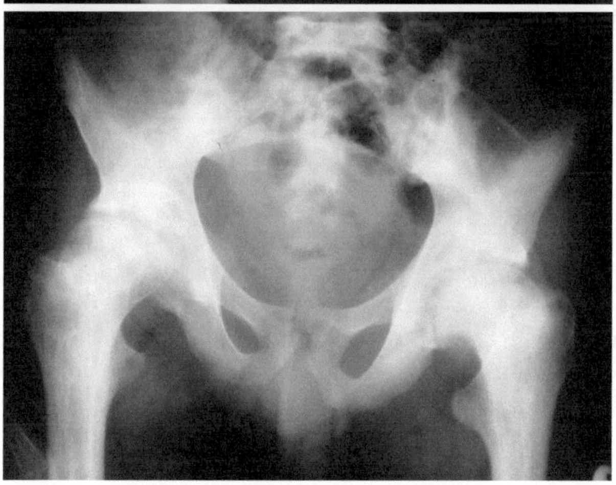

Figs. 8.12 and 8.13 X-rays showing avascular necrosis of the hip joints. Note the extent of the collapse in the femoral heads

- An interesting observation is that patients with HbSS and concomitant alpha thalassemia are at higher risk of developing avascular necrosis (4.5 cases per 100 person-years, compared with 2.4 in those with HbSS without concomitant alpha thalassemia, and 1.9 cases per 100 person-years in those with HbSC disease).
- It was also shown that high levels of HbF have a protective effect against avascular necrosis.

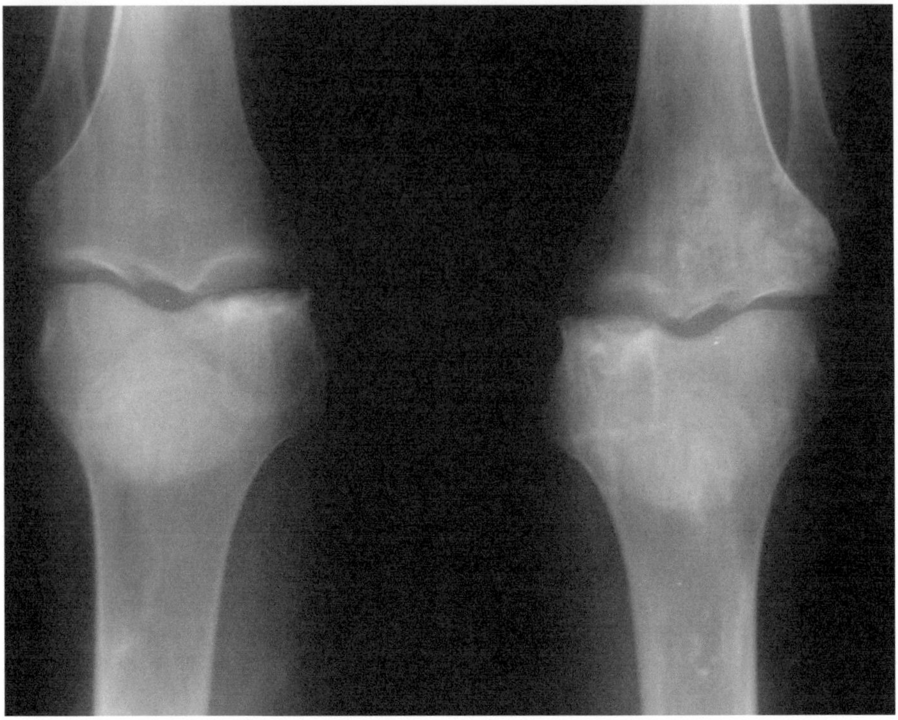

Fig. 8.14 X-ray showing deformity of the knee following avascular necrosis

- The prevalence of avascular necrosis of the femoral head increases with age but was reported in children as young as 5 years of age.
- Avascular necrosis can sometimes be bilateral.
- Asymptomatic avascular necrosis of the femoral head was present simultaneously with symptomatic avascular necrosis of the contralateral hip.
- These findings suggest that radiologic assessment of the contralateral hip should be considered in patients with SCA diagnosed with femoral head avascular necrosis.
- The most common sites of avascular necrosis are (Figs. 8.17, 8.18, 8.19, and 8.20):
  - The femoral heads.
  - The head of the humerus.
  - Knee.
  - Small joints of the hands and feet.
  - There are case reports of avascular necrosis affecting other joints and bony structures, including the mandibular condyle and temporomandibular joint and the elbow.
- Bony infarcts can also occur in unusual locations, including the walls of the orbits (orbital bone infarction and orbital compression syndrome).

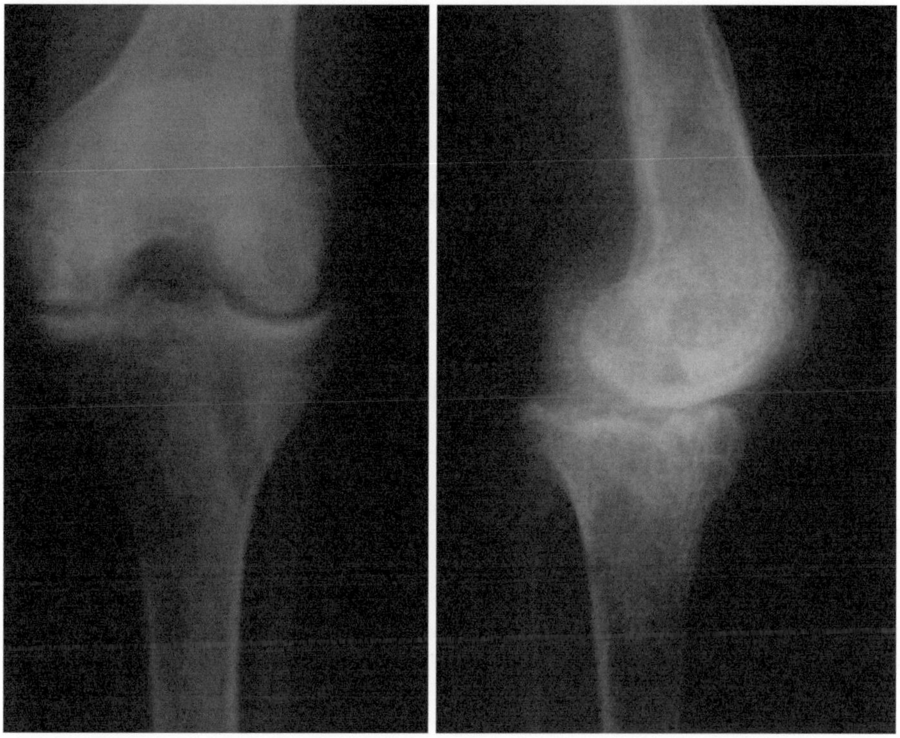

Figs. 8.15 and 8.16 X-rays showing degenerative changes in the knee following avascular necrosis

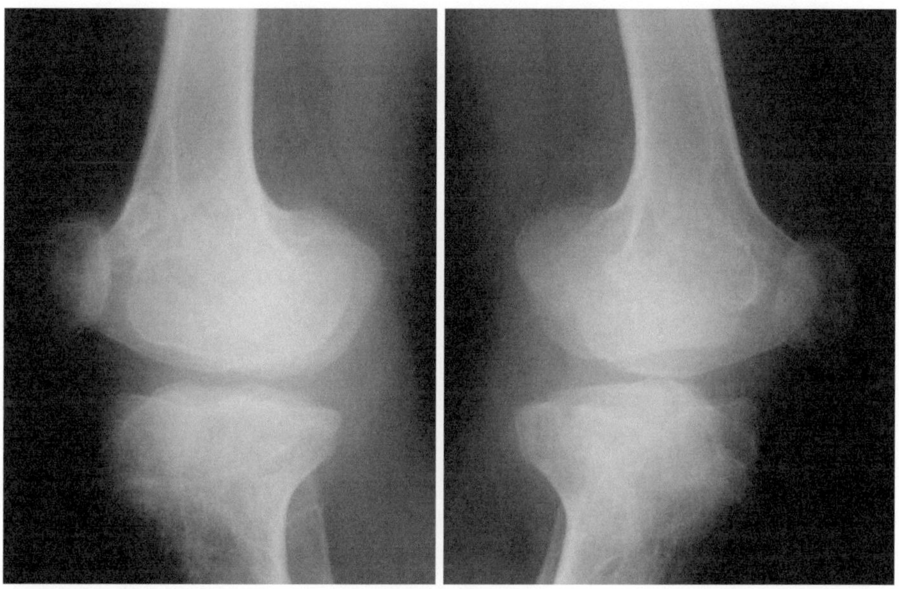

Figs. 8.17 and 8.18 X-rays showing degenerative changes of the knee following avascular necrosis

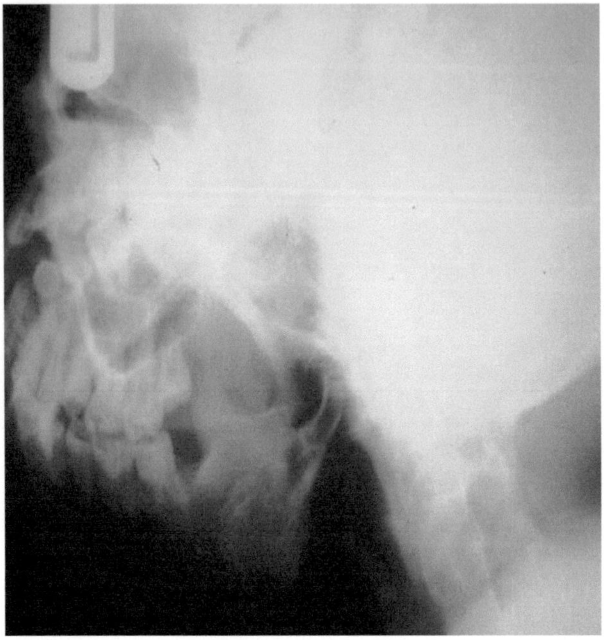

Fig. 8.19 X-ray showing changes in the mandible in a patient with sickle cell anemia

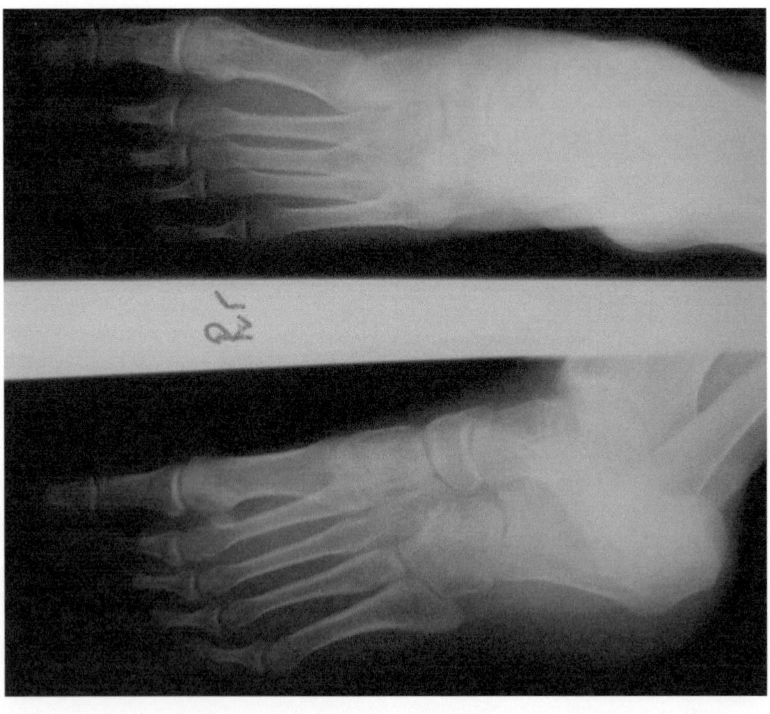

Fig. 8.20 X-rays of the feet showing changes in the small joints following avascular necrosis

- This is characterized by acute periorbital pain and swelling and can be accompanied by the formation of subperiosteal or intracranial hematomas.
- The orbital compression syndrome is characterized by:
  - Proptosis.
  - Limitation of extraocular movement.
  - Corneal hyperesthesia.
  - Optic nerve dysfunction.
  - This condition can be mistaken for orbital cellulitis, but it will not respond to antibiotic therapy.
- Treatment of the orbital compression syndrome is conservative. Significant hematomas or optic nerve compromise necessitates urgent surgical drainage of the hematoma.
- It is common to have multiple joints affected:
  - >50 % of patients with an affected hip have bilateral disease.
  - 74 % of those with an affected shoulder will also have avascular necrosis of the femoral head.
- In the spine, avascular necrosis of the end plate produces a sharp central step in the vertebral body end plate, causing the H-shaped vertebra.
- This can be easily differentiated from the smooth concavity seen with bone softening (Figs. 8.21 and 8.22).
- Clinical features:
  - Symptomatic patients complain of painful, limited motion of the affected joint.
  - Avascular necrosis of the femoral head is characterized by hip pain with weight bearing.
  - Occasionally they complain of pain at rest.
  - Avascular necrosis can also be asymptomatic discovered incidentally.
  - Untreated, 87 % of affected femoral heads will collapse within 5 years of diagnosis.
- Diagnosis:
  - Early avascular necrosis is difficult to diagnose by plain X-rays.
  - Advanced avascular necrosis may be easily diagnosed with plain radiographs.
  - These will show (Figs. 8.23, 8.24, 8.25, 8.26, and 8.27):
    - Mottled attenuation of the epiphysis
    - Subchondral lucent areas
    - Flattening/collapse of the articular surfaces
    - Narrowing of the joint space
    - Articular sclerosis
    - Osteophyte formation
  - MRI is the best investigation to diagnose early avascular necrosis.
- Staging of avascular necrosis of the hip joint:
  - There are several staging systems, and now all are based on a combination of plain films and MRI findings. These include:
  - Extent of the femoral head lesion on MRI:
    - <15 %
    - 15–30 %
    - >30 %

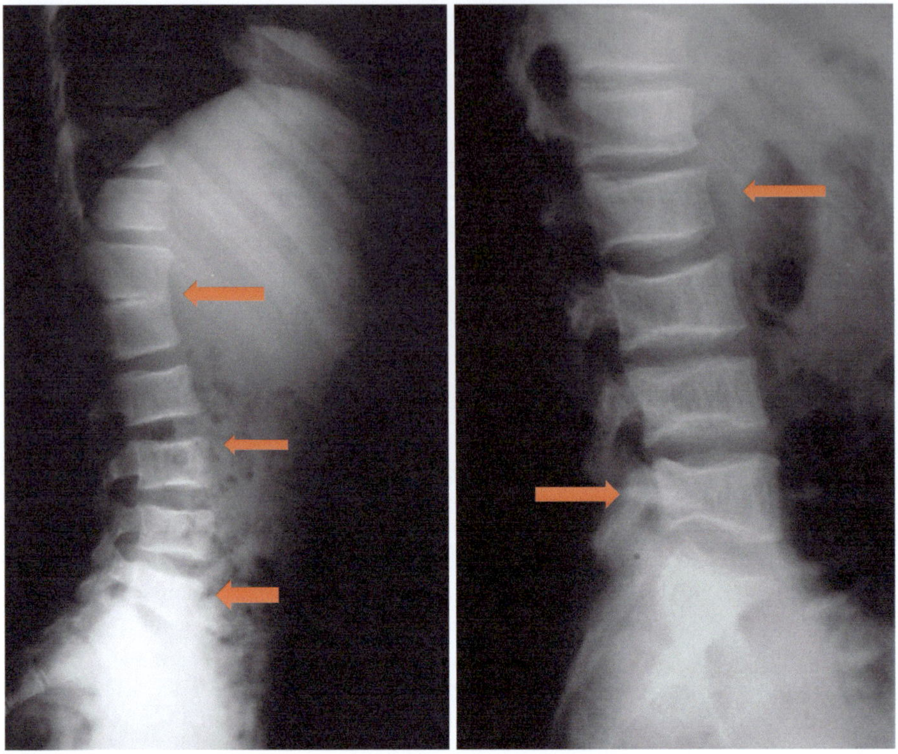

Figs. 8.21 and 8.22 X-rays showing vertebral changes following avascular necrosis including collapse, fish mouth deformity, and fusion of adjacent vertebrae

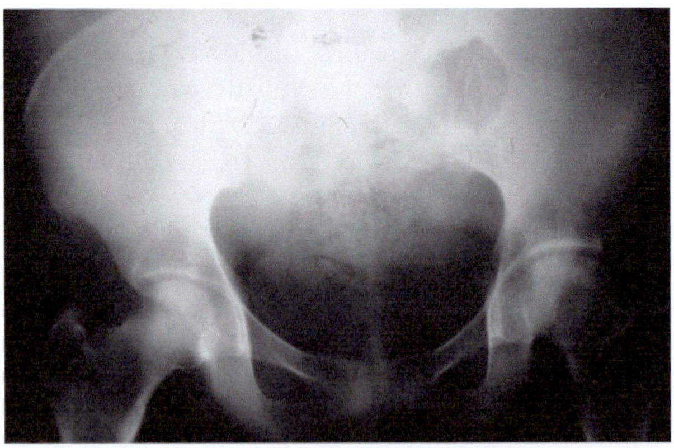

Fig. 8.23 X-ray of the hip joints showing avascular necrosis of the left hip joint. Note the early changes of the head of the femur and narrowing of the joint space

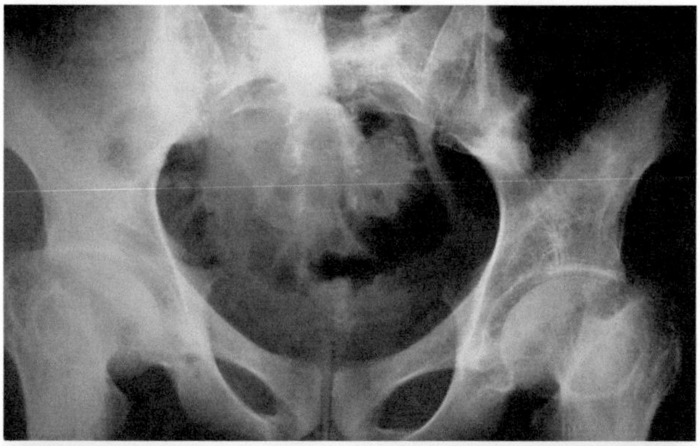

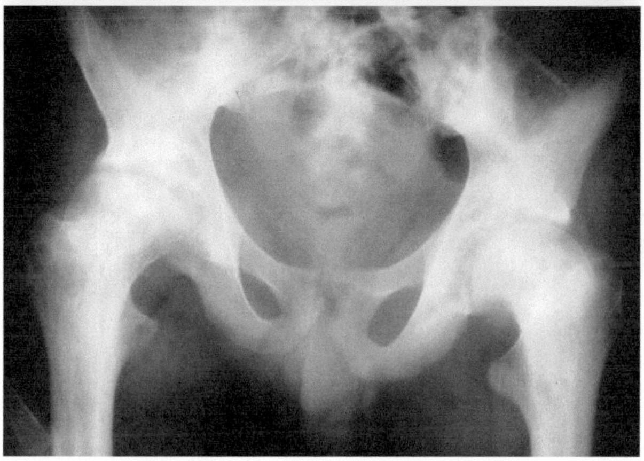

Figs. 8.24 and 8.25 X-rays of the hip joints showing avascular necrosis involving both hip joints. Note the extent of involvement which is different in both joints

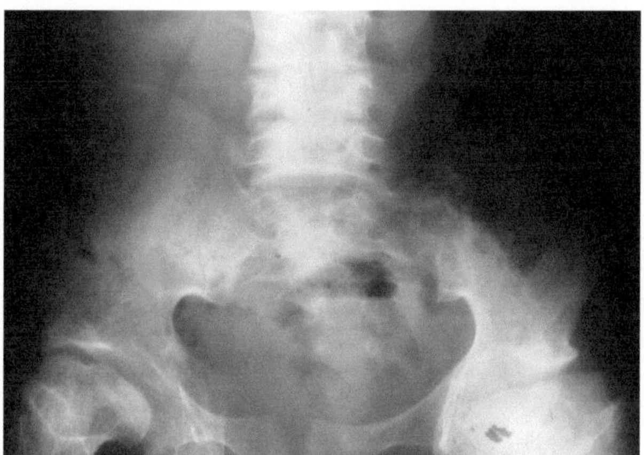

Fig. 8.26 X-ray of the hip joints showing severe bilateral avascular necrosis

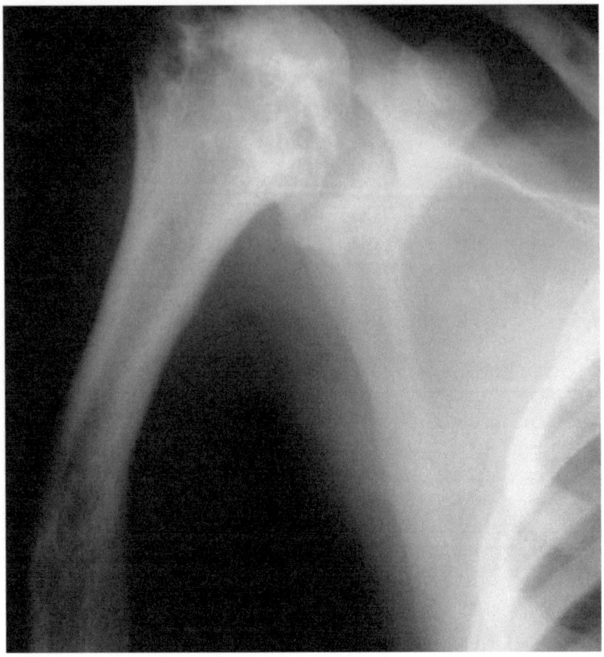

Fig. 8.27 X-ray of the shoulder joint showing avascular necrosis. Note also the lucent areas seen in the head of the humerus

  - Extent of involvement of the articular surface:
    - <15 %
    - 15–30 %
    - >30 %
  - Acetabular changes:
    - Mild
    - Moderate
    - Severe
  - Extent of femoral head collapse or depression:
    - <15 % or 2 mm
    - 15–30 % or 2–4 mm
    - >30 % or 4 mm
  - Other radiographic findings:
    - Sclerosis
    - Cysts
    - Crescent sign
- Treatment:
  - These patients should be treated in specialized centers with experience in sickle cell anemia. This is to avoid the well-known perioperative complications in these patients.
  - The management of patients with avascular necrosis is challenging as there are no clear guidelines regarding the choice between conservative and operative treatment.

- Early diagnosis and conservative management are important to avoid progression.
- Conservative management has been advocated for those with early avascular necrosis.
- Bed rest, in order to avoid weight bearing, is considered the most effective methods of preventing progression of joint damage.
- This however may not be acceptable for many patients as it is not practical and limits their daily activities. These patients can be mobilized on crutches or a wheelchair.
- Conservative measures include:
  - Analgesics to relieve pain.
  - Reduced or non-weight bearing.
  - Bed rest.
  - Mobilization with crutches or a wheelchair.
  - Physiotherapy is important:
    - To maintain the range of motion in the joint
    - To strengthen the muscles
    - To provide gait training
- The majority of patients however require surgery for pain relief and functional improvement.
- Early disease may improve with conservative treatment, and decompression coring and osteotomy should be reserved for those who are not benefitting.
- The failure rates in some studies of this approach are as high as 50 % at 5 years.
- Patients with advanced disease and those who fail core decompression require joint replacement.
- Core decompression:
  - This procedure consists of removal of necrotic tissue from the joint, with or without a bone graft to fill the "cored" area.
- Arthroplasty (joint replacement) (Figs. 8.28, 8.29, and 8.30):

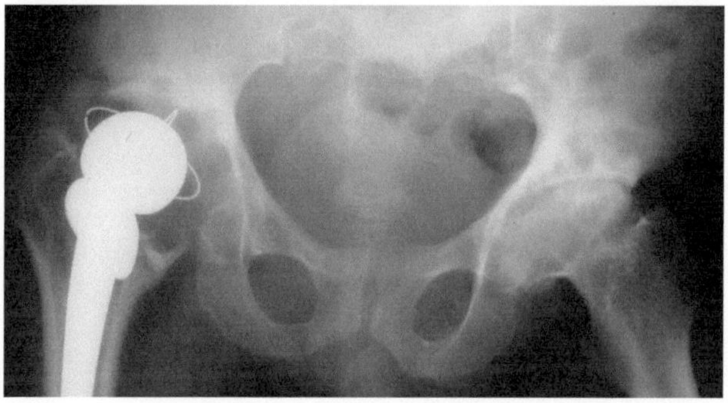

Fig. 8.28 X-ray showing hip replacement on the right side. Note also the avascular necrosis on the left side in a patient with sickle cell anemia

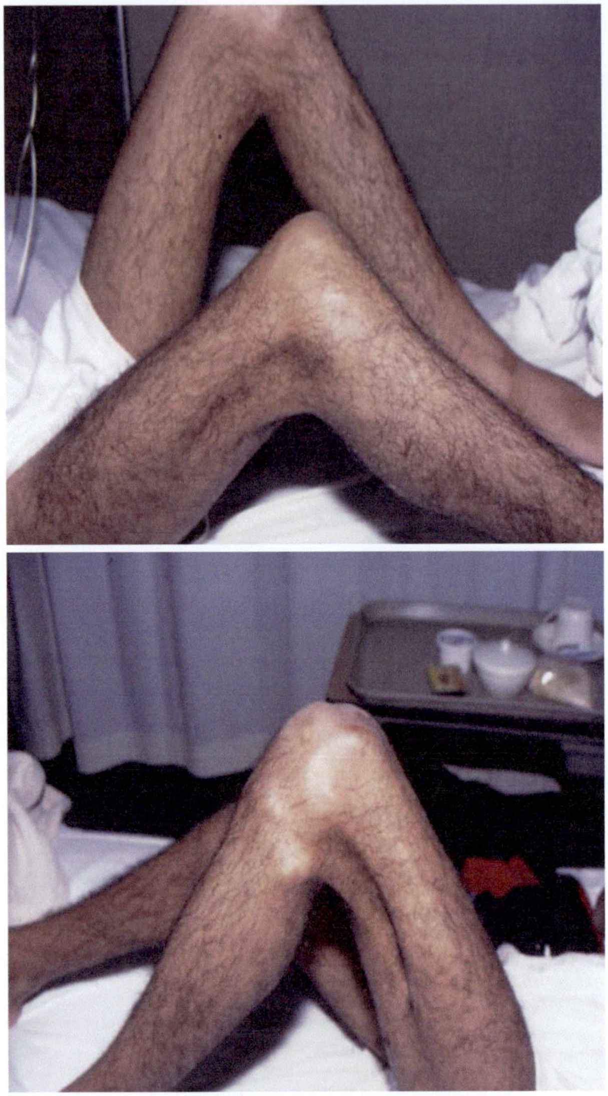

Figs. 8.29 and 8.30 Clinical photographs showing severe deformity of the knee joints in a patient with sickle cell anemia. This was following avascular necrosis that was neglected

- This is reserved for those who are not benefiting from conservative measures and/or core decompression.
- Arthroplasty has 20–30 % failure rate, and those younger than 21 years may have better outcomes.

8.5 Osteopenia and Osteoporosis (Fig. 8.31)

- Patients with sickle cell anemia are known to have an overall reduction in bone mineral density.
- This is attributed to bone marrow hyperplasia.
- The vertebrae in patients with sickle cell anemia are prone to several changes induced by:
  - Bone marrow hyperplasia
  - Osteopenia
  - Vaso-occlusive crisis
  - Avascular necrosis

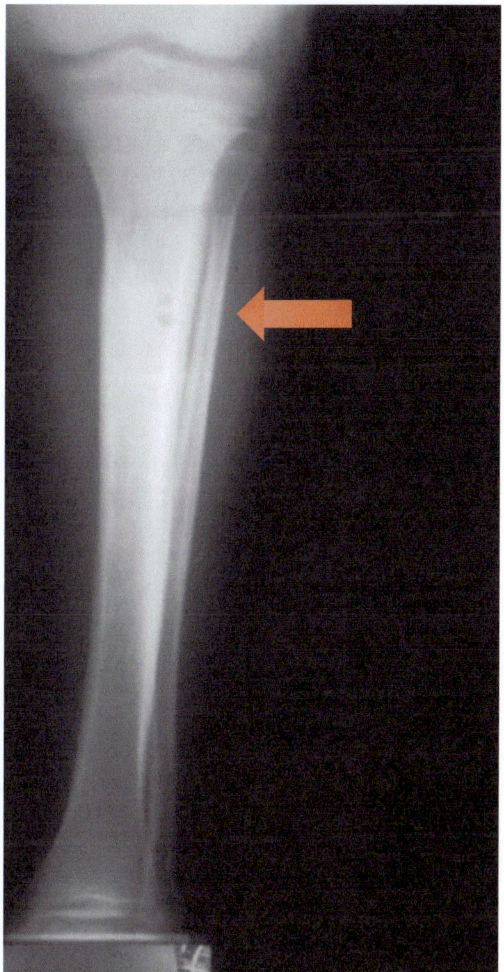

Fig. 8.31 X-rays showing increased density of the bones in a patient with sickle cell anemia

- Vertebral osteoporosis is particularly common in patients with sickle cell anemia.
- Radiological findings in the spine include:
  - An increased radiolucency of the vertebral bodies.
  - Prominence of vertebral trabeculae.
  - A smooth, biconcave deformity of the vertebrae known as "fish mouth" vertebrae, which forms as a result of compression by the adjacent intervertebral disks.
  - "Tower vertebrae" (vertebrae with compensatory elongation located next to infarcted short vertebrae). There is an increase in the height of the vertebral bodies without an associated increase in the girth.
  - These patients may go on to develop vertebral collapse either from the osteoporosis or as a result of vertebral infarction.
- Vertebral collapse is often asymptomatic but may cause acute and/or chronic pain.
- Vitamin D deficiency is a common finding among children and adults with sickle cell anemia.
- This may play a role in the development of bony changes in patients with sickle cell anemia.
- It is still not clear that supplements of vitamin D and calcium can help prevent or reduce the incidence of chronic bone disease in patients with sickle cell anemia.
- Treatment with vitamin D and calcium supplements can improve bone mineral density in these patients.

8.6 Abnormal Growth and Development (Fig. 8.32)

- Patients with sickle cell anemia have reduced growth and height and generally smaller than age-related healthy children.
- This effect is more pronounced in weight and sexual development.
- This is believed to be due to bone marrow hyperplasia, but many think it is multifactorial including:
  - Chronic anemia.
  - Systemic infections.
  - Episodic acute illnesses.
  - Endocrine dysfunction and central hypogonadism.
  - Micronutrient deficiencies. Several studies have shown that children with sickle cell anemia have lower levels of vitamins A, B6, and D.
- Bones are generally shorter. This the result of:
  - Epiphyseal shortening and compromise to the growth plate secondary to ischemia/infarction
  - Premature closure of growth plates
- It was also shown that levels of growth hormone and insulin-like growth factor 1 (IGF-1), as well as IGF binding protein-3 (IGFBP-3), were lower in patients with sickle cell anemia.

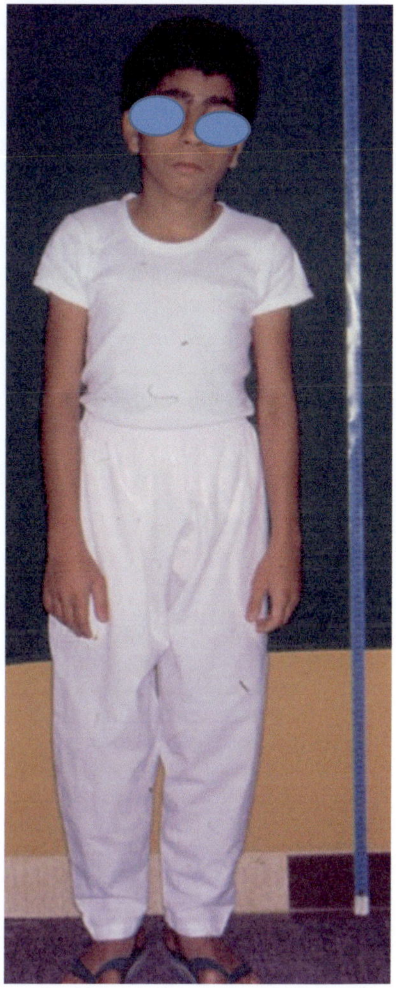

Fig. 8.32 A clinical photograph showing an adolescent patient with sickle cell anemia. Note the growth retardation with reduced growth and height

8.7 Soft Tissue Abnormalities

- In patients with sickle cell anemia, sickling leads to occlusion of blood vessels in the muscles. This will lead to inflammation and myonecrosis with subsequent fluid collection and hematoma formation. Superadded infection will lead to pyomyositis and abscess formation.
- Pyomyositis is a purulent infection of skeletal muscle that can rapidly lead to abscess formation.
- Pyomyositis usually presents with fever and muscle pain. This is commonly seen in the lower extremity.

- The most common causative organism is *Staphylococcus aureus.*
- The diagnosis of pyomyositis in patients with sickle cell anemia is usually delayed as initially this may resemble acute vaso-occlusive crisis. A high index of suspicion is important for early diagnosis.
- MRI is a valuable investigation to confirm the diagnosis. It is also valuable in differentiating this from osteomyelitis.
- Treatment:
  - This comprises a combination of intravenous antibiotics and surgical or percutaneous drainage of the collection.
  - The antibiotic coverage should be broad-spectrum and include antibiotics against *Staphylococcus aureus* and *Salmonella.*
  - There is no consensus regarding the duration of antibiotics but a 3–4 weeks course of parenteral antibiotics is recommended.

Further Reading

Almeida A, Roberts I. Bone involvement in sickle cell disease. Br J Haematol. 2005;129(4):482–90.

Burnett MW, Bass JW, Cook BA. Etiology of osteomyelitis complicating sickle cell disease. Pediatrics. 1998;101(2):296–7.

Ejindu VC, Hine AL, Mashayekhi M, Shorvon PJ, Misra RR. Musculoskeletal manifestations of sickle cell disease. Radiographics. 2007;27(4):1005–21.

Keeley K, Buchanan GR. Acute infarction of long bones in children with sickle cell anemia. J Pediatr. 1982;101(2):170–5.

Platt OS, Rosenstock W, Espeland MA. Influence of sickle hemoglobinopathies on growth and development. N Engl J Med. 1984;311(1):7–12.

Umans H, Haramati N, Flusser G. The diagnostic role of gadolinium enhanced MRI in distinguishing between acute medullary bone infarct and osteomyelitis. Magn Reson Imaging. 2000;18(3):255–62.

Ware HE, Brooks AP, Toye R, Berney SI. Sickle cell disease and silent avascular necrosis of the hip. J Bone Joint Surg Br. 1991;73(6):947–9.

9 Gastrointestinal Complications of Sickle Cell Anemia

9.1 Introduction

- Sickle cell anemia is one of the most common inherited hemoglobinopathies worldwide.
- Painful vaso-occlusive crisis is the leading cause of emergency room visits and hospitalization of these patients.
- These attacks commonly affect the skeletal system and can be localized or generalized affecting more than one site of the body.
- Abdominal pain is an important part of these painful attacks.
- It can occur in isolation or more commonly as part of a generalized vaso-occlusive crisis.
- Other sickle cell anemia-related abdominal complications that may be present with abdominal pain include:
  - Cholelithiasis with or without cholecystitis
  - Choledocholithiasis with or without cholangitis
  - Acute splenic sequestration crisis
  - Splenic infarction
  - Splenic abscess
  - Acute pancreatitis
  - Peptic ulcer disease
  - Acute appendicitis
  - Hepatic infarction
  - Hepatic abscess
  - Ischemic colitis
  - Hepatic crisis
  - Mesenteric lymphadenitis

A. Al-Salem, *Medical and Surgical Complications of Sickle Cell Anemia*,
DOI 10.1007/978-3-319-24762-5_9

9.2 Abdominal Vaso-Occlusive Crisis

- This is one of the causes of acute presentation of patients with sickle cell anemia.
- It can present in isolation or more commonly as part of a generalized vaso-occlusive crisis.
- Abdominal pain due to sickle cell vaso-occlusive crisis often represents a diagnostic challenge as it is often indistinguishable from other causes of acute abdomen.
- It is estimated that approximately 10 % of patients with sickle cell anemia are admitted to the hospital each year due to acute abdominal pain.
- These episodes of abdominal vaso-occlusive crisis are often attributed to microvessel occlusion and infarcts of the mesentery and abdominal viscera. This causes severe abdominal pain and signs of peritoneal irritation, and abdominal X-ray often shows a generalized ileus (Figs. 9.1 and 9.2).
- Other causes of abdominal pain in patients with sickle cell anemia include bone marrow infarction of the vertebral bodies with nerve root entrapment, acute pancreatitis, and enlarged mesenteric and retroperitoneal lymph nodes with infarction.
- In the majority of cases, however, no specific cause is identified and spontaneous resolution occurs.
- The fact that many of these patients present to the emergency room with attacks of abdominal pain that resolve spontaneously should not be taken lightly in order not to miss a surgical cause. On the other hand, these patients should not be rushed to the operation room for the fear of missing an acute surgical abdomen.
- It is important to evaluate these patients properly with a careful history, frequent clinical evaluations, and investigations. Patients with moderate and sever attacks of abdominal vaso-occlusive crisis should be admitted to the hospital for further evaluation and observation.

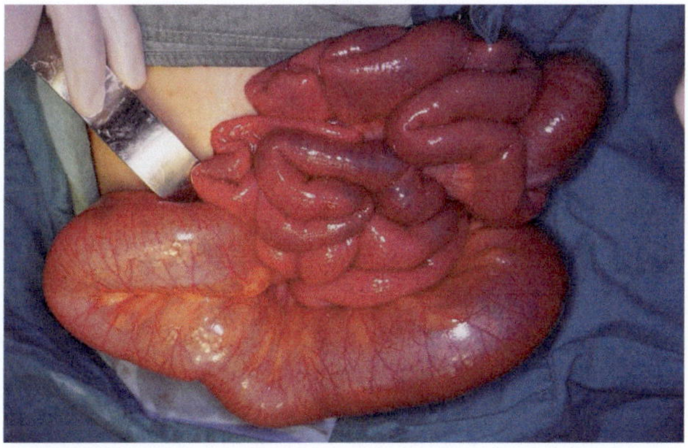

Fig. 9.1 Intraoperative photograph of a child with abdominal vaso-occlusive crisis. Note the congestion and ileus of the affected bowel which is slightly dilated

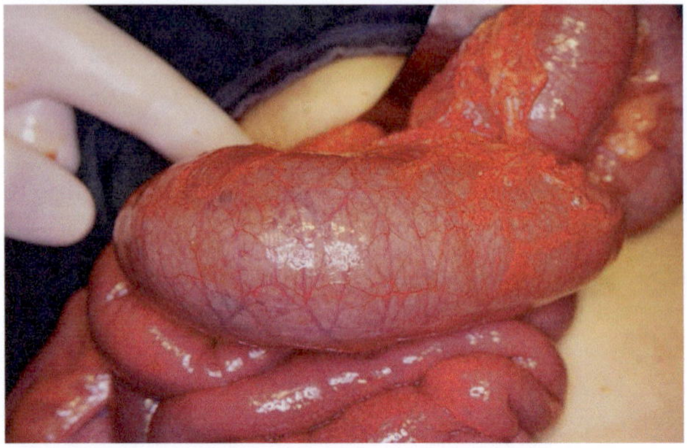

Fig. 9.2 Intraoperative photograph of a child with abdominal vaso-occlusive crisis. Note the dilated small intestine and also small areas of hemorrhage in the bowel wall

- The presence of vaso-occlusive crisis at other sites of the body makes the abdominal pain part of the vaso-occlusive crisis rather than secondary to an acute surgical emergency.
- The management of patients with abdominal vaso-occlusive crisis is conservative and includes:
  - Admission for close observation and frequent evaluation.
  - Nothing by mouth.
  - Intravenous hydration.
  - Investigations including CBC, electrolytes, BUN, creatinine, abdominal X-rays, and abdominal ultrasound.
  - Analgesics should be given once the diagnosis of acute surgical conditions was ruled out.
  - Packed RBC blood transfusion should be given when there is an associated anemia (Hb < 9 g/dl).
- The majority of abdominal vaso-occlusive crisis attacks resolve spontaneously without the need for surgical exploration. The time interval for complete resolution is however variable.

9.3 Peptic Ulcer Disease

- The exact incidence of peptic ulcer disease in patients with sickle cell anemia is not known, and there is no study documenting the prevalence of peptic ulcers in SCA.
- It is estimated that one-third of patients with sickle cell anemia who present with chronic epigastric pain have endoscopic evidence of peptic ulcer (Figs. 9.3 and 9.4).
- In one study, peptic ulcer disease was found in 35 % of patients with sickle cell anemia presenting with epigastric pain.

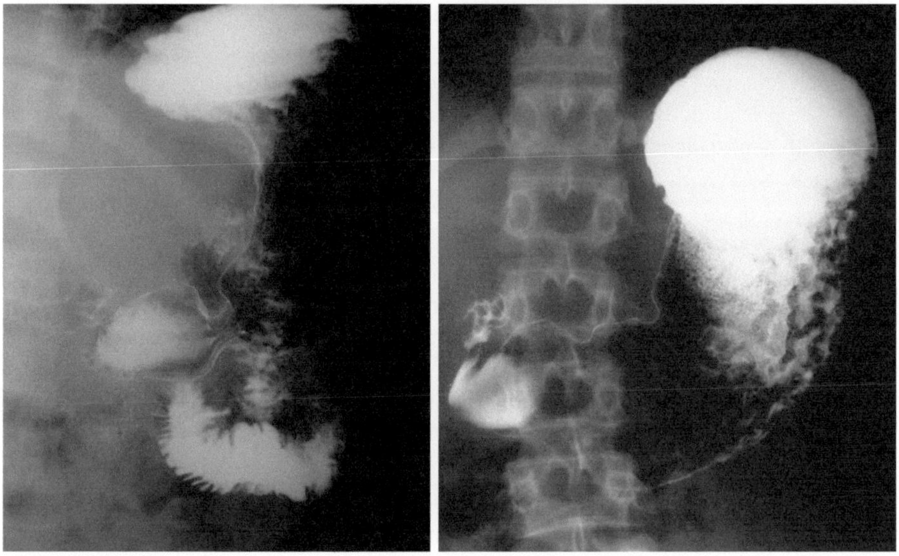

Figs. 9.3 and 9.4 Barium meal showing peptic ulcer disease in two patients with sickle cell anemia

  - Duodenal ulcer (27 %)
  - Gastric ulcer (8 %)
- This high rate of peptic ulcer disease in patients with sickle cell anemia is attributed to mucosal hypoxemia and ischemia as a result of repeated sickling and microvascular occlusion. This may lead to gastroduodenal perforation in the absence of previous epigastric symptoms.
- A much lower incidence of duodenal ulcer (7.6 %) was reported from Jamaica.
- In another study and based on endoscopic findings, 20 out of 51 patients (39.2 %) with chronic epigastric pain were found to have peptic ulcer disease:
  - Duodenal ulcer (27.5 %)
  - Gastric ulcer (8 %)
  - Gastritis (4 %)
- It was also found that patients with higher total hemoglobin and fetal hemoglobin levels are at lesser risk of developing peptic ulcer disease.
- Pathogenesis:
  - The pathogenesis of peptic ulcer disease is different in patients with sickle cell anemia:
  - In patients with sickle cell anemia, duodenal ulcers are not associated with high acid outputs.
  - Several studies have shown that sickle cell anemia patients have low or normal gastric acid secretion. The basal and peak gastric acid output was shown to be similar in sickle cell patients with and without peptic ulcer disease.
  - This suggests that these ulcers might, instead, be due to reduced mucosal resistance, possibly from repeated ischemia.

- The decreased mucosal resistance due to ischemia and use of NSAIDs has also been hypothesized to cause peptic ulcer disease in patients with sickle cell anemia.
- The prevalence of *Helicobacter pylori* infection in sickle cell anemia patients with peptic ulcer disease is not known. These patients however are at increased risk of *Helicobacter pylori* infection because of chronic anemia and increased use of nonsteroidal anti-inflammatory drugs to relief their pains. The role of *Helicobacter pylori* infection in the pathogenesis of peptic ulcer disease in patients with sickle cell anemia is not clear.
- Healing of these ulcers is also impaired due to vascular impairment.
- The rate of complications such as stenosis, hemorrhage, and perforation is also high in these patients.
- Ulcer healing may be promoted by monthly packed red cell transfusions over 6 months.

- Management:
  - Once the diagnosis of peptic ulcer disease is made, medical treatment should be started immediately.
  - This is to avoid subsequent complications such as stenosis, hemorrhage, and perforation.
  - The diagnosis should be confirmed by endoscopy. This should be repeated after 6–8 weeks of medical therapy to monitor the progress and healing of the ulcer.
  - These patients are usually anemic and also have poor healing of these ulcers. To overcome this and promote healing, it was suggested to transfuse these patients every 3–4 weeks with packed RBCs.
  - Surgery should be offered early for poorly healing ulcers as assessed endoscopically. This is to avoid the risk of complications including bleeding and perforation.

9.4 Acute Pancreatitis

- In patients with sickle cell anemia, acute pancreatitis can develop:
  - Idiopathically with no apparent cause.
  - As a result of sickling and microvascular occlusion and ischemic injury to the pancreas.
  - Secondary to cholelithiasis and choledocholithiasis. Sickle cell anemia patients are known to have a high incidence of gallstones and common bile duct stones which may be complicated by acute pancreatitis (Figs. 9.5 and 9.6).
  - Following endoscopic retrograde cholangiopancreatography (ERCP) for the investigation of obstructive jaundice. Acute pancreatitis in these patients can develop even in those who do not have invasive procedures like sphincterotomy. This is usually a mild, transient pancreatitis that resolves quickly (Figs. 9.7 and 9.8).

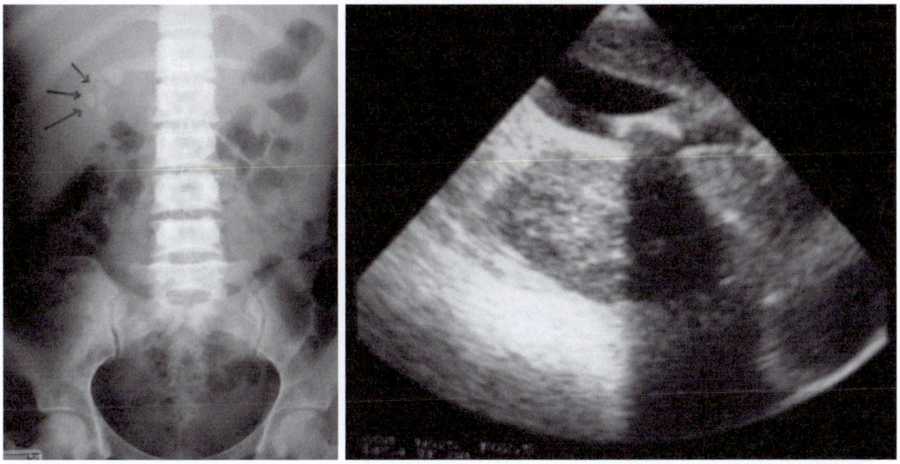

Figs. 9.5 and 9.6 Plain abdominal X-ray and abdominal ultrasound showing gallstones. Gallstones are known to cause abdominal pain and may be complicated by choledocholithiasis and acute pancreatitis

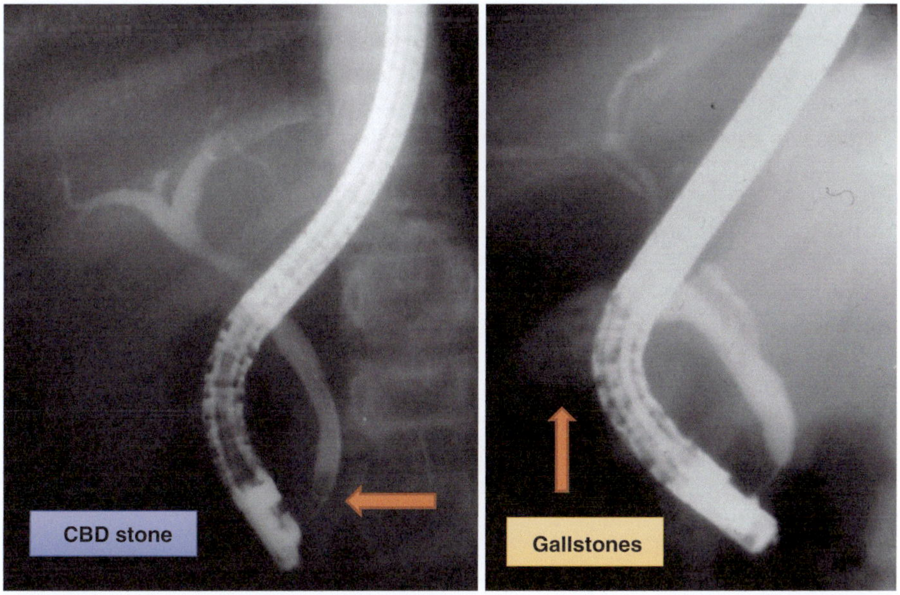

Figs. 9.7 and 9.8 ERCP showing a retained CBD stone. CBD stones are well-known causes of acute pancreatitis. It is also known that ERCP may be complicated by acute pancreatitis. Another ERCP showing gallstones but no CBD stones

- Acute pancreatitis must be kept in mind in sickle cell anemia patients who present with abdominal pain.
- It is also important to remember that sickle cell anemia patients who present with acute pancreatitis might develop acute chest syndrome.

9.5 Ischemic Colitis

- Abdominal pain is a common presentation of patients with sickle cell anemia.
- This is especially during an attack of vaso-occlusive crisis.
- It represents a diagnostic challenge to the treating physician as it mimics a wide spectrum of surgical emergencies and if not evaluated properly may result in unnecessary surgical exploration.
- One of the rare but serious complications of sickle cell anemia is ischemic colitis.
- This seen in patients with sickle cell anemia as a result of massive intravascular sickling.
- Ischemic colitis has been reported in sickle cell anemia patients as young as 18 years of age.
- Ischemic colitis in SCA patients is fortunately rare, and this is attributed to the presence of an extensive collateral circulation in the mesentery and in the bowel wall.
- The exact cause of ischemic colitis is not known.
- Sickle cell anemia patients are liable to develop abdominal vaso-occlusive crisis which in some of them represents a "pre-shock" state leading to vascular spasm, mesenteric arterial thrombosis, and subsequent vascular necrosis.
- It was suggested that ischemic colitis occurs secondary to mesenteric vascular thrombosis with subsequent vascular necrosis to the bowel.
- Cytokines such as interleukin and tumor necrosis factor may play an important role in the etiology of ischemic colitis.
- Pseudomembranous colitis without *Clostridium difficile* has been described in association with SCA and was treated successfully with exchange blood transfusions.
- Diagnosis:
  - Although rare, ischemic colitis should be considered in the differential diagnosis of acute abdominal pain in a patient with sickle cell anemia.
  - This is specially so if the patient presents with:
    - Severe abdominal pain
    - Rectal bleeding
    - Signs of localized peritonism
  - These patients are usually febrile and CBC will show leukocytosis.
  - These patients should be monitored and examined at close interval.
  - Plain abdominal X-ray may show dilated bowel loops with thumb printing.

  - A barium enema should be avoided in these patients as it may cause bowel perforation.
  - Abdominal CT scan may be helpful in establishing the diagnosis.
- Treatment:
  - Keep the patient NPO.
  - Nasogastric aspiration.
  - Intravenous fluid hydration and resuscitation.
  - Broad-spectrum antibiotics.
  - Blood grouping and crossmatching.
  - Blood transfusion in those with anemia (<9 g/dl). These patients may require surgical intervention and should be prepared including correction of pre-existing anemia which may be exacerbated by the ischemic colitis. This may also necessitate exchange blood transfusion.
  - Surgical intervention should not be delayed in these patients. This is indicated in those with:
    - High fever
    - Leukocytosis
    - Signs of peritonitis whether localized or generalized

Further Reading

Baruchet S, Delifer JC, Sigalet D, Hong A, Oudjhane K, Chen MF. Pseudomembraneous colitis in sickle cell disease responding to exchange transfusion. J Pediatr. 1992;121:915–7.

Ebert EC, Nagar M, Hagspiel KD. Gastrointestinal and hepatic complications of sickle cell disease. Clin Gastroenterol Hepatol. 2010;8(6):483–9.

Engelhardt T, Pulitzer DR, Etheredge EE. Ischemic intestinal necrosis as a cause of atypical abdominal pain in a sickle cell patient. J Natl Med Assoc. 1989;81(10):1077–88.

Gange TP, Gagnier M. Ischemic colitis complicating sickle cell crisis. Gastroenterology. 1983;84:171–4.

Karim A, Ahmed S, Rossoff LJ, Siddiqui R, Fuchs A, Multz AS. Fulminant ischaemic colitis with atypical clinical features complicating sickle cell disease. Postgrad Med J. 2002;78(920):370–2.

Lee MG, Therumalai CHR, Terry SI, Serjeant GR. Endoscopic and gastric acid studies in homozygous sickle cell disease and upper abdominal pain. Gut. 1989;30(5):569–72.

Nazem A, Walker M. Sickle cell crisis and the acute abdomen. J Natl Med Assoc. 1986;78(8):787–8.

Sheehan AG, Machida H, Butzner JD. Acute pancreatitis in a child with sickle cell anemia. J Natl Med Assoc. 1993;85(1):70–2.

Woods KF, Onuoha A, Schade RR, Kutlar A. Helicobacter pylori infection in sickle cell disease. J Natl Med Assoc. 2000;92(7):361–5.

Leg Ulcers in Patients with Sickle Cell Anemia

10

10.1 Introduction

- The clinical manifestations of sickle cell anemia (SCA) are diverse.
- Leg ulcers are a relatively common complication in patients with sickle cell anemia. They are considered as markers of disease severity.
- It is most common in sickle cell anemia (HbSS) and less often seen in HbSC disease or HbS-β thalassemia.
- The incidence of leg ulcers is also variable worldwide. It is commonly seen in African and Jamaican but considered extremely rare in Saudi Arabia. The reason for this variation is not known.
- They cause significant physical disability and negative psychological and social impact.
- Leg ulcers are rarely seen before age of 10 years and commonly affect areas with less subcutaneous fat, thin skin, and decreased blood flow (Fig. 10.1).
- They are more common in males than females.
- The commonest sites for leg ulcers are:
  - The medial and lateral malleoli.
  - Less common sites include the anterior tibial area, dorsum of the foot, and posteriorly at the Achilles tendon (Fig. 10.2).
- The geographical distribution of leg ulcers is variable.
  - In the United States, 2.5 % of patients with SCA have leg ulcers.
  - In Jamaica, more than 40 % of patients with SCA have leg ulcers.
  - In Africa, 1.5–13.5 % of patients with SCA have leg ulcers.
  - In Saudi Arabia, leg ulcers are extremely rare.
- The reason for this variation is not known but leg ulcers are known to be rare in patients with:
  - Associated alpha thalassemia
  - High Hb level
  - High HbF level

A. Al-Salem, *Medical and Surgical Complications of Sickle Cell Anemia*,
DOI 10.1007/978-3-319-24762-5_10

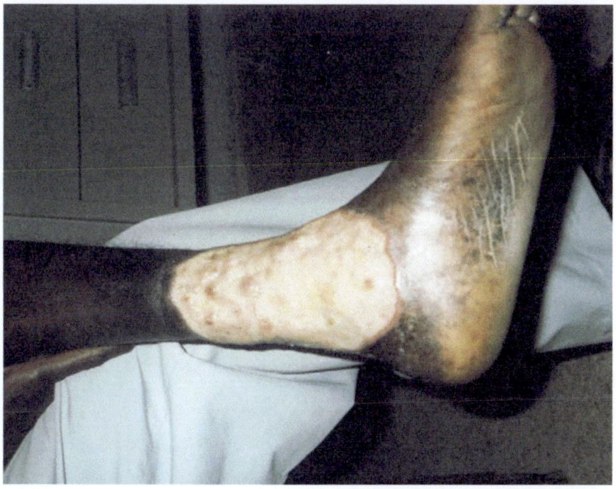

Fig. 10.1 A clinical photograph showing an adult patient with SCA and leg ulcer. Note the site and extent of the ulcer

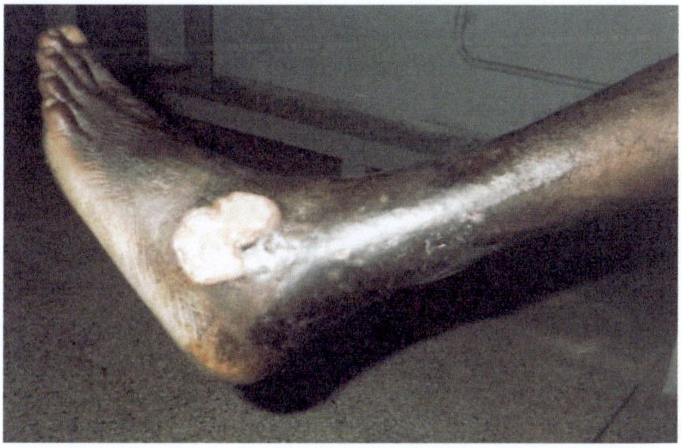

Fig. 10.2 A clinical photograph of an adult with SCA and leg ulcer involving the dorsum of the foot and lateral malleolus

- These factors may contribute to the very low incidence of leg ulcers in SCA patients from Saudi Arabia who are known to have high HbF levels, high Hb levels, and high associated alpha thalassemia.

10.2 Pathogenesis

- The pathogenesis and etiology of leg ulcers in patients with SCA is not exactly known, and several factors may play role in their pathogenesis. These include:
  - Blood vessels obstruction by sickled RBC
  - Venous congestion

  - Trauma
  - Infection
  - Anemia
  - Thrombosis
  - Decreased NO bioavailability
  - Arteriovenous shunting
- The fact that leg ulcers are known to be associated with priapism and pulmonary hypertension supports the role of decreased NO bioavailability in the pathogenesis of leg ulcers.

10.3 Classification

- Leg ulcers are classified depending on the duration of the ulcer into:
  - Acute
  - Chronic
- Although there is no cut point to differentiate between acute and chronic ulcers, an ulcer that does not heal in one month is considered to be chronic.
- Leg ulcers are also classified based on the size, depth, and duration.
- Leg ulcers are also staged according to the depth of the ulcer into four stages:
  - Stage I: erythema of the intact skin.
  - Stage II: superficial ulcer with partial thickness skin loss involving epidermis, dermis, or both.
  - Stage III: this is characterized by full-thickness skin loss extending to the subcutaneous tissue but not through the underlying fascia.
  - Stage IV: this is a deep ulcer with full-thickness skin loss and extends deep to involve the underlying structures (muscles, tendons, bone) (Figs. 10.3 and 10.4).

10.4 Treatment

- The treatment of leg ulcers should be simple and conservative to start with. This should include:
  - Gentle debridement for those with necrotic tissue, eschar and purulent exudate.
  - Control of edema.
  - Wet-to-dry dressing.
  - DuoDERM dressing. DuoDERM is useful for debridement of contaminated ulcers, facilitating their healing.
  - Hydrotherapy.
  - Zinc sulfate 200 mg twice daily.
  - Antibiotics for those with cellulitis, lymphadenitis, or osteomyelitis.
  - Leg elevation.
  - Hypertonic saline dressing.

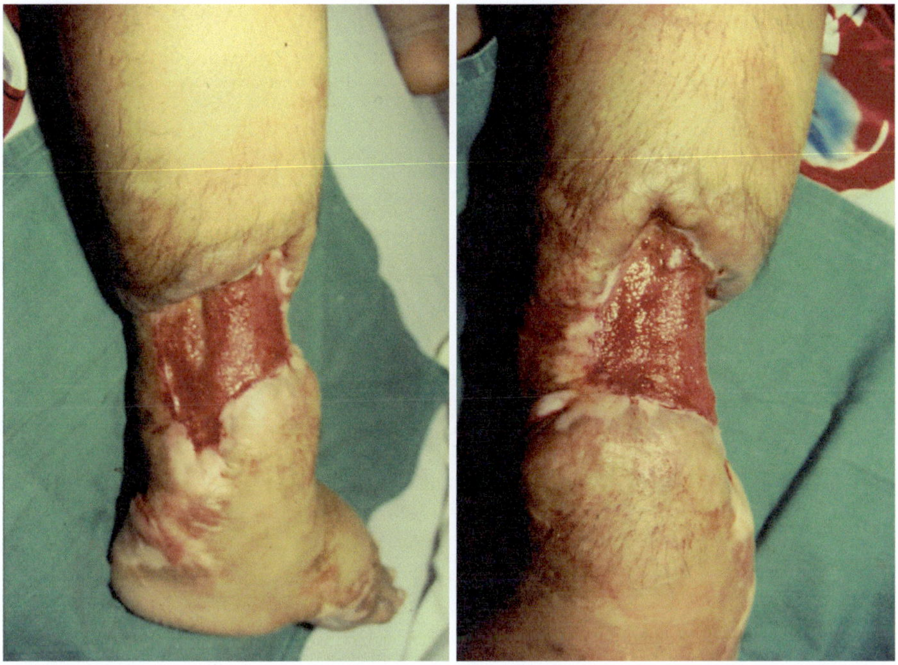

Figs. 10.3 and 10.4 Clinical photographs showing deep leg ulcers. Note the extent and depth of the ulcer

  - Unna boot for those with good granulation dressing and to decrease associated edema. The boot is changed once a week until healing occurs.
  - Compression stockings to decrease associated edema.
  - Zinc oxide impregnated gauze dressing.
  - Arginine butyrate. Arginine butyrate, a fatty acid that aids in the synthesis of fetal hemoglobin.
- The management of chronic resistant ulcers is challenging. This should involve hematologists, dermatologists, and plastic surgeons.
  - Transfusion therapy:
    - The goals of transfusion therapy are to transfuse packed RBCs at intervals to increase the Hb to around 10 g/dl, maintain the hematocrit between 30 and 35 vol percent, reduce the hemoglobin S to less than 30 %, and increase the percentage of Hb A at > 70 %.
    - This however is associated with a 20–30 % risk of alloimmunization.
  - Skin grafts are reserved for large or resistant ulcers.
  - Hydroxyurea:
    - The role of hydroxyurea in the management of leg ulcers is not clear, and so far there is no evidence to suggest that hydroxyurea speeds healing of leg ulcers in these patients.
    - There are also reports of hydroxyurea-induced leg ulcers.

Further Reading

Akinyanju O, Akinsete I. Leg ulceration in sickle cell disease in Nigeria. Trop Geogr Med. 1979;31:87–91.

Eckman JR. Leg ulcers in sickle cell disease. Hematol Oncol Clin North Am. 1996;10:1333–44.

Heckler FR, Dibbell DG, McCraw JB. Successful use of muscle flaps or myocutaneous flaps in patients with sickle cell disease. Plast Reconstr Surg. 1977;59:902–8.

Kersgard C, Osswald MB. Hydroxyurea and sickle cell leg ulcers. Am J Hematol. 2001;68:215–6.

Koshy M, Entsuah R, Koranda A. Leg ulcers in patients with sickle cell disease. Blood. 1989;74:1403–8.

Mack AK, Kato GJ. Sickle cell disease and nitric oxide: a paradigm shift? Int J Biochem Cell Biol. 2006;38:1237–43.

Richards RS, Bowen CVA, Glynn MFX. Microsurgical free flap transfer in sickle cell disease. Ann Plast Surg. 1992;29:278–81.

Serjeant GR, Serjeant BE, Mohan JS, Clare A. Leg ulceration in sickle cell disease: medieval medicine in a modern world. Hematol Oncol Clin North Am. 2005;19:943–56. viii–ix.

Sher GD, Olivieri NF. Rapid healing of chronic leg ulcers during arginine butyrate therapy in patients with sickle cell disease and thalassemia. Blood. 1994;84:2378–80.

Trent JT, Kirsner RS. Leg ulcers in sickle cell disease. Adv Skin Wound Care. 2004;17:410–6.

11 The Hand-Foot Syndrome in Patients with Sickle Cell Anemia

11.1 Introduction

- Sickle cell anemia is a chronic hemolytic anemia which can affect any part of the body including the musculoskeletal system.
- One of the skeletal manifestations of SCA is the hand-foot syndrome. This is also called dactylitis (Figs. 11.1 and 11.2).
- Dactylitis commonly occurs in patients with:
  - Homozygous hemoglobin S disease (sickle cell anemia)
  - Sickle cell-hemoglobin C disease
  - Sickle cell-beta-thalassemia
  - Extremely rare in those with sickle cell trait
- In 1941 Danford, Marr and Elsey reported the first case of dactylitis in a child with sickle cell anemia.
- Tori in 1954 described the radiological changes in dactylitis including destruction and a periosteal reaction in the metacarpals of both hands.
- Smith in 1953 used the term "hand-foot syndrome" to describe the acute swelling in the hands and feet of children with sickle cell anemia.
- The hand-foot syndrome is a relatively common complication of sickle cell anemia and has been reported to occur in 10–20 % of patients with sickle cell anemia
- The hand-foot syndrome commonly affects infants and children between 6 months and 3 years of age.
- It is extremely rare after the age of 5 years, and the reason for this is that hematopoiesis in the small bones of the hand and feet ceases at this age.
- The usual presentation is pain and soft tissue swelling of the dorsum of the hand and feet usually without erythema.
- It usually starts suddenly and it is a self-limiting condition and usually disappears in 1–2 weeks.
- The main differential diagnosis is osteomyelitis.

A. Al-Salem, *Medical and Surgical Complications of Sickle Cell Anemia*,
DOI 10.1007/978-3-319-24762-5_11

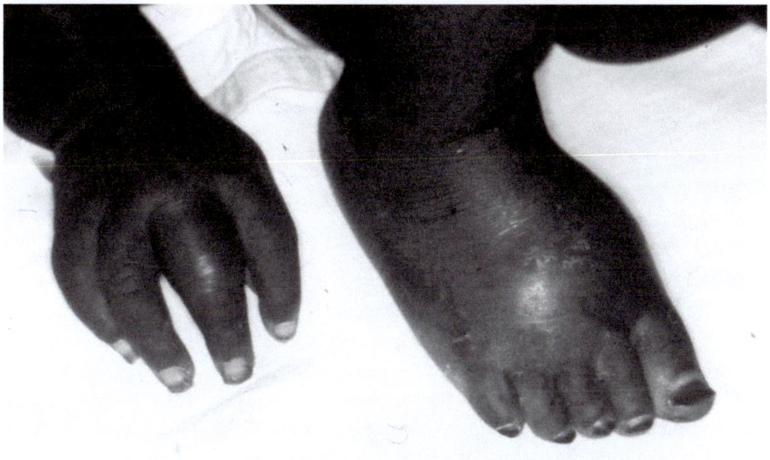

Fig. 11.1 A clinical photograph showing the hand-foot syndrome in a child with sickle cell anemia

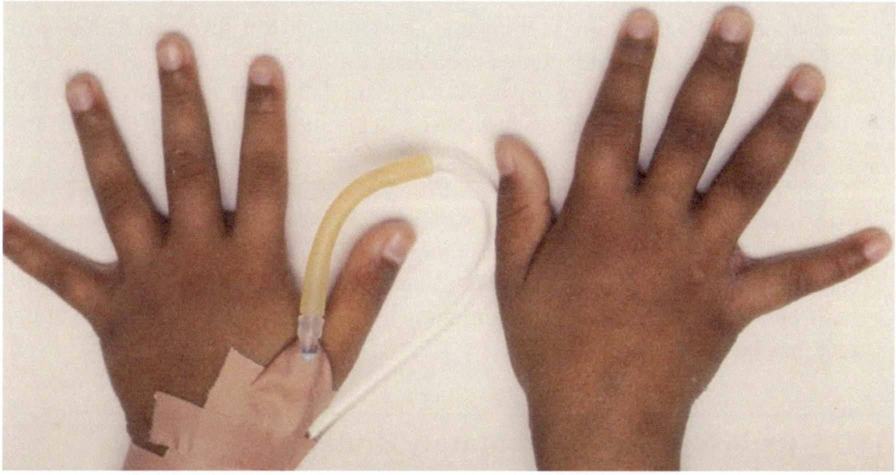

Fig. 11.2 A clinical photograph showing a mild attack of dactylitis involving the right hand. Note the slight swelling of the dorsum of the hand and phalanges when compared to the left hand

11.2 Etiology

- Dactylitis is thought to occur as a result of vaso-occlusive crises within the nutrient arteries of the metacarpals/metatarsals. This results in tender swelling of the digits of the hands and or feet.
- The sequelae of dactylitis include cortical bone thinning and destruction which becomes evident 3–6 weeks after vaso-occlusive crisis.

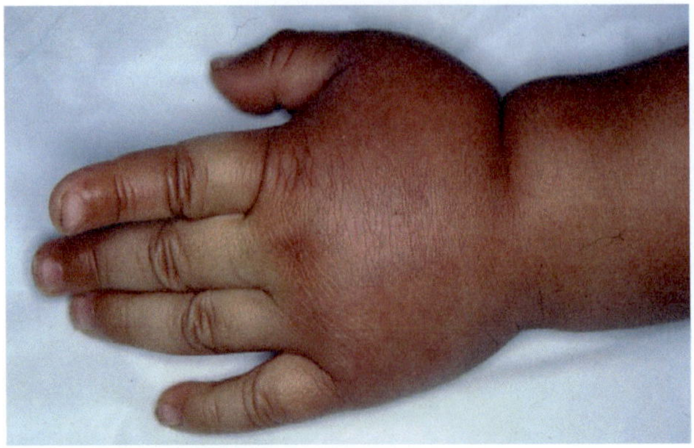

Fig. 11.3 A clinical photograph of *Salmonella* osteomyelitis of the hand in a child with sickle cell anemia. Note the swelling and redness of the dorsum of the hand

- It may be difficult to distinguish dactylitis from acute osteomyelitis, and this is the main differential diagnosis.
- The main differentiating points between the two are that:
  - Osteomyelitis is usually accompanied by leukocytosis, fever, erythema, positive blood cultures, and a lytic appearance on X-rays.
  - In dactylitis, the swelling usually involves all five digits symmetrically, while osteomyelitis usually affects a single digit, but the swelling may involve other digits (Fig. 11.3).
- It is important to note that patients with sickle cell anemia are prone to develop osteomyelitis due to *Salmonella typhimurium*, *Staphylococcus aureus*, and *Escherichia coli.* This must be kept in mind when evaluating children with sickle cell anemia and the hand-foot syndrome. *Salmonella* osteomyelitis affecting both hands simultaneously and simulating the hand-foot syndrome, although rare, has been reported also.

11.3 Radiological and Laboratory Findings

- Usually, there is no leukocytosis in patients with the hand-foot syndrome, and if leukocytosis is present it is part of a generalized vaso-occlusive crisis.
- The radiological changes appear late around 2–5 weeks after the onset of the swelling.
  - The earliest radiological change is the appearance of subperiosteal new bone in one or more of the metacarpal and metatarsal bones.
  - Cortical thinning.
  - Multiple irregular intramedullary deposits.
  - Areas of spot destruction and formation of periosteal new bone giving a moth-eaten appearance.
  - The bones of the hand and foot become rectangular in shape.

11.4 Management

- The hand-foot syndrome is a benign self-limiting condition seen in infants and young children with sickle cell anemia, usually at the time of a crisis.
- Treatment is conservative and supportive including:
  - Analgesics
  - Antibiotics
  - Folic acid
  - Intravenous hydration
  - Blood transfusion when necessary

Further Reading

Babhulkar SS, Pande K, Babhulkar S. The hand-foot syndrome in sickle-cell haemoglobinopathy. J Bone Joint Surg Br. 1995;77(2):310–2.

Bennett OM. Salmonella osteomyelitis and the hand-foot syndrome in sickle cell disease. J Pediatr Orthop. 1992;12(4):534–8.

Rosner F. Hand-foot syndrome in sickle cell disease. J Clin Oncol. 1998;16(2):808–9.

Acute Appendicitis and Sickle Cell Anemia

12

12.1 Introduction

- Patients with sickle cell anemia (SCA), often present with abdominal pain, which is usually attributable to SCA abdominal vaso-occlusive crisis, and based on this, conservative therapy is advocated in the majority of patients with SCA who present with acute abdominal pain.
- This however does not exclude the possibility of other common surgical conditions, namely, cholelithiasis, acute cholecystitis, peptic ulcer disease, and acute appendicitis which may be difficult to differentiate clinically from simple abdominal vaso-occlusive crisis.
- Acute appendicitis remains the most common cause of acute abdomen requiring emergency abdominal operation. This however may not be the case in patients with SCA, where acute appendicitis is reported not only to be rare but also has a rapid course with a high incidence of perforation (Fig. 12.1).
- Acute appendicitis in patients with SCA has been reported not only to be rare but also different.
- The reason for this low incidence of acute appendicitis in patients with SCA is not exactly known.
- Based on this and the risks associated with surgery and anesthesia, it is advocated to limit surgical exploration to those with clear evidence of potential surgical pathology or progressive findings during a period of observation.

12.2 Pathology

- The exact pathogenesis of acute appendicitis is not known, and inflammation is often said to be precipitated by obstruction, but in a large number of acutely inflamed appendices, there was no evidence of luminal obstruction.

A. Al-Salem, *Medical and Surgical Complications of Sickle Cell Anemia*,
DOI 10.1007/978-3-319-24762-5_12

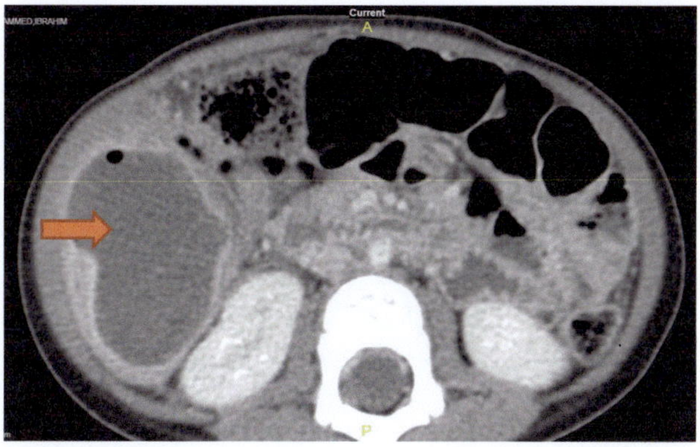

Fig. 12.1 Abdominal CT scan showing acute perforated appendicitis with abscess formation

- About 15–25 % of appendices removed from patients with suspected appendicitis appear normal on histologic examination.
- This however may not be the case always as new distinct pathological entities have now emerged in those with clinically suspected acute appendicitis but normally looking appendix at the time of surgery.
- These include neurogenic appendicopathy, a disease caused by proliferation of nerve fibers and hyperplasia of endocrine cells in the submucosa of the appendix, and pathological changes of the epithelium and lymphatic tissue of the appendix. This may explain the dramatic symptomatic relief following appendectomy in those with clinically diagnosed acute appendicitis but negative appendectomy.
- In patients with SCA, and because of difficulties in distinguishing painful abdominal vaso-occlusive crisis which is common from other surgical conditions, namely, acute appendicitis, it is expected to find a high rate of negative (normally looking appendix) appendectomy. This however is not the case.
- It was found that in the majority of SCA patients operated on for acute appendicitis had moderate to severe inflammation of the appendix with a high incidence of perforation. This was in spite of a short duration of symptoms (Fig. 12.2).
- Acute appendicitis in patients with SCA is not only rare but also tends to have a rapid course with a high incidence of perforation.
- Another interesting feature of acute appendicitis in patients with SCA is the histological absence of acute inflammatory cell infiltrate in some of these patients. This is seen sometimes in patients with clinically acute appendicitis and intraoperative finding of an enlarged, congested, and acutely inflamed appendix (Fig. 12.3).
- Histologically, however, the appendix in these patients will show no evidence of acute inflammatory cell infiltrate. The mucosa is intact, but there is an extensive transmural hemorrhage and the blood vessels are also congested and packed with sickled RBCs (Figs. 12.4, 12.5, and 12.6).
- These changes are attributed to SCA, and with further progression, there will be evidence of mucosal ulceration and acute inflammatory cell infiltrate.

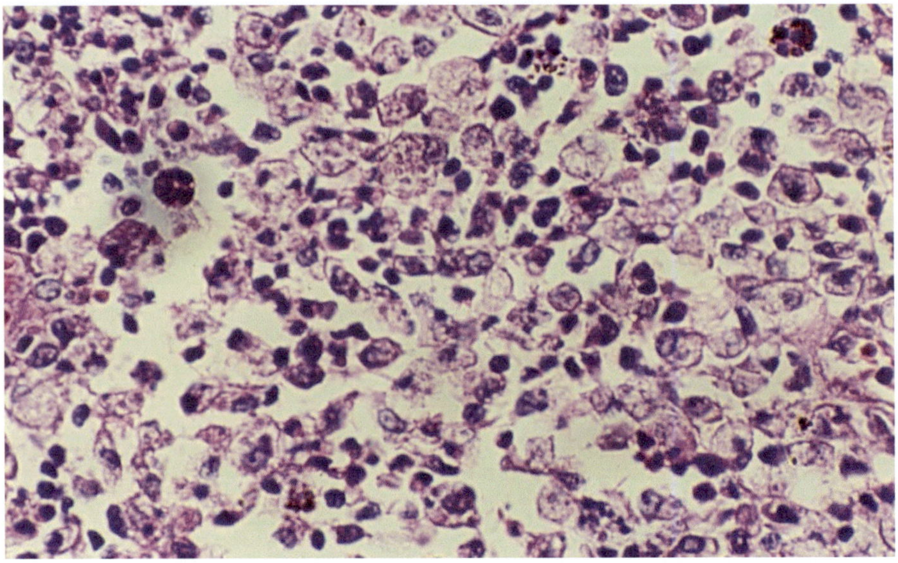

Fig. 12.2 A histological picture showing severe acute inflammatory cell infiltrate in a patient with SCA and acute appendicitis

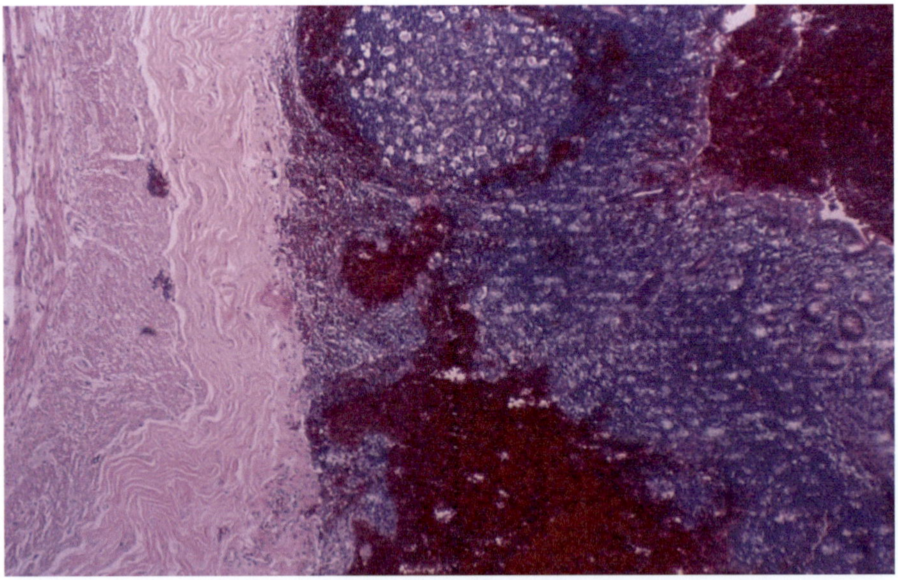

Fig. 12.3 A histological picture showing intact mucosa with severe congestion and hemorrhage of the appendix in a patient with SCA and acute appendicitis

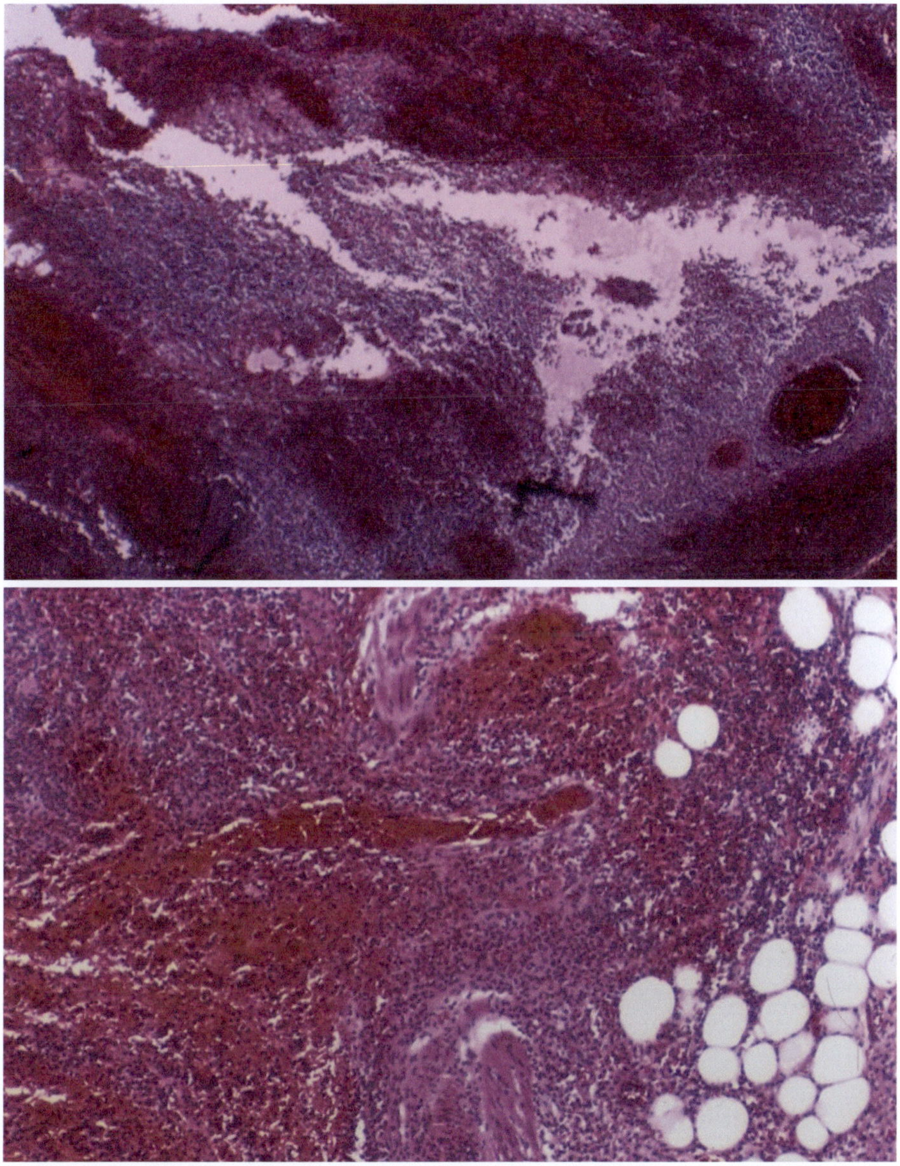

Figs. 12.4 and 12.5 Histological pictures showing sever hemorrhage and congestion of the appendix with inflammatory cell infiltrate in a patient with SCA and acute appendicitis

- In the majority of patients with SCA, there is moderate to severe mucosal ulceration, changes in blood vessels which are packed with sickled RBCs, and high incidence of perforation in spite of short duration of symptoms, as complicated appendicitis is primarily associated with a longer delay before first medical consultation.

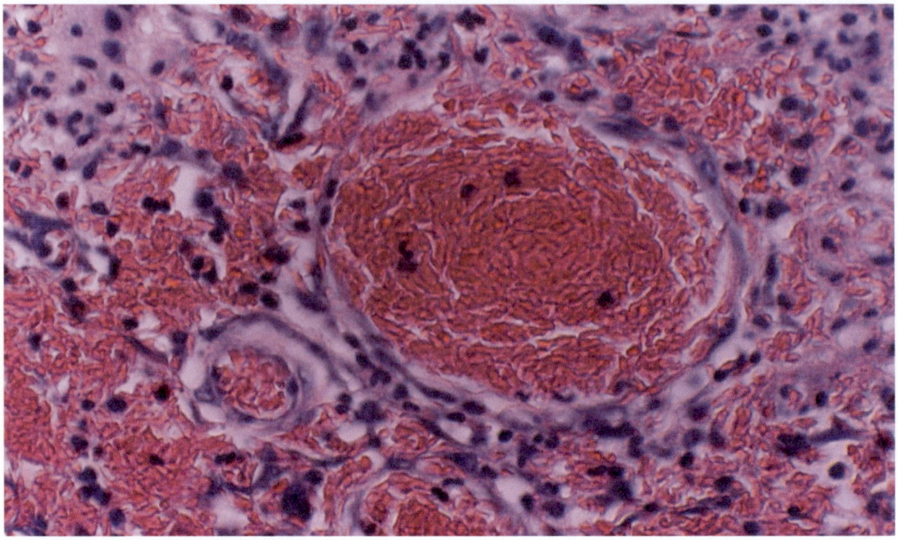

Fig. 12.6 Histological picture showing appendicular vessels packed with sickled RBCs in a patient with acute appendicitis and sickle cell anemia

- Acute appendicitis in patients with SCA is rare and it occurs following blockage of appendiceal blood vessels by sickled RBCs leading to congestion, edema, and ischemia with mucosal ulceration and subsequently a marked inflammatory cell infiltrate.
- Acute appendicitis in patients with SCA has a rapid progressive course with a high incidence of perforation.
- This calls for early and close observation of patients with SCA who present with acute abdominal pain. These patients should be evaluated early and in doubtful cases, abdominal ultrasound, or CT scan should be ordered. Surgical intervention should not be delayed in those with suspected acute appendicitis whether via the open or laparoscopic approach.

Further Reading

Al-Nazer M, Al-Saeed H, Al-Salem AH. Acute appendicitis in patients with Sickle cell disease. Saudi Med J. 2003;24(9):974–7.

Al-Salem AH, Qureshi ZS, Qaisarudin S, Varma KK. Is acute appendicitis different in patients with sickle cell disease? Pediatr Surg Int. 1998;13:265–7.

Antal P, Gauderer M, Koshy M, Berman B. Is the incidence of appendicitis reduced in patients with sickle cell disease? Pediatrics. 1998;101:E7.

Bandio WA. Clinical features of abdominal painful crisis in sickle cell anemia. J Pediatr Surg. 1990;25:301–2.

Ophthalmologic Manifestations of Sickle Cell Anemia

13

13.1 Introduction

- The pathophysiology of sickle cell anemia is basically related to abnormalities of RBCs leading to sickling, aggregation of sickled RBCs, and blockage of terminal arterioles, but other factors play an important role as well including:
- Endothelial activation
- Inflammation
- Nitric oxide bioavailability
- Oxidative stress
- Regulation of the adhesiveness of several types of blood cells including platelets and WBC
- Blockage of blood flow in the terminal arterioles by sickled RBCs will lead to sluggish blood flow, tissue hypoxia, and acidosis. This causes further sickling, increased blood viscosity, and decreased blood flow.
- All of these factors are important in the pathogenesis of ophthalmic manifestation of sickle cell anemia.
- The exact frequency of sickle cell-related complications is not known but visual abnormalities in any stage of life of a patient with sickle cell anemia is reported to be 10–20 %.
- The frequency of sickle cell retinopathy is greatest in adulthood, but retinopathy has also been described in children.
- A meticulous eye examination is necessary in these patients to detect the early changes of sickle cell anemia.
- This ophthalmic assessment should be periodic and include:
  - Measurement of visual acuity
  - Measurement of intraocular pressure
  - Evaluation of the anterior/posterior segment structures by fluorescein angiography

A. Al-Salem, *Medical and Surgical Complications of Sickle Cell Anemia*,
DOI 10.1007/978-3-319-24762-5_13

- Ophthalmic manifestation of sickle cell anemia can affect the:
  - Orbit
  - Conjunctiva
  - Iris
  - Uvea
  - Papillary and retinal changes
- The most relevant anterior segment abnormalities are:
  - The conjunctival sign
  - Iris atrophy
  - Hyphema
- The retinal manifestations of sickle cell anemia can be:
  - Nonproliferative
  - Proliferative
- The proliferative changes are more serious and associated with a real risk of ocular morbidity.
- Nonproliferative retinopathy includes venous tortuosity which is nonspecific, but it is seen in about 50 % of patients with SCA.
- The ocular manifestations of sickle cell anemia result from vascular occlusion. Sickle cell vaso-occlusive events can affect every vascular bed in the eye and may occur in the conjunctiva, iris, retina, and choroid.
- These changes are however not unique to sickle cell anemia and can be seen with other diseases such as diabetes mellitus, central retinal artery or vein thrombosis, familial exudative vitreoretinopathy, polycythemia vera, and uveitis.
- Angioid streaks:
  - Angioid streaks occur in association with sickle cell anemia, with an overall incidence of less than 6 %.
  - The changes are age dependent, occurring in 2 % of sickle cell anemia patients less than 40 years of age versus 22 % in those who are more than 40 years of age.
- Epiretinal membranes:
  - Epiretinal membranes may produce visual loss in patients with sickle cell anemia.
  - Macular epiretinal membranes are seen more frequently in those with retinal neovascularization, retinal tears, and vitreous hemorrhage, as well as those that have had laser treatment or surgery of the retina or vitreous.
  - Progressive visual loss from macular distortion is well known seen in up to 30 % of these patients.
  - Peripheral neovascularization may stimulate formation of epiretinal membranes by transudation of plasma and RBCs into the vitreous, disrupting the vitreous cortex and inducing posterior vitreous detachment.
  - Successful treatment of the neovascular tissue reduces the risk of epiretinal membrane development by approximately 30 %.
  - Although spontaneous separation of epiretinal membranes following treatment of peripheral neovascularization has been observed, surgical removal may be considered when patients exhibit moderate to severe visual loss.
  - Traction across the macula from peripheral neovascularization is thought to contribute to the formation of macular holes in sickle cell retinopathy.

- Conjunctival sickle sign:
  - Abnormalities of the bulbar conjunctival blood vessels are believed to be the result of flow obstruction by sickled cells.
  - These abnormalities include:
    - Linear dilatations, interrupted, dilated, and truncated vascular segments
- Iris atrophy and neovascularization:
  - Occlusions of the iris vessels can result in atrophy, and patients may present with asymptomatic white patches of the iris.
  - Iris neovascularization may develop in eyes with chronic retinal detachment or major arteriole occlusions and can in rare cases cause a secondary neovascular glaucoma.
- Hyphema:
  - Sickle cell patients are susceptible to develop central retinal artery occlusions and optic atrophy secondary to elevated intraocular pressure.
- Retinal artery occlusions:
  - Occlusions of the central retinal artery and major arteriolar branches are seen most frequent in young patients with sickle cell anemia.
  - They may cause permanent or transient visual loss and can occur simultaneously in both eyes.
  - Arterial occlusion has also been reported to occur as a complication of retrobulbar anesthesia and following compression of the eye during photocoagulation.
- Retinal venous occlusions:
  - Retinal venous occlusions are surprisingly uncommon in patients with sickle cell anemia.
  - The reason for this is not known but anemia and low blood pressure present in sickle cell patients may be protective against venous occlusions.
  - An underlying systemic disease associated with a higher incidence of venous occlusions (e.g., hypertension) should be suspected when a venous occlusion occurs in a patient with sickle cell anemia.
- Macular small vessel occlusions:
  - Occlusions of the fine vasculature of the macular and perimacular area have been reported in 10–40 % of patients with sickle cell anemia.
  - In the acute phase, the occluded vessel will have a dark red appearance and may appear as a dark line on fluorescein angiography.
  - Nerve fiber layer infarcts (cotton-wool spots) are also seen.
  - Other macular and perimacular changes include:
    - Microaneurysm-like dots
    - Dark and enlarged segments of arterioles
    - Hairpin-shaped venular loops
    - Pathologic avascular zones
    - Widening and irregularities of the foveal avascular zone
  - Careful examination by fluorescein angiograph, is often necessary to identify these macular changes.
  - These changes may be transient, and the macula may appear normal on subsequent fluorescein angiograms.

  - A loss of the inner retinal layers results in an ophthalmoscopic focal concavity with an abnormal reflex (retinal depression sign). These changes are usually permanent.
  - The retinal depression sign is not pathognomonic of sickle cell anemia and may be seen with other arteriolar occlusive diseases, such as embolic retinopathy, vasculitis, and hypertension.
- Macular function tests in sickle cell anemia:
  - The visual acuity in patients with sickle cell anemia is often normal, despite the presence of an enlarged foveal avascular zone or other evidence of sickle cell maculopathy.
  - In addition, patients with sickle cell maculopathy have a remarkable absence of visual complaints.
  - Automated visual field analysis has demonstrated significantly larger scotomas in patients with abnormally enlarged foveal avascular zone.
  - Color vision testing has revealed a greater incidence of blue-yellow defects in patients with sickle cell retinopathy; however, no significant correlation has been demonstrated between color vision defects and the presence of sickle cell maculopathy.
- Choroidal vascular occlusions:
  - Choroidal vascular occlusions may occur focally at the level of the choroidal precapillary arteriole or capillary bed (Elschnig's spots) or from posterior ciliary artery occlusion.
  - Although focal precapillary arteriole occlusions have not been specifically identified in patients with sickle cell anemia, clinical and histopathologic evidence of spontaneous posterior ciliary artery occlusions have been reported in sickle cell anemia.
  - The findings are similar to those described following compression of the eye during general anesthesia and after peripheral photocoagulation.
  - In the acute phase, the occlusions appear as white, circumscribed, triangular patches at the level of the retinal pigment epithelium and outer retina.
  - Subsequently, the white lesions fade and retinal pigment epithelial mottling develops.
  - Patients with acute ciliary artery occlusions may be asymptomatic and the diagnosis is often based solely on the appearance of peripheral pigment mottling.
  - In sickle cell anemia, it has been suggested that choroidal ischemia plays a role in the development of angioid streaks.
- Retinal hemorrhages, iridescent spots, and black sunbursts:
  - When an arteriole of intermediate size is occluded by sickled erythrocytes, hemorrhage may occur.
  - The hemorrhages typically appear adjacent or distal to an intraluminal obstruction. It is likely that ischemic necrosis causes a weakening of the vessel wall and that reperfusion of the vessel causes a rupture of the damaged vessel wall, resulting in a hemorrhage.

- This type of hemorrhage is round or oval shaped and bright red and measures 1/4–1 disk diameter.
- Retinal hemorrhages ("salmon patches"), found most commonly in the equatorial periphery.
- These hemorrhages are bright red, but after several days, the partially degenerated blood acquires a characteristic orange-red color (hence the name salmon patch).
- In most cases, these hemorrhages are asymptomatic.
- The majority of these hemorrhages remain confined to the sensory retina; however, blood may leak through the internal limiting membrane into the vitreous or dissect deeper into the subretinal space.
- Resolution occurs over days to weeks and may result in a focal area of atrophic split retina (a "schisis" cavity), a pigmented retinal scar, or a grayish-white vitreous deposit, depending on the location of the hemorrhage. The blood is slowly cleared by macrophages.
- Over time, hemoglobin degradation occurs. The hemorrhagic defect then appears as bright yellow dots at several levels of the sensory retina; these are known as iridescent bodies.
- If the hemorrhage occurs in the outer retinal layers, it appear as dark, oval or round, 1/4–2 disk-diameter chorioretinal lesions. These lesions, which are similar in appearance to chorioretinitis scars, are known as black sunbursts.
- The hemorrhages are temporary, and those that occur in the posterior part of the eye are difficult to diagnose. Their late signs, such as iridescent bodies and black sunbursts, can be observed in approximately 25–40 % of cases and are seen more frequent in SCA.
- Intraretinal blood breakdown products, either extracellular or within macrophages, may appear as refractile copper-colored granules ("iridescent spots"). Macular iridescent schisis lesions have not been described clinically, but they have been observed on histologic examination.
- The occluded vessels may reopen, and the capillary network in the area of a schisis cavity may appear normal; however, more commonly, the vessels will remain closed. In rare cases, an area of retinal neovascularization may be found within a schisis cavity.
- Black pigmented spiculate or stellate chorioretinal lesions ("black sunbursts") are typically found around or anterior to the equator and adjacent to an arteriole.
- Occasionally, a pigmented lesion may be seen trailing from an arteriole or as a cuff of pigment overlying the vessel. Additionally, the overlying arteriole may be occluded.
- Refractile deposits are often seen interspersed with the pigment.
- Black sunbursts are believed to be due to deep retinal blood stimulating pigment epithelial migration, hyperplasia, and hypertrophy.
- Histopathologic findings support this hypothesis, and the development of black sunbursts has been documented in an area of previous intraretinal and subretinal hemorrhage.
- An alternative explanation for black sunbursts is the occurrence of choroidal ischemia and aborted choroidal neovascularization.

- Dark- and white-without-pressure fundus lesions:
  - Flat, geographic dark brown areas have been identified in the posterior pole or midperiphery of the retina in patients with sickle cell anemia without any signs of a previous hemorrhage or definite evidence of retinal or choroidal vascular occlusion.
  - These dark-without-pressure lesions are transient, changing shape or disappearing over weeks to months.
  - Areas of white-without-pressure, which are possibly secondary to condensation of the overlying basal vitreous, also have been described.
- Peripheral retinal manifestations:
  - The peripheral retinal capillary network thins to a single layer approximately 1 mm from the ora serrata.
  - A similar thinning of the retinal capillary network occurs around the foveal avascular zone.
  - These two areas appear to be the most susceptible to vascular occlusions from sickle cell retinopathy.
  - Peripheral vascular occlusions are seen more frequently on the temporal side, tend to be more rapidly progressive in children and adolescents than in adults, and are significantly more common in sickle cell anemia.
  - Redirection of blood flow results in the formation of arteriolar-venular anastomosis at the border of the perfused and nonperfused peripheral retina.
- The ophthalmic changes are also divided according to the site.
- Posterior segment abnormalities:
- The abnormalities of the posterior segment can be divided into six categories, as follows:
  - Optic disk changes
  - Posterior retinal and macular vascular occlusion
  - Chronic macular changes (sickling maculopathy)
  - Choroidal vascular occlusions
  - Nonproliferative retinal changes
  - Proliferative retinal changes
- Optic disk changes:
  - They result from intravascular occlusions on the surface of the optic disk.
  - Vascular changes in the optic nerve are transient and consist of dark, small and red dilated capillaries that show occlusion in fluorescein angiography, without any impact on visual acuity.
  - Transient dark red spots, representing plugs of sickled erythrocytes within superficial capillaries, may be seen on the surface of the optic disk.
  - These disk changes are found in 30 % of all patients with sickle cell anemia and include dilated loops and multiple comma-shaped vascular segments.
  - They appear as dark red intravascular spots.
  - These changes are usually transient and do not produce any clinical impairment.
- Posterior retinal and macular vascular occlusions:
  - Retinal artery occlusions are either central or involve only a branch.
  - These are rare.

- Retinal vein occlusions also are rare in patients with SCA.
- Dilation and tortuosity of the retinal veins was one of the first recognized abnormalities of sickle cell eye disease seen in up to 47 % of patients with sickle cell anemia.

• Chronic macular changes:
  - Chronic macular vascular occlusions occur in SCA.
  - These are manifested by microaneurysms resembling dots, hairpin-shaped vascular loops, and abnormal foveal avascular zone.
  - Sickle cell maculopathy occurs as a result of chronic changes in the perifoveal capillary network.
  - It may be present in 10–40 % of sickle cell anemia patients.
  - Another finding in sickle cell maculopathy is the formation of microaneurysm-like dots and vascular loops.
  - Ischemic macular changes associated with sickle hemoglobinopathy are due to the occlusion of arteriolar circulation around the foveal avascular zone and branches that supply the temporal horizontal raphe. The end result is macular infarction.
  - Angioid streaks are seen in about 1–2 % of patients with SCA.
  - Occlusion of the central retinal artery may rarely occur in patients with SCA.
• Choroidal vascular occlusions:
  - This is an extremely rare manifestation of SCA.
• Nonproliferative retinal changes:
  - Nonproliferative or background sickle retinopathy includes the following manifestations:
    • Venous tortuosity
    • Salmon-patch hemorrhage
    • Schisis cavity
    • The black sunburst
  - Venous tortuosity probably is due to arteriovenous shunting from the retinal periphery.
  - Salmon-patch hemorrhages are superficial intraretinal hemorrhages. They are usually seen in the mid periphery of the retina adjacent to a retinal arteriole.
  - The schisis cavity is a space caused by the disappearance of the intraretinal hemorrhage.
  - Nonproliferative sickle retinopathy features iridescent spots and glistening refractive bodies in the schisis cavity.
  - The black sunburst consists of round chorioretinal scars usually located in the equatorial fundus. These lesions result from pigment accumulated around the vessels. They do not cause any visual symptoms.
• Proliferative retinopathy:
  - This is the primary cause of visual acuity reduction in patients with SCA.
  - Proliferative sickle retinopathy is the most severe ocular change in patients with SCA.
  - The exact incidence of proliferative retinopathy is not known but it is estimated to be 0.5 cases/year per 100 patients with sickle cell anemia.

- Proliferative retinopathy remains asymptomatic and the changes are slow until complications such as vitreous hemorrhage or retinal detachment occur.
- This is typically seen in those 20–30 years of age.
- In 20–60 % of patients with proliferative retinopathy, there is spontaneous regression of the neovascular complexes.
- The peripheral retina, especially the temporal portion, is characterized by very thin vascular channels with small diameter which makes them highly susceptible to the effects of intravascular sickling and subsequent occlusion.
- The occluded segment can display a "silver wire" appearance, but the ischemic phenomenon and the degree of perfusion are more easily observed by fluorescein angiography.
- It was estimated that vitreous hemorrhage occurs in approximately 5 % of proliferative retinopathy cases which contribute to the development of retinal detachment (traction retinoschisis).
- The association between retinal atrophy (post-ischemic) and vitreous traction can lead to the formation of retinal tears. These are typically followed by retinal detachment.
- Goldberg in 1971 classified proliferative sickle cell retinopathy into the following five stages:
  1. Peripheral arteriolar occlusions
  2. Arteriolar-venular anastomosis
  3. Neovascular proliferation
  4. Vitreous hemorrhage
  5. Retinal detachment
- Stage I is characterized by occlusion of the peripheral arteriolar vessels. They appear as dark-red lines, but eventually they turn into silver-wire-appearing vessels.
- Stage II is characterized by peripheral arteriolar-venular anastomosis, and peripheral to these anastomoses, no perfusion is present.
- Stage III is characterized by new vessel formation at the junction of the vascular and avascular retina. These neovascular tufts resemble sea fans.
- Stage IV and V: Subsequently, the sea fan grows in size and may acquire a glial and fibrotic tissue envelope. This envelope may pull on the vitreous leading to vitreous hemorrhage, and retinal detachment may occur.

Classification of Proliferative Sickle Retinopathy (Goldberg 1971)

Stage	Peripheral retinal findings
I	Peripheral arteriolar occlusions
II	Peripheral arteriolar-venular anastomosis
III	Neovascular and fibrous proliferation
IV	Vitreous hemorrhage
V	Retinal detachment

- This classification was modified by Penman et al. in 1994.

New Classification of Sickle Retinopathy (Penman et al. 1994)

Stage	Peripheral retinal vascular pattern
I	Qualitatively normal; continuous arteriolar-venular loops with thinned capillary bed
II	Qualitatively abnormal
A	Capillary stumps extending into nonperfused retina
B	Irregular capillary border without arteriolar-venular loops or capillary stumps
III	Indeterminant

- Anterior segment abnormalities:
  - Anterior segment abnormalities include the following:
    - Segmentation "corkscrew" conjunctival vessels: Best observed in the inferior bulbar conjunctiva
    - Iris infarct and atrophy
    - Cataracts
    - Phthisis bulbi
    - Hyphema

13.2 Management

- Therapeutic intervention is not indicated for the peripheral manifestations of stage I or stage II sickle cell retinopathy.
- There is no proven benefit in treating these stages, nor is there any way at present to predict which patients will progress to the proliferative stage.
- For patients with sickle cell anemia, frequent examinations of the peripheral retina with periodic fluorescein angiography are indicated in an effort to identify neovascular tissue in the early stages of evolution.
- Treatment of vascular occlusions of the posterior pole should focus on promoting increased blood flow and preventing further sickling.
- Hyperbaric oxygen increases inner retinal oxygen levels and could potentially prove useful in treating retinal vascular occlusions associated with sickle cell anemia.
- Exchange transfusions have been used, but the true benefit of this is not well established because the natural history of these occlusions is not well documented.
- In view of the potential complications of exchange blood transfusion and variable outcome, routine use of exchange blood transfusions for retinal vascular occlusions in sickle cell anemia is not recommended.

- The aim of treatment should be directed toward preventing vision loss from:
  - Vitreous hemorrhage
  - Retinal detachment
  - Epiretinal membranes
- Carbonic anhydrase inhibitors should be avoided because they may cause further sickling and worsen the outflow obstruction.
- If the intraocular pressure remains elevated after a trial of medical therapy, surgical intervention with an anterior chamber lavage is indicated.
- Modalities to treat proliferative sickle retinopathy include:
  - Diathermy
  - Cryotherapy
  - Xenon arc photocoagulation
  - Argon laser photocoagulation
    - Various modalities have been utilized, including diathermy, cryotherapy, xenon arc photocoagulation, and various techniques of laser photocoagulation, such as feeder vessel, local scatter, and peripheral circumferential scatter. Laser photocoagulation is the treatment modality most commonly used.
    - Patients with recent vitreous hemorrhage and visual acuity impairment are usually followed for at least six months to allow spontaneous clearing.
    - Photocoagulation or cryotherapy can be performed when the visibility permits it.
    - Sickling in the anterior chamber can result in elevated intraocular pressure due to blockage of the trabecular meshwork. Blood in the anterior chamber in patients with sickle cell disease is a medical emergency.
    - Patients with sickle cell anemia are prone to central retinal artery occlusion and optic atrophy. Close monitoring of the intraocular pressure is warranted in these patients.
    - Vitreous hemorrhage is treated conservatively for about 6 months hoping for reabsorption, and if this fails it is treated with laser or cryotherapy. This however is associated with the risk of retinal detachment and secondary glaucoma.
    - Pars plana vitrectomy is considered when the vitreous hemorrhage is massive and long-standing or in those who developed retinal detachment or glaucoma as complications.

13.3 Perioperative Management

- These patients must be prepared for surgery.
- Exchange blood transfusion or erythrocytapheresis is performed 48–72 h prior to surgery. The aim should be to reduce HbS level to 40–50 % and to achieve a final hematocrit of no higher than 35–39 % to prevent elevated whole-blood viscosity. Other benefits of partial exchange transfusions are enhancement of perfusion and oxygen delivery and minimization of intraoperative and early postoperative sickling. This proved to reduce postoperative complications in these patients.

- The use of supplemental oxygen.
- Local anesthesia should be used whenever possible.
- Phenylephrine drops to dilate the pupils should be avoided as they cause vasoconstriction.
- It is important to decrease the intraocular pressure.
- The following are additional ways to reduce potential complications, particularly anterior segment ischemia:
  - Use no sympathomimetics with local anesthesia.
  - Use topical sympathomimetics minimally.
  - Use supplemental 100 % oxygen for 48 h after surgery.
  - Avoid excessive manipulation of extraocular muscles.
  - Use transscleral diathermy or cryotherapy minimally and avoid the long ciliary arteries.
  - Avoid the use of wide encircling scleral buckling elements.
  - Limit the use of expansile concentrations of intraocular gases.
  - Utilize internal drainage of subretinal fluid.
  - Close monitoring and treating elevated intraocular pressure.
  - Avoid the use of carbonic anhydrase inhibitors.

Further Reading

Downes SM, Hambleton IR, Chuang EL, Lois N, Serjeant GR, Bird AC. Incidence and natural history of proliferative sickle cell retinopathy: observations from a cohort study. Ophthalmology. 2005;112(11):1869–75.

Elagouz M, Jyothi S, Gupta B, Sivaprasad S. Sickle cell disease and the eye: old and new concepts. Surv Ophthalmol. 2010;55(4):359–77.

Emerson GG, Lutty GA. Effects of sickle cell disease on the eye: clinical features and treatment. Hematol Oncol Clin North Am. 2005;19(5):957–73, ix.

Fine LC, Petrovic V, Irvine AR, Bhisitkul RB. Spontaneous central retinal artery occlusion in hemoglobin sickle cell disease. Am J Ophthalmol. 2000;129(5):680–1.

Fox PD, Dunn DT, Morris JS, Serjeant GR. Risk factors for proliferative sickle retinopathy. Br J Ophthalmol. 1990a;74:172.

Fox PD, Dunn DT, Morris JS, Serjeant GR. Risk factors for proliferative sickle retinopathy. Br J Ophthalmol. 1990b;74(3):172–6.

Fox PD, Acheson RW, Serjeant GR. Outcome of iatrogenic choroidal neovascularisation in sickle cell disease. Br J Ophthalmol. 1990c;74(7):417–20.

Gill HS, Lam WC. A screening strategy for the detection of sickle cell retinopathy in pediatric patients. Can J Ophthalmol. 2008;43(2):188–91.

Leen JS, Ratnakaram R, Del Priore LV, Bhagat N, Zarbin MA. Anterior segment ischemia after vitrectomy in sickle cell disease. Retina. 2002;22(2):216–9.

Liem RI, Calamaras DM, Chhabra MS, Files B, Minniti CP, Thompson AA. Sudden-onset blindness in sickle cell disease due to retinal artery occlusion. Pediatr Blood Cancer. 2008;50(3):624–7.

Penman AD, Talbot JF, Chuang EL, Thomas P, Serjeant GR, Bird AC. New classification of peripheral retinal vascular changes in sickle cell disease. Br J Ophthalmol. 1994;78(9):681–9.

Sokol JA, Baron E, Lantos G, Kazim M. Orbital compression syndrome in sickle cell disease. Ophthal Plast Reconstr Surg. 2008;24(3):181–4.

Cardiovascular Complications of Sickle Cell Anemia

14

14.1 Introduction

- Sickle cell anemia is an autosomal recessive disorder that results from a change of a single amino acid in the beta chain of hemoglobin.
- In sickle cell anemia, the amino acid glutamic acid at the 6th position of the 146 amino acids of the beta chain of hemoglobin is replaced by valine.
- Although this single change of one amino acid is the underlying defect of sickle cell anemia, it does not explain the heterogeneity of SCA that is observed clinically.
- In the recent years, two sub-phenotypes of SCA have been described.
  - The "viscosity-vaso-occlusion" sub-phenotype. This is responsible for the erythrocyte sickling related complications such as:
    - Painful vaso-occlusive crisis
    - Acute chest syndrome
    - Avascular necrosis
  - The "hemolysis-endothelial dysfunction" sub-phenotype. This is responsible for the sickle cell anemia vasculopathy that involves:
    - Pulmonary hypertension
    - Priapism
    - Leg ulcers
    - Sudden death
    - Stroke
    - Asthma
  - In the clinical setting, there may be an overlap between these two sub-types.
  - This, however, is of clinical and therapeutic importance and may help when considering therapies for a specific sub-phenotype.
- The pathophysiology of sickle cell anemia is complex, and several factors may play a role.

A. Al-Salem, *Medical and Surgical Complications of Sickle Cell Anemia*,
DOI 10.1007/978-3-319-24762-5_14

- Recently, it was shown that dysfunction of the vascular endothelium in these patients plays a major role in the pathophysiology of sickle cell anemia, and impaired nitric oxide (NO) bioavailability represents the central feature of endothelial dysfunction.
- NO is an endogenous vasodilator.
- It is synthesized by endothelial cells from L-arginine, which is converted to citrulline by the NO synthases enzymes.
- It is well known that NO generated by healthy endothelial cells has several functions:
  - Vasorelaxant
  - Anti-inflammatory
  - Antithrombotic
- Deficiency of NO in patients with SCA is an important factor in the pathogenesis of SCA vasculopathy.
- Decreased NO bioavailability has several adverse effects including:
  - Endothelial cell activation
  - Upregulation of the potent vasoconstrictor endothelin-1
  - Vasoconstriction
  - Platelet activation
  - Increased tissue factor
  - Activation of coagulation
- All of these contribute to the clinical manifestations seen in patients with sickle cell anemia.
- Pathophysiology of sickle cell vasculopathy:
  - Normally, the hemoglobin is stored in the red blood cells, but when hemolysis occurs, it is released into the plasma where it rapidly reacts with and destroys NO.
  - It is the heme part of the hemoglobin that reacts with NO leading to its consumption.
  - Add to this the NO scavenging by vascular superoxide anion.
  - NO consumption and the formation of reactive oxygen species ultimately inhibit vasodilatation.
  - Red blood cell hemolysis will also lead to the simultaneous release of erythrocyte arginase.
  - This will limit the availability of arginine to NO synthase to form NO, contributing also to the deficiency of NO.
  - Arginase will redirect the metabolism of arginine away from NO to ornithine and the formation of polyamines and proline, which are essential for smooth muscle cell growth and collagen synthesis.

- With the shift away from NO toward ornithine metabolism, arginase contributes to the proliferative vasculopathy common to sickle cell anemia, pulmonary hypertension, and cardiovascular disease.
- The levels of asymmetric dimethylarginine (an arginine analog) are also elevated in SCA, associated with hemolysis, pulmonary hypertension, and mortality, and will also affect the overall global arginine bioavailability.
- Low arginine bioavailability may further compromise NO generation due to NO synthase uncoupling.
- NO inhibits platelet activation, tissue factor expression, and thrombin generation, and intravascular hemolysis has the potential to drive a procoagulant state in these patients.
- Hemolysis in patients with SCA leads to deficiency of NO for the following reasons:
  • NO scavenging by the heme of sickle hemoglobin released into the plasma by the hemolyzed RBCs
  • NO scavenging by vascular superoxide anion
  • Depletion of plasma arginine by arginase released by lysed RBCs
  • Endogenous NO synthesis inhibitors
  • Inactivation of tetrahydrobiopterin, a NO cofactor leading to the production of superoxide anion rather than NO

14.2 Pulmonary Artery Hypertension (PAH)

• The normal pulmonary artery pressure is 15 mmHg.
• PAH is defined as mean pulmonary artery pressure > 25 mmHg at rest or > 30 mmHg during exercise.
• There are several causes for pulmonary artery hypertension which include primary and secondary causes.
• The exact cause of primary PAH is not known.
• Secondary PAH can be caused by several conditions including:
  - Chronic lung disease and heart disease
  - Collagen vascular disease
  - Thromboembolism
  - HIV
  - Liver cirrhosis
  - Anorexic agents
  - Sickle cell anemia

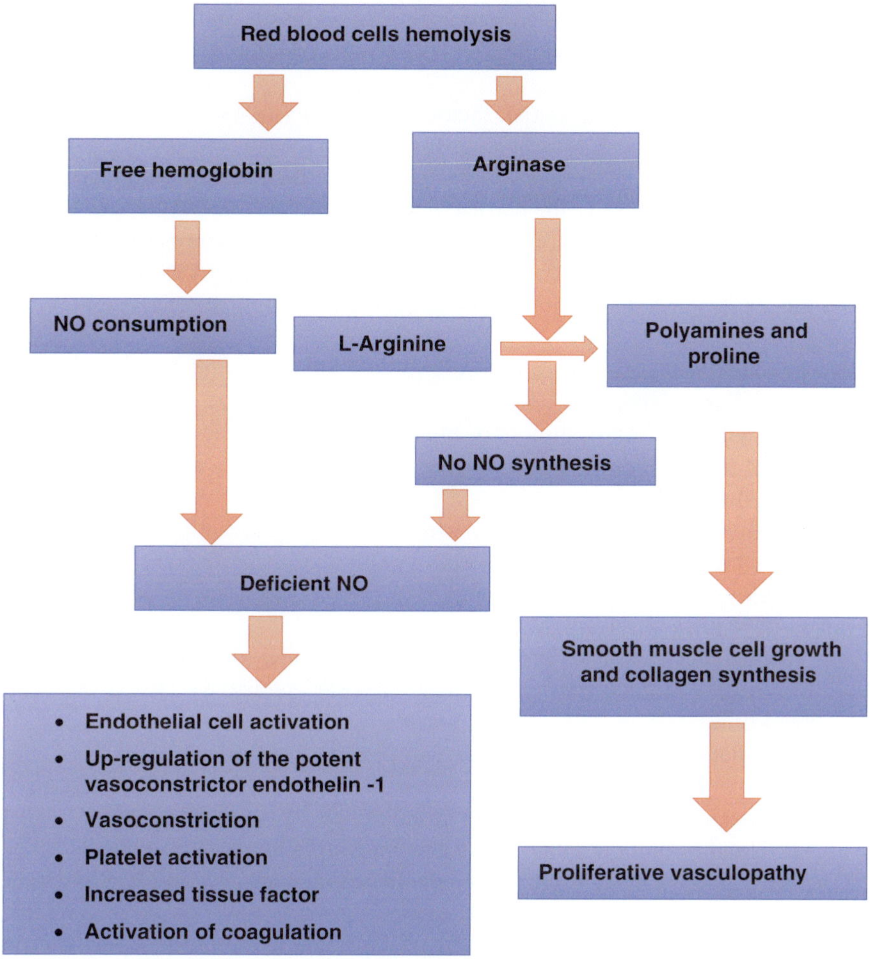

14.3 Pathophysiology of PAH

- Intravascular hemolysis leading to NO deficiency is considered the main etiological factor of PAH in patients with SCA.
- A relative deficiency of NO will lead to vasoconstriction and eventual remodeling of pulmonary vessels by smooth muscle cell growth and collagen synthesis.
- Add to this platelet aggregation and attachment, release of growth factors, and procoagulant factors.
- Thickening of the media and intima of small pulmonary vessels.
- Medial thickening of muscular arteries and extension of muscle cells into non-muscular arterioles.

- Thickening, concentric non-laminar intimal hyperplasia, and fibrosis.
- Pulmonary artery hypertension (PAH) is a relatively common and severe complication of sickle cell anemia.
- PAH is also an independent risk factor for mortality in patients with sickle cell anemia.
- Patients with SCA are known to have an anemia secondary to hemolysis. This will lead to an increase in the cardiac out.
- This increase in cardiac output requires precapillary pulmonary microcirculation vasodilatation in order to accommodate the increased flow of blood.
- Failure of this vasodilatation for any reason will result in an increase in pulmonary pressure.
- It was shown that patients with SCA have high pulmonary pressures and pulmonary vascular resistance.
- Patients with SCA and pulmonary hypertension have a significantly increased mortality rate when compared with SCA patients without pulmonary hypertension.
- A mortality as high as 40 % was reported in SCA patients with pulmonary hypertension when compared to those without pulmonary hypertension.
- The etiology of PAH in patients with SCA is multifactorial, and several mechanisms have been proposed including:
  - Intravascular hemolysis leading to nitric oxide (NO) deficiency
  - Progressive interstitial pulmonary fibrosis secondary to acute chest syndrome
  - Pulmonary vasculopathy secondary to platelet activation
  - Pulmonary vascular intimal thickening
  - Hypoperfusion of the pulmonary vascular bed
  - Recurrent thromboembolic disease and in situ pulmonary thrombosis
- The prevalence of PAH in SCA patients increases with age, and it is associated with a high risk for death.
- The high prevalence is also attributed to the fact that with improved care and new modalities of treatment, more children and young adults with SCA are surviving to an older age group and developing this complication later.
- The risk factors for PAH in patients with SCA include:
  - Older age
  - Degree of hemolysis
  - Increased blood pressure
  - History of renal or heart disease
  - Iron overload
  - Cholestasis
- The risk for PAH is not related to:
  - The level of HbF
  - The frequency of ACS
  - The frequency of painful vaso-occlusive crisis
  - Hydroxyurea treatment

14.4 Clinical Features of PAH

- The clinical features of PAH are variable ranging from asymptomatic in those with mid-elevation of the pressure to those with severe symptoms.
- The symptoms include:
  - Exertional dyspnea is a clue to the presence of PAH.
  - Chronic dyspnea.
  - Hypoxemia.
  - Increased P2 or tricuspid regurgitation.
  - Cor pulmonale in severe PAH.
  - Arrhythmias.
  - Syncope.
  - Sudden death.
  - Fatigue on exertion.

14.5 Investigations of PAH

- Chest X-ray.
- EKG.
- Doppler echocardiography.
- A six-minute walk test.
- Definitive diagnosis requires right heart catheterization (RHC) with demonstration of a resting mean pulmonary arterial pressure (PAP) ≥25 mmHg.
- A less invasive investigation is Doppler echocardiographic assessment of the tricuspid valve regurgitant jet velocity (TRV).
- Doppler echocardiographic assessment of the tricuspid valve regurgitant jet velocity (TRV) has become a less invasive way to detect PAH and a valuable screening modality.
- PAH on ECHO was defined as a TRV of 2.5 m/s or greater.
- Using these criteria, the PAH was assessed and defined as:
  - Mild (TRV = 2.5–2.9 m/s).
  - Severe (TRV > 2.9 m/s).
  - It was also estimated that 25–30 % of the patients have mild PAH and 5–10 % have severe PAH.

14.6 Treatment of SCA-Related PAH

- Fluid hydration.
- Oxygenation.
- Blood transfusion.
- Pulmonary vasodilators.
- Anticoagulants.
- Hydroxyurea with or without erythropoietin.
- Inhaled NO and L-arginine are still being investigated as possible therapy for PAH.

14.7 Cardiac Complications

- It is well known that there is improvement in the care of patients with SCA. This as well as development of new treatment modalities including hydroxyurea have contributed to a significant increase in longevity for SCA patients.
- This however contributed to an increase in the mortality rate from cardiovascular and pulmonary complications.
- Patients with PAH and diastolic LV dysfunction represent a particularly high-risk subgroup.
- These cardiopulmonary complications contribute to a markedly low functional capacity and associated high risk of both sudden death and severe multi-organ dysfunction.
- Cardiac complications are common among patients with sickle cell anemia.
- They are an important cause of the morbidity and mortality in patients with sickle cell anemia.
- Sickle cell anemia is associated with hemolysis both acute and chronic leading to anemia. The anemia results in an increase in cardiac output.
- As a result, the left ventricular stroke volume increases with significant dilation of the LV.
- The dilated LV subsequently hypertrophies as a result of eccentric hypertrophy in which the wall thickening is increased and myofibers are elongated.
- The end result is an increase in LV mass and impaired LV filling and diastolic dysfunction.
- It was shown that these diastolic abnormalities are associated with:
  - Older age
  - Hypertension
  - Increased LV mass
  - Increased creatinine levels
- Direct myocardial damage from microvascular disease and iron deposition has also been postulated as etiologies for the cardiac abnormalities.
- Invasive right heart catheterization measurements of patients with PAH show evidence of diastolic dysfunction in approximately one-half of the patients.
- Although "heart disease" and "heart failure" have been considered common in adult SCA patients, recent studies indicate that LV systolic function is preserved in the majority of patients.
- LV dysfunction is seen particularly in older patients with hypertension and renal disease.
- Patients with SCA also have dilated right heart chambers without significant right ventricular dysfunction.
- Patients with evidence of right ventricular dysfunction are most likely to develop acute right heart failure.
- Myocardial ischemia and infarction have been reported to occur in patients with SCA, but in almost all cases, coronary angiography reveals normal coronary arteries.
  - These findings have been attributed to acute and chronic microvascular occlusion on top of chronic endothelial damage, a procoagulant state, and the systemic vasculopathy.

- Marked abnormalities in exercise capacity have consistently been seen in patients with SCA.
- This is attributed to several factors including:
  - Cardiac filling abnormalities
  - Anemia
  - Pulmonary vascular disease
  - Peripheral vascular disease
  - Myopathy
- The 6-min walk test is a useful measure of functional capacity in these patients.
- Myocardial iron deposition has been considered as one etiology for the cardiac abnormalities seen in SCA. This however is not common.
- Electrocardiographic abnormalities, including QT prolongation, are not uncommon in SCA patients. The significance of this is not known.
- Add to this the occurrence of arrhythmias in patients with ventricular dysfunction.
- Sudden death is an increasingly recognized complication in patients with SCA.
- This can be attributed to several causes, but currently it is considered a direct complication of pulmonary vascular and cardiac disease.

14.8 Peripheral Vascular Disease in Patients with Sickle Cell Anemia

- Vascular obstruction is a major cause of morbidity and mortality in patients with sickle cell anemia (Figs. 14.1, 14.2, 14.3, and 14.4).
- This contributes to a variety of complications including:
  - Painful vaso-occlusive crisis
  - Aseptic necrosis of the bone and joints
  - Dactylitis
  - Pulmonary infarction/hypertension
  - Stroke
  - Priapism
  - Renal medullary infarction
  - Leg ulcers
  - Proliferative retinopathy
  - Peripheral vascular disease
- Vascular occlusion in SCA results from a variety of causes including:
  - Microvasculature occlusion by sickle RBCs
  - Vascular intimal hyperplasia
  - Thrombosis and thromboembolism
  - Bone marrow infarction and fat embolism
  - Altered vascular reactivity, manifested by failure of compensatory vasodilation and/or frank vasospasm
  - Abnormal adhesive and procoagulant properties of sickled RBCs

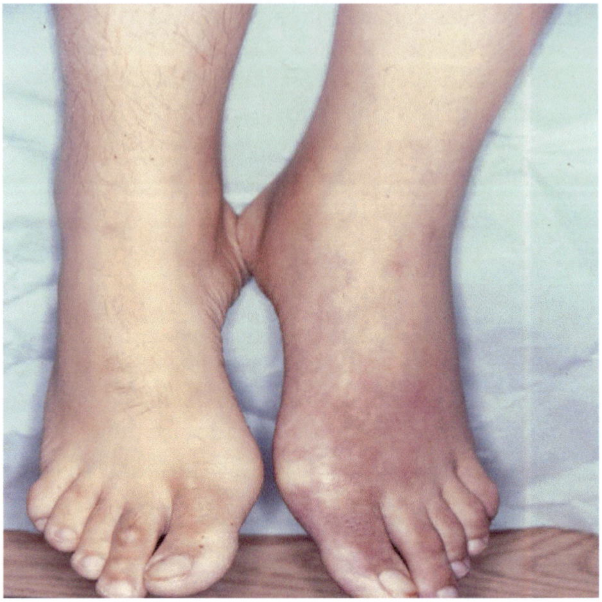

Fig. 14.1 A clinical photograph of a patient with sickle cell anemia and peripheral vascular disease

- Vascular intimal hyperplasia, alone or associated with superimposed thrombosis, is an important cause of peripheral vascular occlusion in patients with SCA.
- In addition to causing direct occlusion and superimposed thrombosis, vascular intimal hyperplasia may also slow microvascular flow and capillary transit time, thereby predisposing to microvascular occlusion by trapping of sickled RBCs.
- Peripheral vascular disease is uncommon in patients with sickle cell anemia.
- Radiological assessment of these patients includes Doppler ultrasonography and CT and MR angiography.
- Doppler ultrasonography is not expensive, noninvasive, and widely available, while MR angiography is expensive.
- Digital subtraction angiography remains the standard investigation to assess peripheral vascular disease (Fig. 14.5).
- Management:
  - The management of sickle cell anemia patients with peripheral vascular disease is difficult.
  - Long-term exchange blood transfusion to correct the anemia and lower the percentage of HbS may prove beneficial in reducing the progress and complications of sickle cell vasculopathy. It will also improve the oxygen-carrying capacity in these patients.
  - Surgical revascularization is not easy in these patients because of the diffuse calcification of the vessels.
  - Endarterectomy rather than bypass is preferable in these patients.

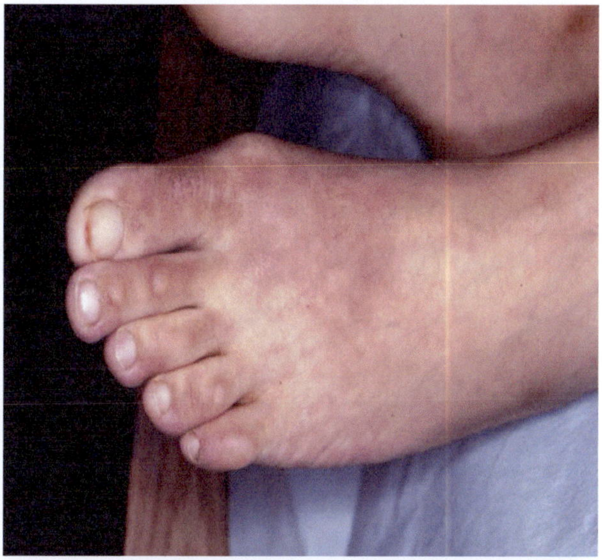

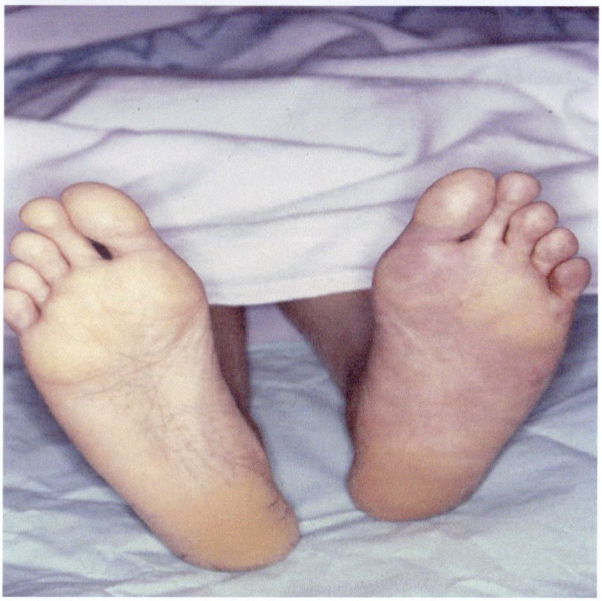

Figs. 14.2 and 14.3 Clinical photographs of a patient with sickle cell anemia and peripheral vascular disease

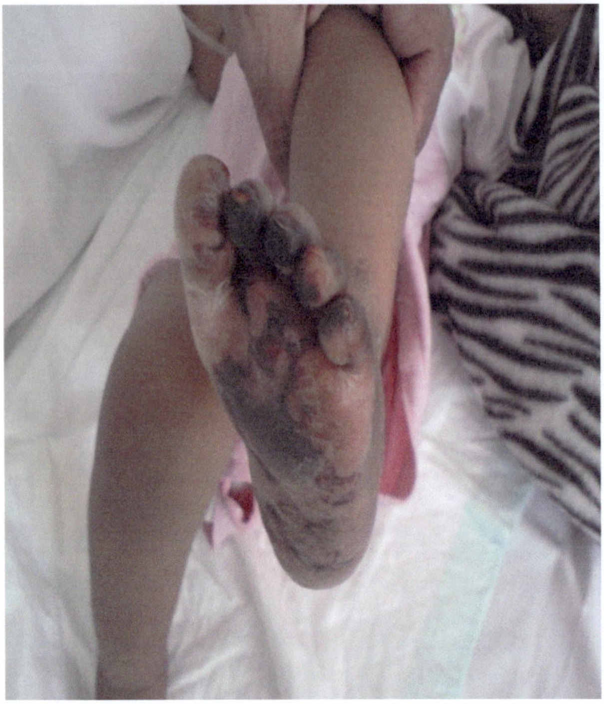

Fig. 14.4 A clinical photograph showing vascular occlusion in a child with sickle cell anemia causing ischemia and gangrene

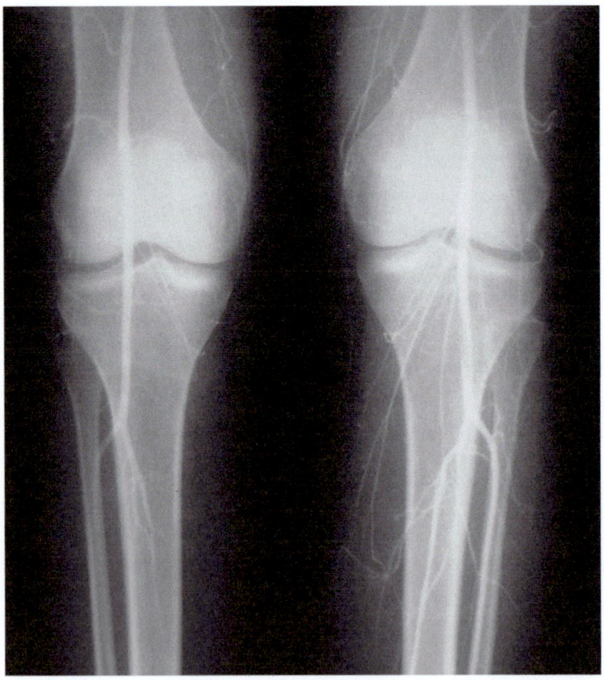

Fig. 14.5 An angiogram of a patient with sickle cell anemia showing thrombosis and obstruction of the popliteal artery

Further Reading

Arteta M, Campbell A, Nouraie M, et al. Abnormal pulmonary function and associated risk factors in children and adolescents with sickle cell anemia. J Pediatr Hematol Oncol. 2014;36:185.

Bayazit AK, Noyan A, Aldudak B, et al. Renal function in children with sickle cell anemia. Clin Nephrol. 2002;57:127.

Falk RJ, Scheinman J, Phillips G, et al. Prevalence and pathologic features of sickle cell nephropathy and response to inhibition of angiotensin-converting enzyme. N Engl J Med. 1992;326:910.

Gladwin MT, Kato GJ. Cardiopulmonary complications of sickle cell disease: role of nitric oxide and hemolytic anemia. Nat Med. 2002;8:1383–9.

Gladwin MT, Vichinsky E. Pulmonary complications of sickle cell disease. N Engl J Med. 2008;359:2254.

Gladwin MT, Sachdev V, Jison ML, et al. Pulmonary hypertension as a risk factor for death in patients with sickle cell disease. N Engl J Med. 2004;350:886–95.

Guasch A, Navarrete J, Nass K, Zayas CF. Glomerular involvement in adults with sickle cell hemoglobinopathies: prevalence and clinical correlates of progressive renal failure. J Am Soc Nephrol. 2006;17:2228.

Halsey C, Roberts IA. The role of hydroxyurea in sickle cell disease. Br J Haematol. 2003;120:177.

Herve P, Humbert M, Sitbon O, et al. Pathobiology of pulmonary hypertension. The role of platelets and thrombosis. Clin Chest Med. 2001;22:451–8.

Klings ES, Anton Bland D, Rosenman D, et al. Pulmonary arterial hypertension and left-sided heart disease in sickle cell disease: clinical characteristics and association with soluble adhesion molecule expression. Am J Hematol. 2008;83:547.

Morris CR. New strategies for the treatment of pulmonary hypertension in sickle cell disease: the rationale for arginine therapy. Treat Respir Med. 2006;5:31–45.

Naik RP, Streiff MB, Lanzkron S. Sickle cell disease and venous thromboembolism: what the anticoagulation expert needs to know. J Thromb Thrombolysis. 2013a;35:352.

Naik RP, Streiff MB, Haywood Jr C, et al. Venous thromboembolism in adults with sickle cell disease: a serious and under-recognized complication. Am J Med. 2013b;126:443.

Pham PT, Pham PC, Wilkinson AH, Lew SQ. Renal abnormalities in sickle cell disease. Kidney Int. 2000;57:1.

Platt OS, Brambilla DJ, Rosse WF, et al. Mortality in sickle cell disease: life expectancy and risk factors for early death. N Engl J Med. 1994;330:1639–44.

Powars DR, Elliott-Mills DD, Chan L, et al. Chronic renal failure in sickle cell disease: risk factors, clinical course, and mortality. Ann Intern Med. 1991;115:614.

Scheinman JI. Sickle cell disease and the kidney. Nat Clin Pract Nephrol. 2009;5(2):78–88.

15 Cerebrovascular Complications of Sickle Cell Anemia

15.1 Introduction

- A variety of neurological complications occur in patients with sickle cell anemia.
- Approximately 25 % of patients with sickle cell anemia have a neurological event in their lifetime, many of these occur in childhood.
- Cerebral infarction, either overt or clinically silent, is one of the major complications of the sickle cell anemia.
- These neurological complications occur most commonly in patients with sickle cell anemia but have been seen in the other hemoglobinopathies, namely:
  - Sickle cell/hemoglobin C disease
  - Sickle cell/beta-thalassemia
- Stroke (infarction or hemorrhagic) is caused by damage to either large or small cerebral vessels.
- Overt stroke is associated with stenosis and occlusion of large cerebral arteries, especially those of the circle of Willis. These vessels may show increased aneurysm formation as an additional manifestation of the sickling-induced cerebral vasculopathy.
- A mass of small friable vessels, similar to moyamoya disease, has been reported to occur as a consequent to the stenosis/occlusion of the cerebral arteries in patients with sickle cell anemia.
- Rupture of aneurysms or of the moyamoya-like vessels results in hemorrhagic stroke, which is commonly subarachnoid but may be intraventricular or intraparenchymal.
- The neurological complications of sickle cell anemia include:
  - Cerebral infarction
  - Intracranial hemorrhage
  - Spinal cord infarction
  - Isolated neuropathies due to anatomical proximity to infarcted bones
  - Lead neuropathy
  - Auditory complications
  - Ocular manifestations

A. Al-Salem, *Medical and Surgical Complications of Sickle Cell Anemia*,
DOI 10.1007/978-3-319-24762-5_15

- The most devastating and most common complication is cerebral infarction.
- There are a number of risk factors for stroke in patients with sickle cell anemia.
- These include:
  - History of transient ischemic attacks
  - High systolic blood pressure
  - Increased steady-state leukocyte count
  - Severe anemia
  - Acute chest syndrome
  - Elevated cerebral blood flow velocity
  - Nocturnal hypoxemia
- The majority of silent cerebral infarcts affect frontal lobe regions.
- It was shown that children with SCA and silent cerebral infarction on neuroimaging commonly have neurocognitive dysfunction.
- These patients suffer from a frontal lobe dysfunction syndrome, which can globally affect executive functioning in areas such as attention, concentration, information processing, and decision-making.
- Those with silent cerebral infarcts have IQs in the low 80s, while those with overt stroke have IQs in the 70s.
- Stroke is a devastating and potentially fatal complication of sickle cell anemia.
- Stroke in patients with sickle cell anemia is usually associated with narrowing or occlusion of the large cerebral arteries including:
  - The internal carotid artery
  - The middle cerebral artery
  - The anterior cerebral artery
  - The basilar artery
- Transcranial Doppler studies of children show that high blood flow velocity through these vessels is associated with higher probabilities of arterial occlusive stroke.
- Children with flow rates of >190 cm/min through the internal carotid artery are at great risk of stroke.
- Chronic blood transfusion therapy in patients identified by transcranial Doppler with increased cerebral blood flow velocity (>200 cm/s) prevented overt stroke.
  - The aim of the transfusion regimen is to maintain the hemoglobin S below 30 %.
  - This showed a relative stroke risk reduction of approximately 85 %.
- Transfusion therapy remains the mainstay of management in the acute phase of cerebral infarction.
- There is considerable evidence to indicate that long-term transfusion programs are effective in the prevention of recurrences.
- This benefit clearly justifies the burden of monthly transfusion, its associated need for deferoxamine chelation therapy to prevent iron overload, and the continuing risk of alloimmunization.
- There is a high recurrence rate of stroke in untreated patients.
- In addition to the potentially devastating effect of stroke with its neurologic sequelae, "silent" infarcts appear to play an important role in the development of cognitive deficits.

15.2 Incidence

- Cerebrovascular accident is defined as any acute neurologic event secondary to arterial occlusion or hemorrhage that results in an ischemic event associated with neurologic signs and/or symptoms.
- Silent cerebral infarcts are defined as abnormal lesion seen on MRI of the brain with increased signal intensity on multiple T2-weighted images but no history or physical finding of a focal neurologic defect lasting more than 24 h.
- A cerebrovascular accident is one of the leading causes of death in both children and adults with sickle cell anemia.
- The reported age-adjusted incidence is 0.61–0.76 per 100 patient-years (i.e., 0.61–0.76 % per year) during the first 20 years of life.
- This rate is approximately 300 times higher than that seen in children without SCA (0.0023 per 100 patient-years).
- Silent cerebral infarcts have been reported to occur in as many as 22 % of patients by 14 years of age.
- Patients with an existing silent cerebral infarct have an increased incidence of a new stroke (1.03 per 100 patient-years) and a marked incidence of new or more extensive silent cerebral infarcts (7.07 per 100 patient-years).
- The frequency of cerebral infarction in patients with sickle cell anemia varies from 6 % to as high as 34 % in different reports.
- The annual incidence of first stroke for those with sickle cell anemia was estimated as 0.6 per 100 patient-years, with the highest rate of 1.02 per 100 patient-years seen in the group aged 2–5 years.
- The cumulative risk of stroke was 11 % by the age 20 years, increasing with age to 24 % by the age 45 years.
- It was also found in the United States that the incidence per 100 patient-years of a first cerebral infarct was 0.70 between ages 2 and 5 years, 0.51 between ages 6 and 9 years, and 0.24 between ages 10 and 19 years and then fall to 0.04 between the ages of 20 and 29.

15.3 Mechanism of Stroke in Sickle Cell Anemia

- The exact etiology of arterial occlusive stroke in patients with sickle cell disease is unknown.
- The arterial lumen is usually occluded by a thrombus that includes red cells, platelets, and fibrin.
- The red cell adherence to the endothelium which is mediated by von Willebrand's protein may be an important factor in arterial occlusive stroke in patients with sickle cell anemia.
- Von Willebrand's protein enhances adherence of sickle red cells to endothelial cells.
- The membranes of sickle red cells are strikingly abnormal. As a result, sickle red cell membranes have procoagulant activity.

- Therefore, a cascade could occur in which von Willebrand's protein promotes sickle red cell/endothelial cell adhesion, which then is a nidus for thrombus formation.
- High rates of blood flow in these patients produce high linear sheer stress through the major cerebral arteries.
- This leads to adherence of these sickled RBCs as well as platelets and fibrin leading to narrowing or occlusion of cerebral blood vessels.
- The involvement of large arteries commonly produces severe neurological deficits.
- Occlusion of the middle cerebral artery causes dense hemiparesis and aphasia if the stroke affects the dominant hemisphere of the brain. Cerebral edema with secondary brain stem compression is often fatal.

15.4 Treatment of Stroke

- Stroke is a life-threatening event for patients with sickle cell anemia.
- Exchange blood transfusion followed by chronic blood transfusion to maintain the level of HbS at <30 % is the treatment of choice.
- Patients with stroke run a risk of recurrence of about 50 % in the absence of chronic transfusion.
- The duration of chronic transfusion needed to prevent recurrent stroke is undefined.
- Clearly, most children do not continue indefinitely with chronic transfusion after a stroke.
- Cessation of chronic transfusion after as long as 5 years was associated with a high incidence of recurrent stroke in some studies.

15.5 Preventive Measures

- Physicians caring for children with sickle cell anemia should consider instituting yearly examinations by transcranial Doppler.
- A chronic transfusion regimen would be considered for children in which the blood flow rate in the assessed artery is >190 cm/min.
- Chronic blood transfusion therapy in patients with sickle cell anemia is beneficial and not only prevents strokes but also has several other clinical advantages including decreased incidence of:
  - Recurrent vaso-occlusive pain necessitating hospitalization
  - Priapism
  - Avascular necrosis
  - Acute chest syndrome
- Chronic blood transfusion therapy is known to be associated with adverse effects including:
  - Transfusion reactions
  - Central venous catheter placement

  - Red cell alloimmunization
  - Burdens regarding monthly clinic visits with associated missed school and work time
  - Transmission of infections including hepatitis B, hepatitis C, and HIV
  - Iron overload
- The duration of blood transfusion therapy for the secondary prevention of silent cerebral infarcts is unknown, but it has been suggested that a minimum of 3 years of therapy should be considered.
- The type of stroke varies with age.
  - An ischemic infarct is most common in children between the ages of 2 and 9, uncommon between the ages of 20 and 29, and has a second peak in adults over age 29.
  - Hemorrhagic stroke can occur in children but is most frequent in individuals between the ages of 20 and 29.
  - It was found that among first cerebrovascular accidents in patients with SCA:
    - 54 % were caused by cerebral infarction
    - 11 % were caused by TIA
    - 34 % were caused by intracranial hemorrhage
    - 1 % had features of both infarction and hemorrhage

15.6 Investigations

- Computed tomographic (CT) scanning and magnetic resonance imaging (MRI) have become the accepted methods for confirming a clinical diagnosis of cerebral infarction or intracranial hemorrhage in patients with sickle cell anemia.
- MRI offers improved resolution and the ability to demonstrate areas of abnormality within 2–4 h following an infarct.
- Transcranial Doppler can be used to identify patients at risk for stroke.
- Magnetic resonance angiography (MRA) can identify vascular disease.
- Positron emission tomography (PET) scan can be used to assess the functional activity of the cerebral tissues and, therefore, microvascular blood flow.
- PET scanning in conjunction with MRI may identify a greater number of patients with silent infarcts than does MRI alone.

15.7 Cerebral Infarction

- Cerebral infarction is defined clinically by the presence of typical symptoms that last for at least 24 h.
- Symptoms of infarctive stroke may include:
  - Hemiparesis
  - Dysphasia
  - Gait disturbance
  - A change in the level of consciousness

- Cerebral infarction is associated largely with occlusion or stenosis of the large intracranial arteries.
- Silent cerebral ischemia is a related condition in which an infarct-like lesion is seen on magnetic resonance imaging (MRI) without a corresponding abnormality on neurologic examination.
- Silent ischemia produces no overt sensorimotor deficits, but it is associated with poor cognitive performance and an increased risk for infarction in children with sickle cell anemia.
- It has been estimated that 11 and 24 % of patients with SCA have a clinically apparent stroke by the ages of 20 and 45 years, respectively.
- Stroke rates at 0.88 events per 100 patient-years were also reported in children with sickle cell anemia.
- High levels of HbF were thought to account for the mild clinical course in patients with sickle cell anemia and may have a protective role against stroke in these patients.
- Recurrent stroke occurs in approximately two-thirds of patients within 2 years of the initial event.
- This risk is age dependent:
  - 6.4 per 100 patient-years in patients with an initial cerebrovascular accident before age 20.
  - This is compared with 1.6 per 100 patient-years in older patients.
- Significant and long-lasting neurologic deficits are much more likely to occur after a second stroke.
- The incidence of silent ischemia appears to be greater than that of cerebral infarction and varies depending on the sensitivity of the imaging modality used.
  - In an MRI/MRA evaluation study of 65 neurologically normal children with SCA (age range, 1.3–5.9 years), it was found that 28 % of them had silent infarcts.
  - Silent ischemic events, defined as an infarct-like lesion seen on MRI without corresponding neurological abnormalities.
  - Silent ischemia may be associated with significant cognitive decline.
- Risk factors for completed infarctive stroke include:
  - Prior transient ischemic attack
  - Low steady-state hemoglobin
  - Rate of acute chest syndrome
  - Episode of acute chest syndrome within the previous 2 weeks
  - Elevated systolic blood pressure
- Transcranial Doppler (TCD), a noninvasive procedure, has become an important tool in predicting the risk for stroke in patients with SCA.
  - It measures the time-averaged mean velocity of blood flow in the large intracranial vessels, which is inversely related to arterial diameter (as documented by cerebral angiography).
  - A focal increase in velocity usually suggests arterial stenosis, whereas a bilateral increase may indicate bilateral arterial disease, increased blood flow, or both.

- In children, a mean transcranial Doppler (TCD) velocity >170 cm/s is worrisome, and values >200 cm/s in the middle cerebral or internal carotid artery are highly associated with an increased risk of stroke, even before lesions become evident on magnetic resonance angiograms (MRA).
- In adults, a time-averaged maximum mean velocity of 123.5 cm/s is highly associated with middle or internal carotid artery intracranial stenosis.
- Patients with abnormal MRA findings and higher TCD velocities are at even higher risk for stroke.
- The use of TCD has become a routine screening tool in many centers that care for children with sickle cell anemia.
- TCD screening of children with SCD after age 2 is effective for assessing stroke risk.
- The optimal frequency of TCD screening has not been established. It was suggested to follow these patients based on the initial result as follows:
  - Flow velocity <170 cm/s: repeat annually
  - Flow velocity >170 cm/s and ≤200 cm/s: repeat in 3 months
  - Flow velocity ≥200 cm/s: repeat in 2–4 weeks
- Children with abnormal flow velocity of ≥200 cm/s in the internal carotid artery or the middle cerebral artery on two repeated studies done by TCD are at high risk of stroke.
- Therefore, patients with two abnormal TCD studies within a 2–4-week period should be entered into a stroke prevention protocol consisting of chronic transfusion therapy.

- G6PD deficiency and hemolysis are two factors that independently increase the risk of cerebral vasculopathy in patients with SCA.
- A prophylactic chronic transfusion program with a goal to lower HbS of less than 30 % of total hemoglobin proved beneficial in preventing stroke and significantly reduced the risk of a new silent infarct in patients with sickle cell anemia.
- Chronic transfusion therapy may also provide benefit to children who have silent ischemia on magnetic resonance imaging (MRI), regardless of findings on TCD.
- The incidence of other vaso-occlusive events was also lower in the transfusion group (e.g., painful episodes, acute chest syndrome, and priapism).
- Chronic transfusion therapy poses certain risks, including alloimmunization, transfusion reactions, transmission of diseases, and iron overload; and although TCD has a high sensitivity for predicting stroke, the specificity is low.
- For families who refuse transfusion therapy, hydroxyurea has been suggested as a second-line option, but its efficacy for primary or secondary prevention of stroke in SCA is not well established.
- The clinical features of cerebral infarction in patients with sickle cell anemia range from the "silent" parenchymal infarct with little or no evidence of large vessel disease to overt stroke with stenosis or arterial occlusion and cortical infarcts.
- Chronic transfusion management of overt stroke has become the "gold standard," but the duration of such therapy is still unsettled.
- Current evidence suggests that transfusion therapy be extended to those with silent cerebral disease as well.

- Still undetermined is the management of patients who decline transfusion for religious reasons, patients who have recurrent stroke despite adequate transfusion, and patients for whom continued transfusion becomes a greater risk.
- Reasons for discontinuance of chronic transfusion therapy include:
  - Erythrocyte alloimmunization such that compatible donor units become difficult to identify and the risk of delayed hemolytic transfusion reactions becomes paramount.
  - Iron overload because of noncompliance with chelation therapy.
  - Hydroxyurea is valuable in prevention of end organ damage, but its full efficacy in preventing recurrence of stroke is not well established.
  - Stem cell transplantation offers the potential for curative therapy.
- Chronic transfusion therapy is the most effective method for both primary and secondary prevention of stroke. The optimal duration of transfusion therapy is uncertain.
  - 80 % of recurrences are known to occur within 3 years of the first event.
  - Thus, attempts have been made at discontinuing transfusion therapy after several years; several case studies have reported a high rate of recurrence within a year of discontinuation of therapy.
  - The duration of transfusion therapy for prevention of stroke in these patients is not well established.
- A prophylactic transfusion program can be stopped in patients without a prior stroke for the following criteria:
  - Treatment with periodic transfusions for a minimum of 30 months with an HbS level <30 % in at least 20 of the 30 months
  - Reversion of TCD velocities to normal (i.e., two normal TCD examinations at least 2 weeks apart while receiving transfusions)
  - No prior stroke
  - No moderate-to-severe arterial lesions on magnetic resonance angiography
- It was suggested that children with SCA identified as being at high risk for stroke will likely be receiving extended, if not lifelong, RBC transfusions for prevention of stroke as well as prevention of silent brain infarcts.

15.8 Acute Stroke Management

- Acute stroke in a patient with SCA is secondary to a vaso-occlusive event, but other causes of stroke should be excluded including:
  - Cardiovascular
  - Drug induced such as cocaine and amphetamine
  - Hypercholesterolemia
  - Diabetes mellitus
- An immediate exchange transfusion to achieve an HbS concentration of <30 % of total hemoglobin and a total hemoglobin level of approximately, but not greater than, 10 g/dL.
- Urgent simple blood transfusion may be appropriate if the patient has severe anemia or if there will be a delay of >4 h to initiate exchange transfusion.

- Exchange transfusion rather than simple transfusion is used in part because it avoids the risk of transfusional volume overload and associated pulmonary edema.
- In addition, exchange transfusion avoids the theoretical risk of increased blood viscosity associated with simple transfusion.
- Another benefit of initial exchange transfusion rather than simple transfusion is a potentially reduced risk of stroke recurrence.
- Additional management includes:
  - Oxygenation.
  - Ventilation.
  - Maintenance of a normoglycemia.
  - Hydration with normal saline rather than hypotonic saline to avoid the potential worsening of cytotoxic cerebral edema that may occur with infusion of hypotonic fluid.
  - The use of thrombolytic agents could increase the risk of intracranial hemorrhage and should be avoided.
  - Aspirin or other antiplatelet agents can be considered, but these may increase the risk of hemorrhage.

15.9 Prevention of Recurrent Stroke

- Patients with SCA who have an initial stroke have a high risk of recurrent stroke.
- Recurrent stroke occurs in approximately two-thirds of patients within 2 years of the initial event, and the risk is particularly high in patients under the age 20 years.
- Significant and long-lasting neurologic deficits are much more likely to occur after a second stroke.
- The risk of recurrence in any patient with SCA who has had a stroke should be reduced.
- This is mainly using chronic blood transfusion protocols.
- Hematopoietic stem cell transplantation should be considered in stabilized patients with available matched donors.
- Although hydroxyurea has been considered as an alternative to chronic transfusion therapy, it is not as effective.
- Chronic transfusion can reduce the incidence of recurrent stroke from approximately two-thirds of patients to below 10 %, when routine monthly red blood cell transfusions are given to maintain the hemoglobin S fraction at less than 30 % of total hemoglobin.

15.10 Intracranial Hemorrhage

- Intracranial hemorrhage (ICH), also called hemorrhagic stroke, accounts for approximately one-third of cerebrovascular events in patients with sickle cell anemia.

- The site of bleeding may be:
  - Subarachnoid
  - Intraparenchymal
  - Intraventricular
  - A combination of these locations
- The peak incidence of ICH is between the ages of 20 and 29 in comparison to cerebral infarction, which is much more common in children.
- Approximately 3 % of children with SCA will have a hemorrhagic stroke by 20 years of age, and 25–50 % will die within 2 weeks of the event.
- Risk factors for hemorrhagic stroke include:
  - Low steady-state hemoglobin
  - Increased steady-state leukocyte count
  - A recent history of hypertension
  - Blood transfusions
  - Corticosteroid therapy
- Clinical manifestations:
  - Typically ICH produces focal deficits such as hemiparesis
  - Severe headache
  - Vomiting
  - Stiff neck
  - Alterations in consciousness
  - Coma and seizures
- Investigations and treatment:
  - Angiography should be considered in all patients with ICH to identify the cause of bleeding and to guide further therapy.
  - Aneurysms should be repaired surgically when possible.
  - When large vessel vasculopathy is present without aneurysm or vascular malformation, chronic transfusion may be recommended.
  - However, in patients for whom the cause of hemorrhage remains unclear, chronic transfusion will not be helpful and is not indicated.
- The mortality rate in patients with ICH is as high as 24–50 %.
- Deaths generally occur within the first 2 weeks of the event, many on the first day.
- In addition, some survivors are left with moderate to severe residual disability.

15.11 Subarachnoid Hemorrhage

- The majority of cases of ICH represent subarachnoid hemorrhage resulting from thc rupture of one or more aneurysms.
- Multiple aneurysms are present in approximately 45 % of patients.
- The etiology of these aneurysms is not exactly known.
- These aneurysms may develop as a result of injury to the endothelium and the high flow rate in SCA.
- The peak incidence of subarachnoid hemorrhage is in young adults.

- Treatment of subarachnoid hemorrhage includes:
  - Intravenous hydration
  - Close monitoring
  - Nimodipine to minimize the incidence of vasospasm
  - Surgery to clip-ligate the aneurysm
  - Careful treatment of hypertension if present as a significant decrease in blood pressure may result in ischemia or infarction

15.12 Intraventricular Hemorrhage

- Intraventricular hemorrhage (IVH) may result from rupture of an anterior cerebral artery aneurysm or from direct extension of intraparenchymal hemorrhage into the lateral or third ventricle.
- Patients who have experienced previous cerebral infarction are at risk for intraventricular and intraparenchymal hemorrhage as a late event, months to years after the ischemic stroke.
- Hemorrhage into the third ventricle or cerebral aqueduct places these patients at high risk for late deterioration.
- Such patients may be awake and alert immediately following such a bleed and then become comatose over the ensuing 48 h because of obstructive hydrocephalus and ventricular dilation.
- Emergency ventricular drainage may be necessary.

15.13 Moyamoya Syndrome

- In approximately 30 % of patients with SCA who develop intracranial hemorrhage, a moyamoya syndrome (sometimes termed "pseudo-moyamoya" or secondary moyamoya pattern) in the basal arteries may be demonstrated by angiography.
- These abnormalities may be the source of hemorrhage.
- This pattern is named for its resemblance to findings in moyamoya disease, a chronic cerebrovascular disease of uncertain etiology that occurs primarily in Japan and other Asian countries and is characterized by severe bilateral stenosis or occlusion of the arteries around the circle of Willis, with prominent collateral circulation.
- Patients with SCA who develop moyamoya syndrome appear to be at risk for recurrence of strokes.
- In children with SCA and moyamoya syndrome, surgical treatment has been used in an effort to restore the circulation of the ischemic brain area, thereby reducing the risk of ischemic stroke.
- Indirect revascularization using encephaloduroarteriosynangiosis (EDAS) is a reasonable option for these patients given their poor outcome without intervention.

15.14 Epidural Hematoma

- Epidural hematoma rarely develops in patients with SCA.
- In these cases, the hematomas were associated with bony infarcts of the skull.
- These should be treated with aggressive surgical intervention.

Further Reading

Adams R, McKie V, Nichols F, et al. The use of transcranial ultrasonography to predict stroke in sickle cell disease. N Engl J Med. 1992a;326:605–10.

Adams RJ, Nichols FT, Figueroa R, et al. Transcranial Doppler correlation with cerebral angiography in sickle cell disease. Stroke. 1992b;23:1073.

Adams RJ, McKie VC, Hsu L, et al. Prevention of a first stroke by transfusions in children with sickle cell anemia and abnormal results on transcranial Doppler ultrasonography. N Engl J Med. 1998;339:5.

Aygun B, McMurray MA, Schultz WH, et al. Chronic transfusion practice for children with sickle cell anaemia and stroke. Br J Haematol. 2009;145:524.

DeBaun MR, Sarnaik SA, Rodeghier MJ, et al. Associated risk factors for silent cerebral infarcts in sickle cell anemia: low baseline hemoglobin, sex, and relative high systolic blood pressure. Blood. 2012;119:3684.

DeBaun MR, Gordon M, McKinstry RC, et al. Controlled trial of transfusions for silent cerebral infarcts in sickle cell anemia. N Engl J Med. 2014;371:699.

Helton KJ, Wang WC, Wynn LW, et al. The effect of hydroxyurea on vasculopathy in a child with sickle cell disease. AJNR Am J Neuroradiol. 2002;23:1692–6.

Jordan LC, Casella JF, DeBaun MR. Prospects for primary stroke prevention in children with sickle cell anaemia. Br J Haematol. 2012;157:14.

Kwiatkowski JL, Zimmerman RA, Pollock AN, et al. Silent infarcts in young children with sickle cell disease. Br J Haematol. 2009;146:300.

Lefèvre N, Dufour D, Gulbis B, et al. Use of hydroxyurea in prevention of stroke in children with sickle cell disease. Blood. 2008;111:963.

Ohene-Frempong K, Weiner SJ, Sleeper LA, et al. Cerebrovascular accidents in sickle cell disease: rates and risk factors. Blood. 1998;91:288.

Pegelow CH, Wang W, Granger S, et al. Silent infarcts in children with sickle cell anemia and abnormal cerebral artery velocity. Arch Neurol. 2001;58:2017–21.

Powars DR. Management of cerebral vasculopathy in children with sickle cell anaemia. Br J Haematol. 2000;108:666.

Quinn CT, McKinstry RC, Dowling MM, et al. Acute silent cerebral ischemic events in children with sickle cell anemia. JAMA Neurol. 2013;70:58.

Schatz J, Brown RT, Pascual JM, et al. Poor school and cognitive functioning with silent cerebral infarcts and sickle cell disease. Neurology. 2001;56:1109–11.

Scothorn DJ, Price C, Schwartz D, et al. Risk of recurrent stroke in children with sickle cell disease receiving blood transfusion therapy for at least five years after initial stroke. J Pediatr. 2002;140:348–54.

Verduzco LA, Nathan DG. Sickle cell disease and stroke. Blood. 2009;114:5117.

Verlhac S, Bernaudin F, Tortrat D, et al. Detection of cerebrovascular disease in patients with sickle cell disease using transcranial Doppler sonography: correlation with MRI, MRA and conventional angiography. Pediatr Radiol. 1995;25 Suppl 1:S14.

Walters MC, Storb R, Patience M, et al. Impact of bone marrow transplantation for symptomatic sickle cell disease: an interim report. Multicenter investigation of bone marrow transplantation for sickle cell disease. Blood. 2000;95:1918–24.

Ware RE, Zimmerman SA, Schultz WH. Hydroxyurea as an alternative to blood transfusion for the prevention of recurrent stroke in children with sickle cell disease. Blood. 1999;94:3022–6.

Renal Complications of Sickle Cell Anemia

16

16.1 Introduction

- Sickle cell anemia is known to be associated with several widespread complications that can affect any part of the body.
- Recently, it was shown that sickle cell anemia vasculopathy plays an important role in the pathogenesis of several of these complications and NO deficiency plays a major role in this.
- Endothelial generation of NO in the body has several important functions including:
  - Vasodilatation
  - Anti-inflammatory
  - Antithrombotic
- Deficiency of NO is an important contributor to the etiology of sickle cell anemia vasculopathy.
- In patients with SCA, deficiency of NO may be due to the following:
  - Scavenging of NO by the heme of sickle hemoglobin released into the plasma by the hemolyzed RBCs
  - Scavenging of NO by vascular superoxide anion
  - Depletion of plasma arginine by arginase released by hemolyzed RBCs
  - The effect of endogenous NO inhibitors
  - Inactivation of tetrahydrobiopterin, a NO cofactor, thereby uncoupling endothelial NO synthase such that superoxide anion, rather than NO, is produced
- Patients with SCA develop renal complications including:
  - Recurrent episodes of hematuria
  - Renal tubular abnormalities:
    - A concentrating defect
    - Impaired potassium excretion
    - Acidification defect

A. Al-Salem, *Medical and Surgical Complications of Sickle Cell Anemia*,
DOI 10.1007/978-3-319-24762-5_16

- It is estimated that about 70 % of patients with sickle cell anemia may develop microalbuminuria.
- It is also estimated that about 26 % of adult patients with sickle cell anemia develop sickle cell related kidney disease. This increases with age.
- The renal complications of sickle cell anemia are variable and include:
  - Functional abnormalities
  - Gross anatomic abnormalities
- The sickle cell anemia renal complications include:
  - Gross hematuria
  - Renal infarction
  - Papillary necrosis
  - Nephrotic syndrome
  - Urine concentration defects
  - Medullary kidney carcinoma
- The renal medulla is relatively hypoxic, hypertonic, and acidotic. This predisposes to sickling of red blood cells (RBCs) leading to vaso-occlusion, which significantly decreases renal medullary blood flow.
- Hematuria is commonly seen in patients with sickle cell nephropathy. It increases venous pressure, which further worsens ischemia of the renal medulla and predisposes the patient to further RBC sickling.
- Proximal tubule dysfunction generally impairs urinary concentration, while more distal tubule dysfunction may impair potassium excretion, leading to hyperkalemia.

Renal Complications of Sickle Cell Anemia

- Gross hematuria
- Renal infarction
- Papillary necrosis
- Nephrotic syndrome
- Urine concentration defects
- Medullary kidney carcinoma

- Hypertension is seen in only 2–6 % of patients with SCA. This is attributed to several factors including:
  - Sodium and water wasting secondary to pathological changes involving the renal medulla
  - Compensatory systemic vasodilatation due to significant reductions in the microcirculation and increased levels of prostaglandins and nitric oxide
- There are several factors involved in the progression of renal complications to end-stage chronic renal failure. These include:
  - Worsening anemia
  - Hypertension
  - The degree of proteinuria
  - Microscopic hematuria

The Frequency of Renal Complications of Sickle Cell Anemia

- About 26 % of adult patients with SCA develop sickle cell related kidney disease.
- 70 % of patients with SCA may develop microalbuminuria.
- Hypertension is seen in only 2–6 % of patients with SCA.
- About 4 % of patients with SCA develop renal failure at a median age of 23 years.
- 5–18 % of patients with SCA develop end-stage renal disease.
- Proteinuria has been estimated to occur in 20–25 % of patients with SCA.
- Renal infarcts and papillary necrosis occur in 30–40 % of patients with SCA.
- Decreased renal function in 5–30 % of patients with SCA.
- 4 % of patients with SCA develop renal failure at a median age of 23 years.
- Acute kidney injury occurs in 5–10 % of patients with SCA.

16.2 Pathophysiology

- The renal medulla is characterized by:
  - Low oxygen tension.
  - Low pH.
  - High osmolality.
- All of these predispose to RBC sickling, leading to increased blood viscosity which contributes to ischemia and eventual infarction that involves the renal microcirculation.
- This will lead to medullary ischemia and infarction that cause papillary necrosis.
- The sloughed papillae may obstruct urinary tract outflow, leading to renal failure.
- It has been estimated that 5–18 % of patients with SCA develop end-stage renal disease.
  - The end-stage renal disease in patients with SCA is more likely to develop in patients with:
  - Hypertension
  - Proteinuria
  - Hematuria
  - Severe anemia
- The recurrent bouts of hematuria and the renal tubular dysfunction arise secondary to renal medullary ischemia.
- This is due to sludging of RBCs in the vasa recta.
- This sludging of RBCs occurs because of:
  - Hypoxia
  - Hypertonicity
  - Acidosis in the medullary environment
  - A relatively low blood flow in the renal medulla

- In patients with SCA, there is hypoperfusion of the renal medulla, while the cortex is often hyperperfused because of decreased renal vascular resistance.
- This increased blood flow in the renal cortex leads to increased glomerular filtration rate.
- An important adverse effect of hyperperfusion of the kidney is glomerulomegaly with subsequent development of glomerulosclerosis.
- Glomerulosclerosis is the most common glomerulopathy in patients with SCA.
- Renal infarcts and papillary necrosis occur in patients with sickle cell anemia with a prevalence of 30–40 %.
- The prevalence of proteinuria among patients with sickle cell anemia has been estimated to be 20–25 %.
- Patients with SCA have decreased kidney function which has been reported in 5–30 %.
- About 4 % of patients with sickle cell anemia develop renal failure at a median age of 23 years. This is seen especially in patients with:
  - Hypertension
  - Proteinuria
  - Hematuria
  - Severe anemia
  - Hyperfiltration
- The histopathological changes seen in renal biopsies include:
- Glomerular hypertrophy.
- Hemosiderin deposits.
- Focal areas of hemorrhage or necrosis.
- Interstitial inflammation, edema, fibrosis, tubular atrophy, and papillary infarcts are seen in advanced stages.
- Glomerular enlargement and focal segmental glomerulosclerosis (perihilar variant being most frequent) are seen in patients who reach end-stage renal disease due to sickle cell anemia.
- The papillary necrosis associated with sickle cell anemia shows destruction of the vasa rectae and vascular congestion of the collecting ducts, inner medulla, and papillae.
- Less often, membrano-proliferative glomerulonephritis with mesangial expansion and basement membrane duplication may be seen, either as an isolated finding or in association with focal segmental glomerulosclerosis.
- The absence of immune complexes and electron-dense deposits differentiates this from idiopathic membrano-proliferative glomerulonephritis.

16.3 Pathogenesis

- The primary event appears to be sickling of RBCs in the vasa recta capillaries in the renal medulla, leading to microthrombotic infarction and extravasation of blood in the renal medulla.
- Sickling is promoted by the low oxygen tension, low pH, and high osmolality in the renal medulla.

- The increased blood viscosity contributes to ischemia and infarction in the renal microcirculation.
- More severe occlusions can lead to renal infarcts and papillary necrosis.
- Glomerular ischemia appears to promote increased renal blood flow and glomerular filtration rate (GFR).

The Renal Histopathological Changes in Patients with Sickle Cell Anemia

- Glomerular hypertrophy.
- Hemosiderin deposits.
- Focal areas of hemorrhage or necrosis.
- Interstitial inflammation, edema, fibrosis, tubular atrophy, and papillary infarcts are seen in advanced stages.
- Glomerular enlargement.
- Perihilar focal segmental glomerulosclerosis.
- Papillary necrosis.
- Destruction of the vasa rectae.
- Vascular congestion of the collecting ducts, inner medulla, and papillae.
- Membrano-proliferative glomerulonephritis.
- Mesangial expansion.
- Basement membrane duplication.

- This is seen as a result of:
  - The vasodilator prostaglandins released presumably to reverse the medullary ischemia
  - Increased glomerular nitric oxide synthesis
  - Glomerular hypertrophy
- Continued glomerular ischemia will lead to progressive renal failure (glomerulosclerosis).
- Glomerular abnormalities:
  - Glomerular abnormalities seen in patients with sickle cell anemia include:
    - Glomerular enlargement
    - Perihilar focal segmental glomerulosclerosis (FSGS)
    - Hemosiderosis
  - Glomerular ischemia seen in these patients leads to a compensatory increase in the renal blood flow and glomerular filtration rate (GFR).
  - This hyperfiltration, combined with glomerular hypertrophy, contributes to glomerulosclerosis.
  - As a result of progression of glomerulosclerosis, the GFR starts to decrease.
  - This will also lead to proteinuria.
- Proximal tubule abnormalities:
  - Increased resorption of phosphate and beta2-microglobulin
  - Increased secretion of ureic acid and creatinine
- Distal tubule abnormalities:
  - Red blood cells sickling in the vasa rectae are believed to interfere with the countercurrent exchange mechanism in the inner medulla.

- The resulting impairment of free water resorption manifests clinically as nocturia or polyuria.
- The impaired ability to concentrate urine (isosthenuria) is the earliest manifestation of sickle cell nephropathy.
- The ability to dilute urine remains intact, and antidiuretic hormone (ADH) secretion remains normal in sickle cell nephropathy patients with isosthenuria.
- This is because the vaso-occlusive process spares the superficial loops of the loop of Henle which are supplied by peritubular capillaries rather than by the vasa rectae.
- These changes are age dependent.
  - In patients aged 10–15 years, urinary concentrating capacity may be restored with multiple transfusions of normal RBCs.
  - Conversely, in patients older than 15 years, the concentration defect is often irreversible.
- Other processes that occur in the renal medulla include urinary acidification and the excretion of potassium.

16.4 Renal Manifestations of SCA

- Hematuria:
  - Painless microscopic or gross hematuria (due to papillary infarcts) is commonly seen in patients with sickle cell anemia and sickle cell trait.
  - The hematuria is typically mild and unilateral (and predominantly left sided).
  - This is attributed to the greater length of the left renal vein and the "nutcracker phenomenon" which further increase the relative hypoxia in the renal medulla promoting further sickling.
  - Hematuria is also self-limited.
- Renal infarction and papillary necrosis:
  - More severe ischemia can lead to renal infarcts and papillary necrosis.
  - Papillary necrosis commonly presents as painless gross hematuria and may be complicated by urinary tract infection or obstruction.
  - Acute segmental or total renal infarcts may present with:
    - Nausea
    - Vomiting
    - Flank or abdominal pain
    - Fever
    - Hypertension
- Diminished concentrating ability:
  - An impairment in concentrating ability (hyposthenuria) is a common manifestation in SCA.
  - This will lead to nocturia and polyuria.
  - Sickling in the vasa rectae interferes with countercurrent exchange in the inner medulla, thereby leading to impairment of free water reabsorption.

  - This defect is reversible by blood transfusions below the age of 10 years but is irreversible in older patients.
  - The net effect is that the maximum urine osmolality at the age 10 years is only 400–450 mosmol/kg, as compared with 900–1200 mosmol/kg in individuals without sickle cell anemia.
- Renal tubular acidosis:
  - Impaired distal hydrogen and potassium secretion can lead to an incomplete form of distal renal tubular acidosis.
  - This can be associated with aldosterone-independent hyperkalemia.
- Abnormal proximal tubular function:
  - The proximal tubular function is supranormal in sickle cell anemia.
  - The reason for this is not known.
  - This may manifest both by hyperphosphatemia (due to increased phosphate reabsorption) and by an elevated creatinine clearance (due to enhanced creatinine secretion) in relation to the true glomerular filtration rate.
  - There is also increased secretion of uric acid in patients with sickle cell anemia.
- Acute kidney injury:
  - The incidence of acute kidney injury in patients with SCA is variable ranging from 5 to 10 %.
  - There are several causes for acute kidney injury among patients with sickle cell anemia. These include:
    - Prerenal failure secondary to intravascular volume depletion
    - Rhabdomyolysis, sepsis, drug nephrotoxicity, renal vein thrombosis, and hepatorenal syndrome (hemosiderosis-induced hepatic failure)
    - Postrenal urinary tract obstruction secondary to blood clots
    - Papillary necrosis
- It is interesting to note that the glomerular filtration rate (GFR) and renal blood flow in patients with renal disease due to sickle cell anemia are age dependent.
- The GFR and renal blood flow are greater than normal in young patients.
- The GFR and renal blood flow are below normal in patients over the age of 30 years.
- The GFR and renal blood flow may progressively fall thereafter, leading to end-stage renal failure.
- This progressive decline in GFR is often associated with increasing proteinuria and evidence of glomerular injury.
- Rarely, these patients may develop nephrotic syndrome due to membranoproliferative glomerulonephritis.
- Renal medullary carcinoma is found almost exclusively in young, black patients with sickle cell trait and, less commonly, sickle cell anemia.
  - Most patients are younger than 20 years of age at presentation.
  - It is more common in males.
  - It may be associated with various chromosomal anomalies.
  - The usual presentation is with:
    - Gross hematuria.
    - Urinary tract infection.

- Flank pain.
- An abdominal mass.
- Weight loss.
- Metastatic disease is commonly present at diagnosis.

- Patients with sickle cell anemia and secondary to impaired immunity are liable to develop urinary tract infection. This can be predisposed to also by papillary necrosis.
- The incidence of hypertension among patients with sickle cell anemia is markedly lower than the general population, and some patients may have lower than normal blood pressure. This is secondary to the following:
  - Sodium and water wasting due to the renal medullary defect
  - Systemic vasodilatation compensating for microcirculatory flow disturbances
  - Increased production of prostaglandins and nitric oxide
  - Reduced vascular reactivity
- It is important to screen these patients regularly to detect early renal disease.
  - The frequency of this is variable depending on the age of the patients.
  - It was suggested that patients with age 5 years or older should be assessed every 4–6 months, and those older than age 18 years are screened every 2–3 months.
  - The assessment includes:
    - Measurement of the serum creatinine.
    - Estimation of glomerular filtration rate.
    - Urinalysis for blood.
    - Determination of urine albumin to creatinine ratio.
    - Microscopic analysis of urine.
    - Blood pressure measurement.
    - Patients with urine albumin to creatinine ratio >300 should be further tested to determine total urine protein or albumin to creatinine ratio.
    - Individuals who have decreased GFR <60 mL/min per 1.73 m^2, hematuria, or increased albumin to creatinine ratio >300 should undergo additional evaluation.

Renal Manifestations of Sickle Cell Anemia

- Hematuria
- Renal infarction and papillary necrosis
- Diminished concentrating ability
- Renal tubular acidosis
- Abnormal proximal tubular function
- Acute kidney injury
- Renal medullary carcinoma
- Nephrotic syndrome
- Urinary tract infection

16.5 Investigations

- Urinalysis
- Measurement of total proteinuria
- BUN, creatinine, and serum electrolytes
- Renal ultrasound
- CT scan for those presenting with hematuria
- Screening for hepatitis B and C and human immunodeficiency virus (HIV)
- A renal biopsy for patients presenting with massive proteinuria or rapidly progressive renal failure
- Renal Doppler sonography resistive index (RI) and pulsatility index (PI)

16.6 Treatment

- Hematuria in patients with sickle cell anemia is self-limiting and should be treated conservatively.
- Bed rest is recommended to avoid dislodging of blood clots.
- Intravenous hydration in severe cases.
- Diuretics to increase urine flow rate. The use of diuretics should be used with caution as they can cause intravascular volume depletion that may precipitate sickle cell crises.
- Simple packed RBC transfusion to increase the hemoglobin and lower the concentration of hemoglobin S.
- Oral urea in doses high enough to raise the blood urea nitrogen (BUN) to 100 mg/dL (36 mmol/L) or higher was used to treat those presenting with hematuria as it inhibits the gelation of deoxygenated sickle hemoglobin.
- Patients with severe, prolonged hematuria can be treated with epsilon-aminocaproic acid. There is, however, a risk of urinary tract obstruction due to the formation of blood clots within the collecting system.
- Angiographic localization and embolization of the involved renal vessel or balloon tamponade.
- Unilateral nephrectomy should be avoided as bleeding can recur in the contralateral kidney.
- Angiotensin converting enzyme (ACE) inhibitors (or angiotensin II receptor blockers [ARBs]) are used to lower protein excretion.
- The addition of hydroxyurea to an ACE or ARB may lead to further reduction of proteinuria.
- Although nonsteroidal anti-inflammatory drugs (NSAIDs) prevent hyperfiltration, they should be avoided since they also reduce renal plasma flow and GFR in patients with sickle cell anemia.
- Hemodialysis for those with end-stage renal disease.
- Renal transplantation for those with end-stage renal disease.

Further Reading

Bayazit AK, Noyan A, Aldudak B, et al. Renal function in children with sickle cell anemia. Clin Nephrol. 2002;57:127.

Falk RJ, Scheinman J, Phillips G, et al. Prevalence and pathologic features of sickle cell nephropathy and response to inhibition of angiotensin-converting enzyme. N Engl J Med. 1992;326:910.

Guasch A, Navarrete J, Nass K, Zayas CF. Glomerular involvement in adults with sickle cell hemoglobinopathies: prevalence and clinical correlates of progressive renal failure. J Am Soc Nephrol. 2006;17:2228.

Halsey C, Roberts IA. The role of hydroxyurea in sickle cell disease. Br J Haematol. 2003;120:177.

Pham PT, Pham PC, Wilkinson AH, Lew SQ. Renal abnormalities in sickle cell disease. Kidney Int. 2000;57:1.

Platt OS, Brambilla DJ, Rosse WF, et al. Mortality in sickle cell disease: life expectancy and risk factors for early death. N Engl J Med. 1994;330:1639–44.

Powars DR, Elliott-Mills DD, Chan L, et al. Chronic renal failure in sickle cell disease: risk factors, clinical course, and mortality. Ann Intern Med. 1991;115:614.

Scheinman JI. Sickle cell disease and the kidney. Nat Clin Pract Nephrol. 2009;5(2):78–88.

17 Priapism and Sickle Cell Anemia

17.1 Introduction

- Sickle cell anemia is a common hemoglobinopathy seen in many parts of the world.
- It is characterized by periods of remissions and exacerbations called crisis. These are secondary to deoxygenation which results in aggregation and polymerization of HbS tetramers in the red blood cells, leading to distortion of the red blood cells forming sickle-shaped red blood cells.
- Sickling of RBC is seen more commonly in areas with low blood flow including the splenic sinusoids, the bone marrow, and the penile corpora during an erection. This will result in a vicious cycle of inflammation, hypoxia, and acidosis resulting in more sickling, vessel occlusion, and ischemia. One of these devastating complications is priapism.
- Priapism is a sustained, painful penile erection in the absence of sexual activity or desire (Figs. 17.1 and 17.2, 17.3 and 17.4, 17.5 and 17.6).
- The exact prevalence of priapism in SCA is not known and ranges from 2 to 35 %.
- It has been estimated that up to 35 % of men with sickle cell anemia are affected by priapism.
- Early recognition and appropriate treatment of priapism in males with SCA is critical, as prolonged and/or repeated attacks of priapism can lead to ischemia and fibrosis in the corpora cavernosa of the penis. This ultimately leads to impaired sexual function and impotence.

17.2 Classification

- Priapism is prolonged painful erection of the penis often starting in the early hours of the morning.

A. Al-Salem, *Medical and Surgical Complications of Sickle Cell Anemia*,
DOI 10.1007/978-3-319-24762-5_17

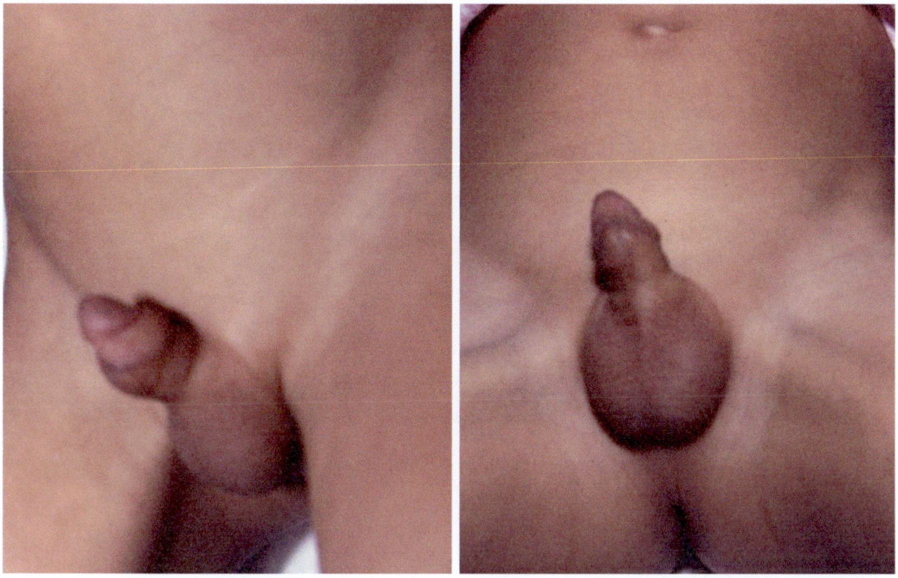

Figs. 17.1 and 17.2 Clinical photographs showing priapism in a child with sickle cell anemia

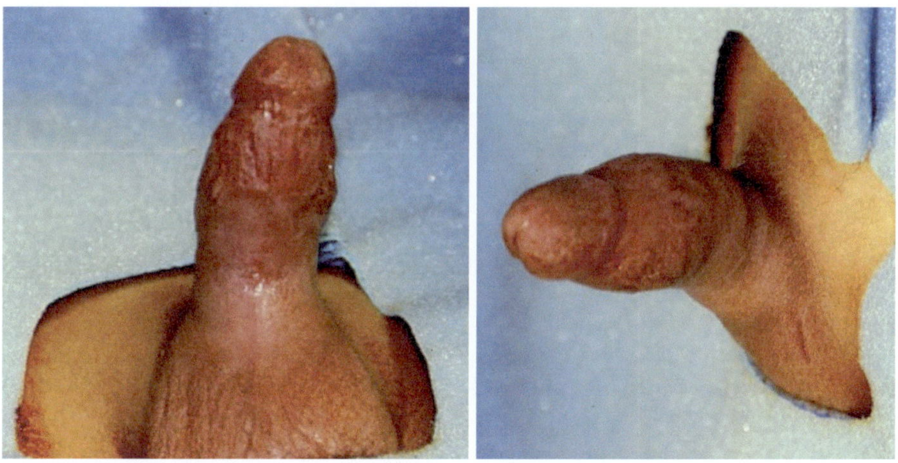

Figs. 17.3 and 17.4 Clinical photographs showing priapism in a child that did not respond to conservative treatment

- Priapism develops when there is excess arterial inflow to the penis or when there is persistent venous outflow obstruction to the penis.
- Priapism is classified into two types:
  - High-flow arterial priapism. This is also called nonischemic priapism.
  - Low-flow priapism. This is also called ischemic priapism.

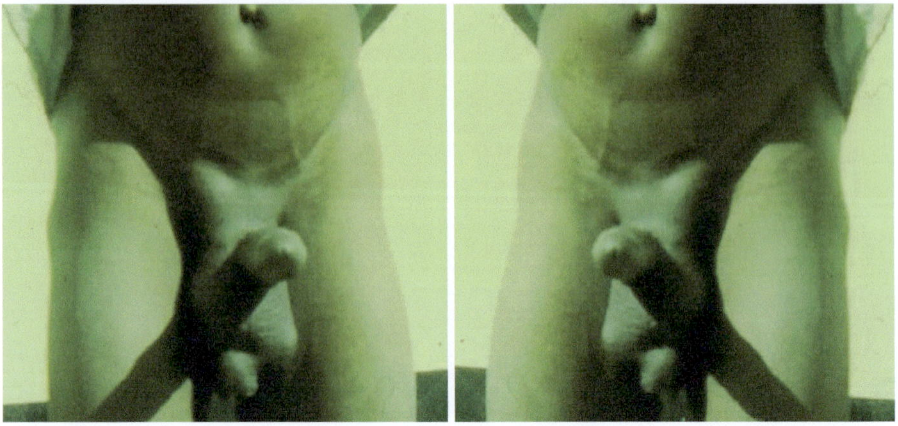

Figs. 17.5 and 17.6 Clinical photographs showing priapism in an adult with sickle cell anemia

- High-flow priapism is usually seen following trauma causing injury to the cavernosal artery.
- The penis in high-flow priapism is neither fully rigid nor painful and does not require an emergency treatment.
- Low-flow priapism is the classic type seen in patients with SCA where there is stasis leading to hypoxia and acidosis of venous blood in a normally erected penis. This will lead to sickling of RBCs within the corpora cavernosa venous sinusoids, venous outflow obstruction, and engorgement of the corpora cavernosa. The corpora spongiosa and glans of the penis are spared.
- The corpora cavernosa becomes rigid and tender to palpation.
- Low-flow priapism is considered a medical and surgical emergency.
- The two types of priapism can be differentiated using color duplex Doppler ultrasonography and analysis of blood aspirated from the corpora cavernosa.
- Color duplex Doppler ultrasonography measures blood flow. This typically shows little or no blood flow in the cavernosal arteries in those with low-flow priapism.
- Analysis of blood aspirated from the corpora cavernosa is done at the time of aspiration and irrigation.
- In patients with high-flow priapism, the aspirated blood is bright red and has a pO_2 >90 % mmHg, pCO_2 <40 mmHg, and a pH of approximately 7.40.
- In patients with low-flow priapism, the aspirated blood is dark in color and has a pO_2 <30 mmHg, pCO_2 >60 mmHg, and a pH <7.25.

• Priapism is also classified in two types:
  - Stuttering priapism: this lasts 2–4 h, often recurrent and may precede a severe attack.
  - Severe priapism: this lasts longer than 4 h and can result in impotence.

17.3 Pathophysiology of Priapism

- Anatomically, the penis is composed of two corpora cavernosa and one corpora spongiosum.
- The two corpora cavernosa are made up of smooth muscles and covered in a tunica albuginea. This is made up of two layers, an inner layer that supports the cavernous tissue and an outer layer that runs longitudinally from the glans to insert onto the pubic rami.
- The inner and outer layers of the tunica albuginea are connected by emissary veins.
- The corpora spongiosum on the other hand has no tunica albuginea and, therefore, serves as an arteriovenous fistula with less rigidity than the corpora cavernosa. The urethra runs within the corpora spongiosum.
- Normally, erection results from corporal smooth muscle relaxation secondary to the release of neurotransmitters.
- The principal neurotransmitter for erection is nitric oxide (NO), which is released by both nerve terminals and endothelial cells. The NO then diffuses into both trabecular cells and arterial smooth muscle cells. This activates guanylate cyclase, which catalyzes the formation of cGMP from GTP, and results in a cascade that decreases intracellular calcium and opens potassium channels to cause smooth muscle relaxation.
- This results in increased blood flow and filling of the corpora cavernosa sinusoids with blood and ultimate compression of venous outflow and trapping of blood.
- Alternative pathways generate cAMP, which enhances this effect.
- Detumescence follows degradation of cGMP and cAMP. cGMP is degraded by phosphodiesterase-5 (PDE5).
- Stasis and low blood flow rates within the sinusoids of the erectile tissue make the penis a site at high risk for developing a veno-occlusive crisis in SCA.
- Typically, in priapism, the corpora cavernosa are tense, congested, and tender to palpation, while the glans and corpus spongiosum are usually soft and uninvolved.
- Classically, in priapism, the primary mechanism is thought to be obstruction of venous drainage resulting in viscous, hypoxic blood leading to interstitial edema and fibrosis of the cavernosa, ultimately resulting in impotence.
- It was shown that the length of time of ischemia directly correlates with the likelihood of return of erectile function, and therefore, ischemic priapism is considered a urologic emergency.
- It was shown that all patients with ischemic priapism episodes of greater than 12 h duration had reduction in erectile function and no patients with priapism lasting greater than 36 h had return of spontaneous erectile function.
- In patients with SCA, several factors contribute to the development of priapism including anatomic factors and a low-flow state.
- In males with SCA, the basic pathology of priapism is venous obstruction of the corpora cavernosa blood flow.
- Recently however it was shown that nitric oxide (NO) plays an important role in the pathogenesis of priapism in these patients.

- RBC hemolysis results in the release of cell-free plasma hemoglobin which scavenges available NO.
- The absence of NO leads to:
  - Increased vascular tone
  - Platelet activation
  - Upregulation of vascular adhesion molecules
- Reduced levels of NO have been implicated in the pathogenesis of pulmonary hypertension, priapism, and leg ulcers in patients with SCA.
- NO is an important smooth muscle relaxant and a potent vasodilator. It mediates this through increasing levels of cyclic GMP (cGMP). This results in smooth muscle relaxation, vasodilatation of penile arteries, increased blood flow, and penile erection. This effect is regulated by phosphodiesterase type 5 (PDE-5) which degrades cGMP.
- SCA patients have elevated free hemoglobin concentrations compared to normal volunteers as a result of hemolysis. This will result in increase in NO scavenging with subsequent prevention of vasodilation.
- Other associated risk factors for priapism include lactate dehydrogenase (LDH), bilirubin, and reticulocyte count which are elevated in patients with SCA and priapism.
- Chronic scavenging of NO results in a decreased expression of downstream regulatory molecules including PDE5 that normally degrades cGMP, the second messenger in NO signaling.
- The combination of chronically decreased PDE5 and normal cGMP generation following nerve stimulation may result in an unregulated, prolonged erection.
- In patients with SCA, there is:
  - Reduction in NO bioavailability.
  - A significant downregulation of PDE-5.
  - Uncontrolled cGMP activity.
  - Elevated levels of adenosine in the penis may also contribute to the pathogenesis of priapism, but this has not been well established.
- Risk factors for priapism in SCA patients include:
  - Prolonged sexual activity
  - Fever
  - Dehydration
  - Exposure to alcohol
  - The use of marijuana
  - The use of cocaine, psychotropic drugs, and testosterone
- Priapism may occur at any age. The mean age of onset is 12–15 years but has been reported in children (Figs. 17.7 and 17.8 and 17.9).
- 70–90 % of affected patients report their first episode prior to 20 years of age.
- The exact prevalence of priapism is not known, but it has been estimated to range from 6 to 45 %.
- Priapism has been reported in various hemoglobinopathies. Commonly it is seen in sickle cell anemia (homozygous sickle cell) but has been reported in patients with hemoglobin SC disease, sickle cell beta-thalassemia, and rarely in those with sickle cell trait.

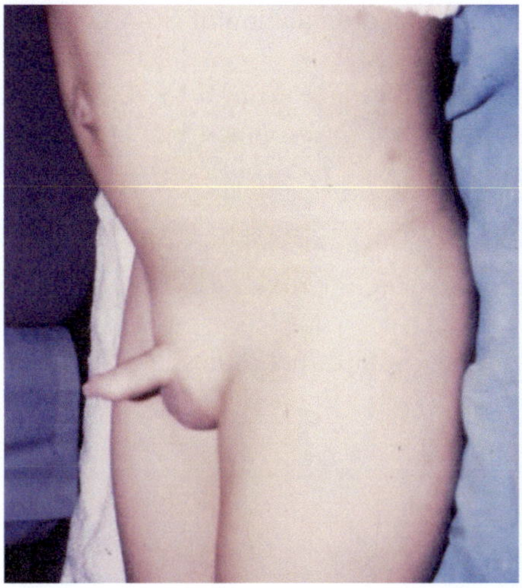

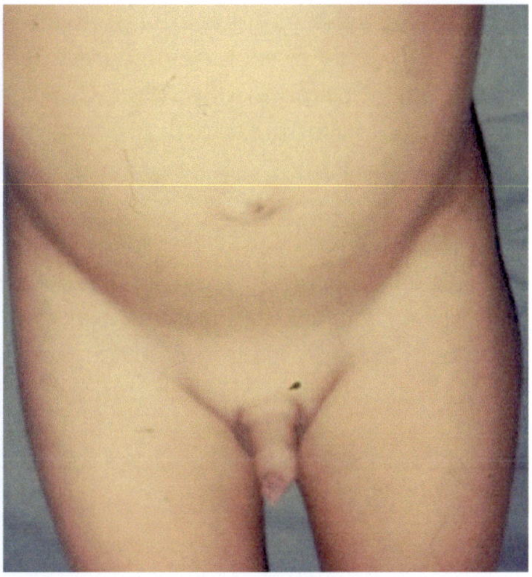

Figs. 17.7 and 17.8 A clinical photograph showing two children with SCA and priapism

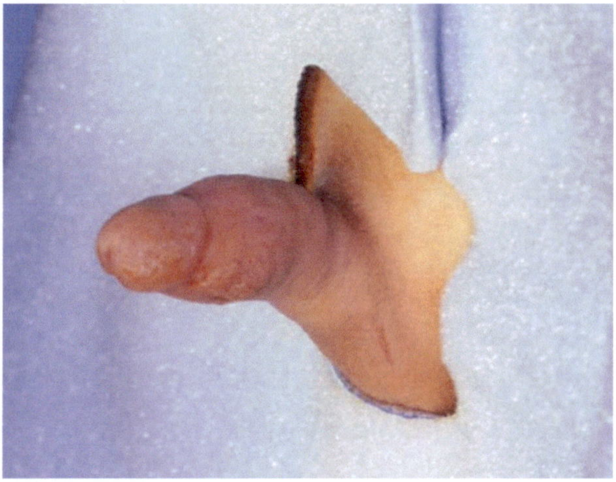

Fig. 17.9 A clinical photograph showing priapism in a child with SCA

17.4 Clinical Features

- Priapism may occur as an isolated episode or as part of generalized SCA vaso-occlusive crisis.
- Priapism may occur also during sleep or following an active sexual intercourse.
- These patients usually present with an erect painful penis, and on palpation, the penis is hard in consistency, while the glans penis is soft.

- Many of these patients are not aware of this as a complication of SCA, and this leads to delay in seeking medical advice.
- The mean duration of symptoms was reported to range from 6 to 70 h (mean 22 h). Some of these patients may resort to sexual intercourse in an attempt to relieve the pain.
- Stuttering priapism:
  - An episode of priapism lasting more than a few minutes but less than 3 h.
  - Stuttering priapism typically occurs in clusters, approximately two to three times per week for several weeks.
  - About 60 % of those who develop stuttering priapism will develop an attack of acute priapism in the future.

17.5 Treatment of Priapism

- There is no well-established treatment protocol of priapism.
- The treatment options depend on the duration of priapism which strongly influences the subsequent development of erectile dysfunction.
- Treatment of priapism <4 h duration:
  - Adequate oral hydration
  - Oral analgesics
  - Attempt to urinate as soon as priapism begins
  - Exercise
  - Warm compressors
  - Masturbation or sexual intercourse
- Treatment of priapism >4 h duration:
  - These patients should be admitted to the hospital and treated in specialized centers with experience in SCA and urologist experience in treating priapism.
  - They should receive intravenous fluid hydration and parenteral analgesia to control pain.
  - This as well as specific treatment which include:
- Exchange blood transfusion:
  - This is done using packed RBCs.
  - This however may be associated with neurological complications including headaches, seizures, and obtundation.
  - These complications may be related to the rapid elevation of Hb to above 12 g/dl and release of procoagulant and vasoactive factors from the corpora cavernosa.
  - To ovoid this, the target of exchange RBC transfusion should be an Hb <10 g/dl and hemoglobin S <50 %.
  - A regular simple packed RBC transfusion was found beneficial for those with stuttering or repeated attacks of priapism. The aim is to reduce HbS level to less than 30 %.

- Aspiration and irrigation of the corpora cavernosa (Figs. 17.10 and 17.11, 17.12, 17.13, and 17.14):
  - This is the standard treatment for priapism lasting more than 4 h.
  - It is done under general anesthesia where aspiration of blood from the corpora is done and irrigation of saline.
  - It can be also done under penile block.
  - Some advocate using alpha- and beta-adrenergic agonists mixed together (epinephrine and etilefrine and the alpha-1 selective adrenergic agonist phenylephrine) into the corpora cavernosa during irrigation.
  - The American Urological Association prefers intracavernous instillation of 1 ml of phenylephrine solution which is diluted with normal saline (100–500 mcg/ml), every 3–5 min, for a total of 3–4 doses. A higher dose of diluted phenylephrine/saline (10 μg/ml) can be used in persistent priapism.
  - Two sizes of 19- or 21-gauge needles are placed through the glans of the penis, one into each corpora cavernosa. One is used for aspiration and the other one is for irrigation.
  - For cases of persistent priapism that are not responding to aspiration and irrigation, a formal surgical shunt procedure should be done.
- Surgical management (Figs. 17.15 and 17.16):
  - This is reserved for those who do not respond after 12 h of first-line treatment (aspiration and irrigation and RBC exchange transfusion).
  - The aim of this is to shunt blood away from the corpora cavernosa to the corpora spongiosum.
  - There are several shunt procedures:
    - Winter or El-Gorab procedure: distal glans-cavernosal shunt. This is the most common procedure.
    - Quackels or Sacher procedure: proximal spongiosal-cavernosal shunt.
    - Grayhack procedure: cavernosal-saphenous shunt.

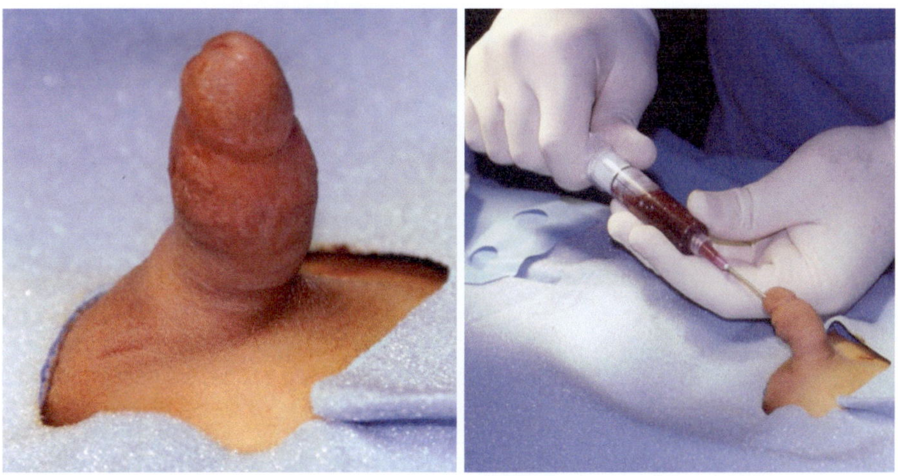

Figs. 17.10 and 17.11 Clinical photographs showing priapism in a child with SCA being treated with aspiration and irrigation

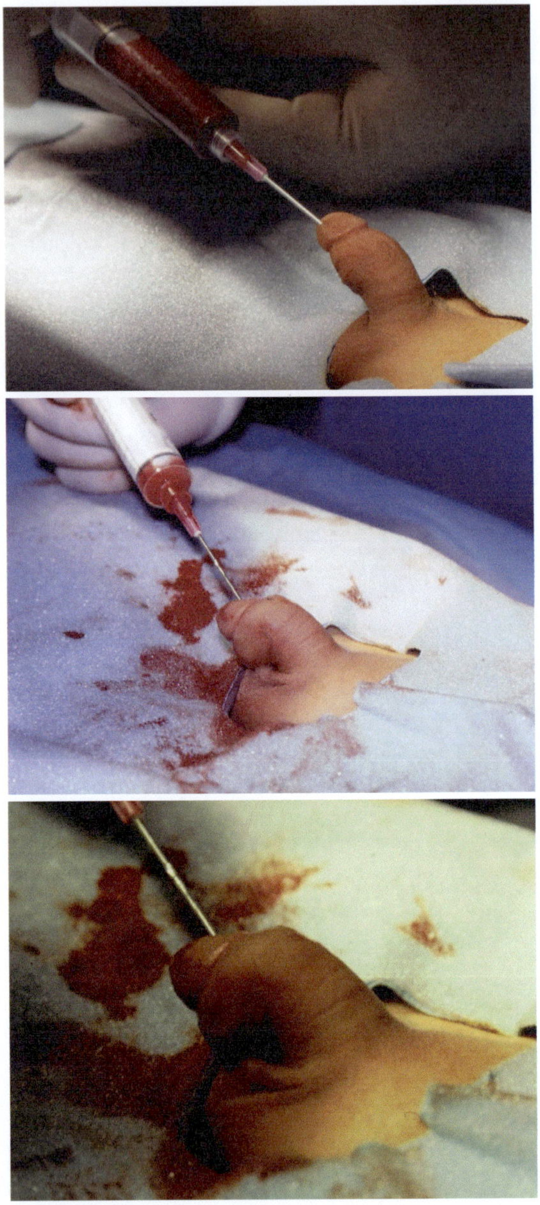

Figs. 17.12, 17.13, and 17.14 Clinical photographs showing priapism in a child with SCA being treated with aspiration and irrigation. Note the response to the treatment with resolution of priapism

- Hydroxyurea:
  - This is used to reduce vaso-occlusive attacks of SCA and to prevent priapism.
  - It has been recommended to those with repeated and stuttering episodes of priapism.
  - Hydroxyurea is given in a daily dose of 10 mg/kg/day, and the dose can be increased up to 30 mg/kg/day as tolerated.

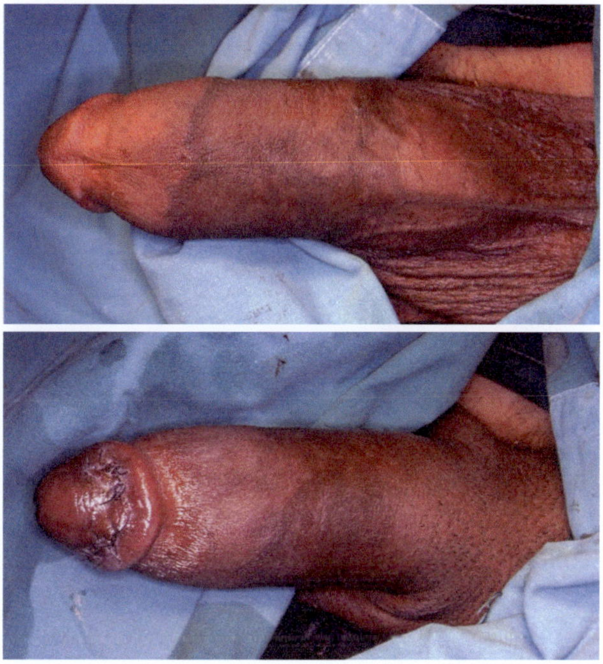

Figs. 17.15 and 17.16 Clinical photograph showing priapism in an adult with SCA being treated with a distal glans-cavernosal shunt

- Drugs and hormonal therapy:
  - Several drugs and hormones (diethylstilbesterol, gonadotropin-releasing hormone, 5-alpha reductase inhibitor, PDE-5 inhibitor) were used to suppress sleep-related erections and so decrease the incidence or prevent priapism.
  - These are however associated with side effects and still no long-term available results.

17.6 Complications of Priapism

- Most episodes of priapism resolve without complications.
- These are usually of short duration.
- Prolonged episodes of priapism on the other hand may lead to fibrotic changes in the corpora cavernosa and subsequently erectile dysfunction.
- These changes are time dependent, and after 24–48 h of priapism, irreversible changes develop leading to erectile dysfunction.
- It has been reported that SCA patients who present with priapism and seek medical advice within 12 h usually retain normal erectile function, while all those who present beyond 36 h after the onset of priapism develop erectile dysfunction.
- If irreversible damage has been done, long-term management of erectile dysfunction may be treated with placement of a penile prosthesis to restore function depending on the preference of the patient.
- A severe and prolonged episode of priapism will result in cavernous smooth muscle necrosis, fibrosis, and ultimately penile shortening. If erectile function is

unlikely to recover, immediate implantation of a penile prosthesis may, therefore, be considered to avoid the complications of penile fibrosis and shortening of the penis.

Further Reading

Adeyoju AB, Olujohungbe ABK, Olujohungbe ABK. Priapism in sickle-cell disease; incidence, risk factors and complications—an international multicentre study. BJU Int. 2002;90(9):898–902.

Bialecki ES, Bridges KR. Sildenafil relieves priapism in patients with sickle cell disease. Am J Med. 2002;113(3):252.

Kato GJ, McGowan V, McGowan V. Lactate dehydrogenase as a biomarker of hemolysis-associated nitric oxide resistance, priapism, leg ulceration, pulmonary hypertension, and death in patients with sickle cell disease. Blood. 2006;107(6):2279–85.

Nolan VG, Wyszynski DF, Farrer LA, Steinberg MH. Hemolysis-associated priapism in sickle cell disease. Blood. 2005;106(9):3264–7.

Rogers ZR. Priapism in sickle cell disease. Hematol Oncol Clin North Am. 2005;19:917.

Salem EA, ElAasser O. Management of ischemic priapism by penile prosthesis insertion: prevention of distal erosion. J Urol. 2010;183:2300–3.

Wen C, Munarriz R, Mcauley I, Goldstein I, Traish A, Kim N. Management of ischemic priapism with high-dose intracavernosal phenylephrine: from bench to bedside. J Sex Med. 2006;3(5):918–22.

18 Perioperative Management of Patients with Sickle Cell Anemia

- Sickle cell anemia (SCA), which is due to homozygous inheritance of the HbS variant, is one of the commonly inherited hemoglobinopathies worldwide.
- Patients with SCA often require operative interventions to treat SCA-related complications.
- This however is associated with an increased risk of perioperative complications particularly vaso-occlusive crisis and acute chest syndrome.
- Anesthesia and surgery are historically associated with an increased incidence of morbidity and mortality.
- Recent multicenter data still found perioperative complications in 22 % of sickle cell patients undergoing elective surgery.
- Optimal surgical outcome requires careful preoperative, intraoperative, and postoperative management by a team consisting of a surgeon, anesthesiologist, and hematologist.
- Acute chest syndrome (ACS) is a well-documented postoperative complication in patients with SCA with an incidence ranging from 0.4 to 10 %.
- The acute chest syndrome can be mild, moderate, or severe (Figs. 18.1, 18.2, and 18.3).
- A high HbF level (HbF level >20 %) has a protective effect and reduces the risk of postoperative ACS.
- For many years, surgery on patients with SCA was associated with an unacceptably high complication rate, sometimes as high as 50 %.
- These complications are part of the disease process and usually develop secondary to intraoperative or immediate postoperative events such as hypoxia, hypovolemia, hypothermia, and acidosis.
- Although these complications can be seen following any operative procedure, they are more commonly seen in those undergoing thoracotomy or laparotomy (Figs. 18.4 and 18.5).
- Nowadays and in spite of better understanding of SCA, improved anesthetic and surgical techniques, and careful perioperative management, the perioperative complication rate in these patients is still high.

A. Al-Salem, *Medical and Surgical Complications of Sickle Cell Anemia*,
DOI 10.1007/978-3-319-24762-5_18

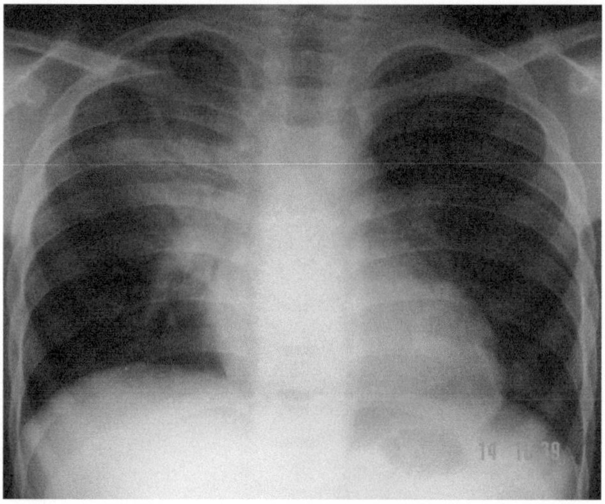

Fig. 18.1 Chest X-ray showing mild postoperative acute chest syndrome

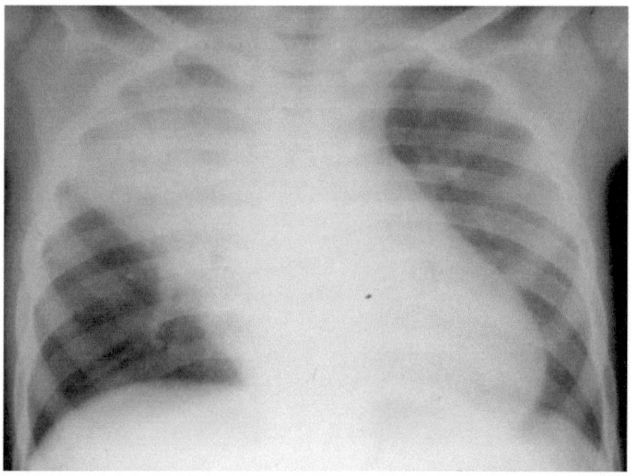

Fig. 18.2 Chest X-ray showing a moderate postoperative acute chest syndrome in patient with sickle cell anemia

- Earlier studies reported a perioperative mortality rate as high as 10 % and a postoperative complication rate of up to 50 %, and because of this unacceptably high complication rate, they advocated against surgery except in symptomatic patients.
- To minimize these risks, a variety of perioperative management protocols, including different preoperative blood transfusion regimens, have been adopted.
- Blood transfusion is considered part of the preoperative management of patients with sickle cell anemia.

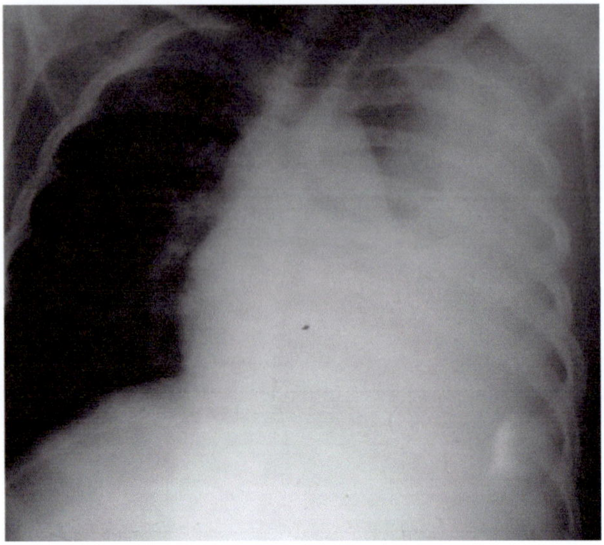

Fig. 18.3 A chest X-ray showing a severe postoperative acute chest syndrome which developed following splenectomy

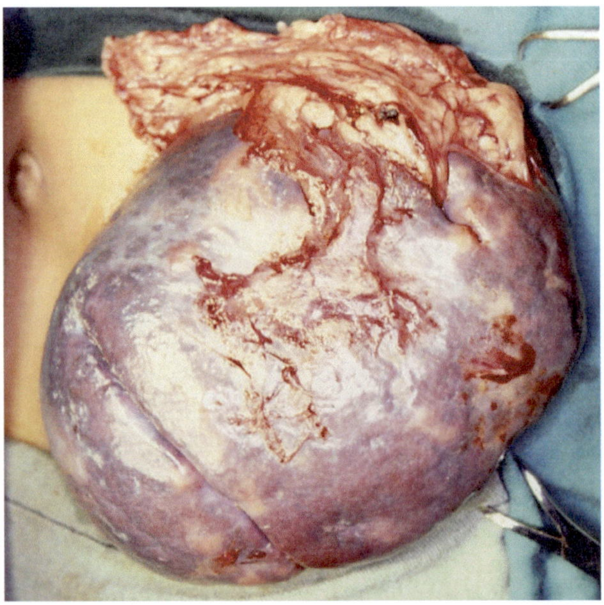

Fig. 18.4 A clinical intraoperative photograph showing laparotomy to remove a large spleen in a child with sickle cell anemia

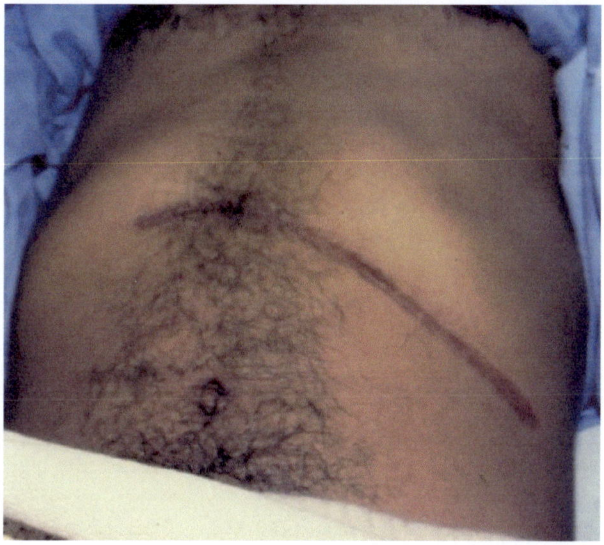

Fig. 18.5 A clinical postoperative photograph showing a large abdominal wound following splenectomy and cholecystectomy. Such a large wound may be complicated by a postoperative acute chest syndrome

- Perioperative blood transfusion to correct the anemia and decrease the percentage of HbS level is beneficial in reducing the rate of SCA-related complications, but the amount of blood transfusion necessary for safe surgery is not known.
- An aggressive blood transfusion regimen to alleviate anemia and reduce HbS level to less than or equal to 30 % was adopted in the past. This is accomplished using either multiple blood transfusions or partial exchange blood transfusion with its attendant risks.
- In a multicenter trial comparing a conservative blood transfusion regimen to increase the Hb level to 10 g/dl to an aggressive blood transfusion regimen designed to lower the HbS level to less than 30 % in a total of 551 patients who underwent 604 operations, the frequency of serious postoperative complications was similar in the two groups, i.e., 35 % in group 1 versus 31 % in group 2. Add to this the fact that the conservative transfusion regimen resulted in only half as many transfusion-related complications. They reported a mortality rate of 0.3 %, and among the serious complications, acute chest syndrome occurred in about 10 % of each group.
- In general, raising the hemoglobin concentration to a level of more than 10 g/dl but less than 12 g/dl provides the patient with approximately 20–30 % hemoglobin A. The presence of this fraction of normal hemoglobin may provide some protection from complications.
- Simple blood transfusion preoperatively to increase the Hb level to 10–12 g/dl was as effective as the traditionally aggressive transfusion therapy or exchange transfusion therapy in reducing postoperative complications in patients with SCA undergoing major surgery.
- Add to this the fact that blood transfusion is not readily available, and in spite of careful blood donor screening, the risk of transmission of blood-borne infections remains a concern in multiple-transfused patients.

- There is also the risk of allosensitization which is reported in 15–20 % of SCA patients, and this increases with the increase in transfusion therapy.
- Whereas preoperative blood transfusion may not be indicated for patients with SCA undergoing minor operative procedures under general anesthesia, blood transfusion is indicated in those undergoing major surgery.
- Simple blood transfusion is as effective as an aggressive transfusion regimen, but the preoperative Hb level is still controversial. A 9–11 g/dl is properly an accepted preoperative Hb level with blood kept ready for possible intraoperative or postoperative blood transfusion.
- This is even so in children undergoing major abdominal surgery. The importance of maintaining an adequate hydration and preventing stimuli for sickling such as hypoxia, hypothermia, acidosis, and stasis intraoperatively cannot be over emphasized.
- More complex operative procedures or operations requiring longer duration of anesthesia times are more likely to lead to acute chest syndrome or other complications. Preoperative blood transfusion in these cases may decrease the risk of postoperative complications.
- It is advocated that patients undergoing complex surgical procedure or operations known to be lengthy should have exchange blood transfusion or erythrocytapheresis to reduce the HbS concentration to 30 %, while keeping the total hemoglobin level at less than 12 g/dl.
- In patients undergoing retinal surgery, brain surgery, cardiac surgery, and vascular surgery, the HbS concentration needs to be reduced to less than 30 %.
- One of the complications of blood transfusion that must be kept in mind is alloimmunization.
- Matching for C, E, Kell, JKB (Kidd), and Fya (Duffy) antigens can significantly reduce alloimmunization.
- In patients with sickle cell anemia, blood transfusion usually consists of:
  - Sickle negative
  - Leuco reduced
  - Phenotypically matched blood for red cell antigens C, E, K, Fy, and Jkb
- Another complication of frequent blood transfusion is iron overload.
- One way to reduce iron overload in those patients receiving exchange blood transfusion is erythrocytapheresis.
- Erythrocytapheresis is an automated red cell exchange procedure that removes blood that contains HbS from the patient while simultaneously replacing that same volume with packed red cells free of HbS.
- Patients with a history of pulmonary or CNS disease, recurrent hospitalization, and/or those who have been previously heavily transfused are at high risk for perioperative complications, especially ASC and vaso-occlusive events.
- Perioperative protocol for patients with SCA undergoing major surgery:
  - Thorough preoperative clinical evaluation.
  - They should be evaluated by the anesthesiologist the day before surgery.
  - Preoperative simple blood transfusion using packed red blood cells to increase the Hb level to 9–11 g/dl.

- Blood transfusion is not necessary in those with a preoperative hemoglobin around 9 g/dl, but blood should be prepared for possible intraoperative or postoperative transfusion.
- Preoperative exchange blood transfusion to lower the percentage of hemoglobin S to less than 30 % is given for certain operations:
  - Neurosurgical operations
  - Cardiac operations
  - Vascular operations
  - Operations on the retina
- Preoperative intravenous hydration. This is started the night before surgery and given at a rate of 1 1/2 their maintenance requirement using either D5% in normal saline or D5% in 1/2 normal saline depending on the age of the patient. This is continued postoperatively till the patient takes adequate oral fluids.
- Intraoperative monitoring, adequate oxygenation, and avoiding hypoxia, hypothermia, and acidosis.
- Postoperative adequate analgesia.
- Early ambulation.
- Chest physiotherapy.

Further Reading

Adams DM, Ware RE, Schultz WH, et al. Successful surgical outcome in children with sickle hemoglobinopathies: the Duke University experience. J Pediatr Surg. 1998;33:428–32.

Bhattacharyya N, Wayne AS, Kevy SV, Shamberger RC. Perioperative management for cholecystectomy in sickle cell disease. J Pediatr Surg. 1993;28:72–5.

Delatte SJ, Hebra A, Tagge EP, et al. Acute chest syndrome in the postoperative sickle cell patient. J Pediatr Surg. 1999;34:188–92.

Griffin TC, Buchanan GR. Elective surgery in children with sickle cell disease without preoperative blood transfusion. J Pediatr Surg. 1993;28:681–5.

Koshy M, Weiner SJ, Miller ST, et al. Surgery and anesthesia in sickle cell disease. Blood. 1995;96:3676–84.

Platt O, Brambilla DJ, Roses WF, et al. Mortality in sickle cell disease: life expectancy and risk factors for early death. N Engl J Med. 1994;330:1639–44.

Rosse WF, Gallagher D, Altman N, et al. Alloimmunization to red blood cell antigens in patients with sickle cell disease, abstracted. Blood. 1985;66:65a.

Scott-Conner CE, Brunson CD. The pathophysiology of the sickle hemoglobinopathies and implications for perioperative management. Am J Surg. 1994;168(3):268–74.

Vichinsky EP, Haberkern CM, Neumayr L, et al. A comparison of conservative and aggressive transfusion regimens in the perioperative management of sickle cell disease. N Engl J Med. 1995;333:206–13.

Recent Advances in the Treatment of Sickle Cell Anemia

19

19.1 Introduction

- Sickle cell anemia is one of the common hemoglobinopathies around the world.
- It results from a single change of one amino acid valine instead of glutamic acid in the sixth position among the 146 amino acids of the beta chain of hemoglobin.
- This change produces abnormally rigid, sickle-shaped red blood cells that hemolyze easily and adhere to each other blocking blood vessels and can lead to life-threatening complications.
- A single change of one amino acid in the hemoglobin beta chain can lead to so much morbidity and sometimes mortality.
- Currently, there is no cure for sickle cell anemia, and for many years, the treatment was symptomatic and directed to relive their pain and anemia. This as well as preventing and treating sickle cell anemia related complications.
- Bone marrow transplantation is the only potential cure for these patients, but this is very expensive and not readily available.
- The treatment of sickle cell anemia is directed:
  - To relieve the pain which is usually secondary to vaso-occlusive crisis
  - To treat associated anemia
  - To prevent infections
  - To prevent and manage various SCA-related complications
- Pain management:
  - Pain is treated depending on its severity.
  - Usually nonsteroidal anti-inflammatory drugs (NSAIDs) are used to treat mild to moderate pain.
  - Sever pain requires the use of opioids.
  - It is important to control the dose of opioids as an overdose can cause respiratory depression and hypoventilation which can be complicated further by atelectasis and acute chest syndrome.

A. Al-Salem, *Medical and Surgical Complications of Sickle Cell Anemia*,
DOI 10.1007/978-3-319-24762-5_19

- It is also important to monitor the use of these strong analgesics as the patients can easily become addicted to them.
- Patient-controlled analgesia is an alternative and effective way to control pain in patients with severe pain.

- Sickle cell anemia patients with high HbF level usually have a milder disease, and it has been suggested that hemoglobin F exhibits its favorable influence through inhibition of hemoglobin S polymerization and thus survival of hemoglobin F containing cells and less sickling.
- It is important to treat these patients at specialized centers with nurses and hematologist experienced in treating sickle cell anemia.
- Antibiotics:
  - Antibiotics are given to treat infections at various sites and also as long-term prophylaxis to infants and children and those who had splenectomy.
  - Penicillin is usually given as a prophylactic antibiotic to prevent infection. It can be given intramuscularly once every 3 weeks or more preferably orally twice daily.
  - The empirical use of antibiotics to treat infections in patients with sickle cell anemia should take in consideration the fact that these patients are prone to develop *Salmonella* infections at various sites. These antibiotics should be broad spectrum and cover *Salmonella* till the result of cultures which must be taken prior to the start of antibiotics.
- Vaccinations:
  - Vaccinations play an important role in the management of patients with sickle cell anemia.
  - All children with sickle cell anemia should receive their normal immunizations regularly.
  - Patients who are going to have splenectomy should be immunized at least 2 weeks before splenectomy for an effective immune response. If splenectomy is performed on an emergency basis, immunization should be given as soon as possible following splenectomy. The immunizations should include:
    - Pneumococcal vaccine
    - Meningococcal vaccine
    - H influenza vaccine
- There are however recent advances in the management of patients with sickle cell anemia. These include:
  - Hydroxyurea
  - Blood transfusion
  - Bone marrow or stem cell transplantation

19.2 Hydroxyurea

- Normally the hemoglobin present in the fetus is called HbF. This is made up of two alfa and two gamma chains ($\alpha_2\gamma_2$).
- This persists in the newborn until about 6 months of age, and subsequently it is replaced by the normal adult hemoglobin.

- The normal adult hemoglobin is made up of two alfa and two beta chains ($\alpha_2\beta_2$).
- In some patients with sickle cell anemia, HbF may persist at higher levels into adulthood.
- Higher levels of fetal hemoglobin in patients with sickle cell anemia were shown to be beneficial, and these patients have a milder disease.
- Fetal hemoglobin production can be reactivated pharmacologically which was shown to be useful in the treatment of sickle cell anemia.
- Hydroxyurea (Droxia) is not a cure for sickle cell anemia but a drug that stimulates the production of HbF.
- Hydroxyurea is recommended to treat adolescents and adults with moderate-to-severe sickle cell anemia. This is defined as a sickle cell crisis occurring three or more times a year.
- Hydroxyurea was shown to reduce the frequency of these attacks and also reduces episodes of acute chest syndrome.
- It is important to know that not all patients with sickle cell anemia respond to hydroxyurea, but the benefits appear to be long lasting.
- There are reports of similar response to hydroxyurea treatment in children with sickle cell anemia, but there are reports of severe side effects, and so it is still being investigated as a therapy for young patients with sickle cell anemia.
- Hydroxyurea however is not without side effects and these include:
  - Constipation
  - Nausea
  - Drowsiness
  - Hair loss
  - Inflammation of the mouth
  - Neutropenia
  - Thrombocytopenia
  - There have been concerns that long-term use of hydroxyurea may increase the risk of developing leukemia, but the significance of this risk remains unclear.
- Hydroxyurea should not be given to pregnant women as it can cause birth defects.

19.3 Blood Transfusion

- The half-life of sickled red blood cells is shorter than normal red blood cells.
- As a result of early red blood cell hemolysis, these patients have chronic anemia, but sometimes excessive hemolysis can lead to acute anemia.
- The normal hemoglobin levels for patients with sickle cell anemia are around 8 g/dL.
- Treating sickle cell-related anemia will improve the low oxygen-carrying capacity caused by the severe anemia, and this in turn will reduce further sickling.
- Blood transfusions are often necessary and form part of the management of patients with sickle cell anemia.
- The indications for blood transfusions in patients with sickle cell anemia can be divided into three main groups:
  - To correct severe anemia

- To treat specific episodes (episodic blood transfusion)
- Chronic transfusion therapy to prevent life-threatening complications

- The aim of blood transfusion should be to increase the hemoglobin level to around 10 g/dL after transfusion.
- A higher Hb level will increase the viscosity of the blood and may precipitate vaso-occlusive crisis.
- Treating severe anemia:
  - In general, patients should be transfused if there is evidence of physiologic derangement, such as heart failure, dyspnea, hypotension, or marked fatigue.
  - There is no universally accepted Hb level at which blood transfusion should be given.
  - A hemoglobin level less than 5 g/dL or a 20 % fall below the baseline during an acute illness is considered common indications for blood transfusion.
  - Simple packed RBC transfusion rather than whole blood is used to treat anemia.
- Episodic blood transfusion:
  - This is indicated to manage sudden acute and severe complications of sickle cell anemia. These include:
    - Acute chest syndrome
    - Stroke
    - Priapism
    - Septicemia
    - Multi-organ failure
    - Acute splenic sequestration crisis
    - Aplastic anemia
    - Preoperative preparation for major surgery
  - Several studies suggested that early transfusion may prevent the progression of acute chest syndrome. For mild cases, simple red blood cell transfusion is used, but in severe cases, exchange blood transfusion/red cell pheresis is recommended.
  - Acute splenic sequestration is a serious complication of sickle cell anemia, and major attacks lead to hypovolemia, cardiovascular decompensation, and death. Early recognition and blood transfusion is important. Since there is hypovolemia, simple packed red blood cell transfusion is recommended. Overtransfusion should be avoided.
  - In patients with severe anemia secondary to excessive hemolysis or aplastic anemia (usually secondary to parvovirus B19 infection), packed red blood cell transfusion is recommended to improve the oxygen-carrying capacity.
  - Acute multi-organ failure is a devastating complication of sickle cell anemia. This is associated with a fall in hemoglobin and platelet count, as well as progressive multi-organ failure. It was suggested that aggressive blood transfusion may improve survival and recovery of organ function.
- Chronic blood transfusion:
  - Chronic blood transfusion was shown to be beneficial in preventing recurrence of serious complications of sickle cell anemia. These include:
    - Stroke
    - Pulmonary hypertension, acute chest syndrome, and chronic lung disease

    - Splenic sequestration crisis
    - Recurrent frequent vaso-occlusive crisis
    - Heart failure
    - Chronic kidney disease
  - The role of blood transfusion in acute stroke is not well established, but it has been suggested that early exchange blood transfusions may improve perfusion and oxygenation to brain tissue, thus limiting damage.
  - It was shown that regular blood transfusion (every 3–4 weeks) can reduce the risk of a first stroke by 90 %.
  - It was also shown that as many as 90 % of patients who have experienced a stroke do not experience another stroke after 5 years of regular blood transfusions.
  - Chronic blood transfusion was also shown to reduce the risk of acute chest syndrome and also splenic sequestration crisis. These however reoccurred when attempts were made to stop the blood transfusion.
- Types of blood transfusions:
  - Blood transfusions may be simple or exchange.
  - Simple blood transfusion:
    - Simple blood transfusions are used to restore blood volume and correct anemia.
    - This involves transfusing packed red blood cells.
    - Simple blood transfusion is used:
      - To correct anemia
      - To treat splenic sequestration crisis
      - To treat acute chest syndrome
      - To prepare patient for major surgery
  - Exchange blood transfusion:
    - Exchange blood transfusion involves drawing out the patient's blood while exchanging it for donor red blood cells.
    - It can be done as manual procedure or as automatic one called erythrocytapheresis.
    - Exchange blood transfusions are used in severe complications of sickle cell anemia including:
      - Stroke
      - Severe acute chest syndrome
      - Priapism not responding to simple blood transfusion
      - Preoperative preparation for certain operations (neurosurgical operations, cardiac operations, vascular operation, operations on the retina)
    - In children, a practical estimate of the volume required for exchange blood transfusion is 50–60 mL/kg.
    - In adults, blood can be removed from the patient in 500 mL aliquots, followed by infusion of 500 mL of reconstituted blood. This may be repeated for 6–8 units of blood transfusion.
    - Alternatively, the following technique can be used:
      - Bleed 1 unit (500 mL) of blood from the patient and infuse 500 mL of saline.

- Bleed a second unit from the patient and infuse 2 units of blood.
- Repeat steps 1 and 2; if the patient has a large red blood cell mass, repeat once more.

- Complications of blood transfusions:
  - Repeated and chronic blood transfusion is not without complications. These must be borne in mind and every effort should be made to reduce them.
  - These complications include:
    - Iron overload.
    - Alloimmunization.
    - Blood-borne infections including hepatitis B, hepatitis C, and HIV.
    - Hyperviscosity and volume overload.
    - Acute hemolytic transfusion reactions occur primarily with major blood group (ABO) mismatches and must be treated aggressively to maintain blood pressure and glomerular filtration.
  - Iron overload is known to increase the risk of damage to the liver, heart, and other organs.
  - Iron overload once detected, usually by a liver biopsy, should be treated with chelation therapy.
  - In the past, deferoxamine (Desferal) was the treatment of choice and must be given by a pump and for 12 h each day.
  - Currently, deferasirox (Exjade), an oral chelating therapy, is used which made it much easier for these patients.
  - Alloimmunization was reported to occur in 5–20 % of sickle cell anemia patients who received regular blood transfusion.
  - Careful screening and matching of donor blood groups before the transfusion is important in this regard as alloimmunization can be life-threatening. Add to this the fact that once alloimmunization develops, it may be difficult to find blood that is suitable to be transfused to the patient on an emergency basis.
  - It is recommended that all sickle cell anemia patients should receive limited blood phenotypic matching for antigens E, C, and Kell. Extensive phenotypic matching is recommended for patients who have formed alloantibodies.
  - Hyperviscosity develops in patients who are overtransfused leading to adherence of normal red blood cells and cells containing HbS. This will lead to increase in blood pressure, altered mental status, seizures, and increased risk of vaso-occlusive crisis.
  - One of the serious complications of blood transfusion is transmission of blood-borne diseases. These include:
    - Hepatitis B
    - Hepatitis C
    - Malaria
    - HIV
    - Other blood-borne viral diseases
  - To avoid this, it is important to screen all donors' blood prior to transfusion.

19.4 Bone Marrow or Stem Cell Transplantation

- For many years, there was no cure for sickle cell anemia.
- At this time, the only chance for cure for sickle cell anemia is bone marrow or stem cell transplantation.
- Transplantation of a healthy bone marrow from a genetically matched donor after destroying the sickle cell patient's diseased bone marrow and stem cells leads to the production of new normal red blood cells.
- With the recent advances in bone marrow transplant, it has been reported that up to 80–85 % of patients who receive a bone marrow transplant remain disease-free.
- Criteria for bone marrow transplant for patients with sickle cell anemia:
  - Age 16 or younger (patients in their 20s have had successful transplants also)
  - Severe symptoms but no long-term organ or neurologic damage
  - A genetically matched brother or sister who will donate their marrow
- Bone marrow transplant, however, carries a significant number of complications.
  - About 10 % of those who receive bone marrow transplants die from the treatment.
  - A graft-versus-host disease (GVHD).
  - Bleeding.
  - Pneumonia.
  - Severe infection.
  - Long-term complications from the drugs used in transplantation.
  - An increased risk for cancer and infertility.
- The umbilical cord blood and cells from placentas are another source for healthy stem cells to patients who do not have genetically matched donors for bone marrow transplant.
- The cord blood has the capacity to produce more cells quickly, and the risk and severity of graft-versus-host disease may be reduced.
- Partial chimerism:
  - This uses a mixture of the patient's and a donor's bone marrow instead of total bone marrow transplantation.
  - The procedure has fewer side effects.
  - Although some sickle blood cells remain, the patients have very mild symptoms and are free of infections and severe vaso-occlusive crisis.

19.5 Gene Therapy

- Sickle cell anemia affects millions of people worldwide.
- The only permanent cure for sickle cell anemia is a successful bone marrow transplant.
- Bone marrow transplant, however, is expensive, and the lack of compatible donors makes it a very limited option.
- Treating sickle cell anemia patients with hydroxyurea encourages the formation of fetal hemoglobin which is known to alleviate disease symptoms.

- Recently, there is progress in research for possible cure for sickle cell anemia using gene transfer to permanently increase fetal hemoglobin levels.
- This depends on a technique to insert the gene for gamma-globin into blood-forming cells using a harmless viral carrier. It is hoped that those cells would permanently generate red blood cells containing fetal hemoglobin, which alleviate the disease.
- These results are encouraging, and hopefully it will be possible to correct sickle cell anemia with genetic therapy to produce fetal hemoglobin.

19.6 Family Counseling

- Sickle cell anemia is an autosomal recessive disorder that is transmitted from parents to children.
- One way to prevent it is to council patients prior to marriage and do an electrophoresis for each of them to determine whether there are diseased or carriers. This is important for the carriers who are usually asymptomatic.
- This is important in areas known to have a high frequency of sickle cell anemia.
- A couple who are both sicklers (homozygous SS) should not get married as there is 100 % chance that their children will have sickle cell anemia.
- If one of the couple is a sickler (homozygous SS) and the other has sickle cell trait (heterozygous AS), then there is a chance that 50 % of their children will be sicklers and the other 50 % will have sickle cell trait. These also should not get married from each other.
- If one of the couple is a sickler (homozygous SS) and the other is normal (AA), there is 100 % chance that all their children will be carriers. These can get married to each other as none of their children will have sickle cell anemia.
- If both couples are carriers (heterozygous AS), there is 50 % chance that their children will have sickle cell anemia and so should not get married.
- This pre-marriage testing and counseling is important in diluting the sickle cell gene and decreasing the frequency of those affected.
- In Saudi Arabia, there was a royal decree stating that marriage arrangers (the religiously appointed, equivalent of the registrar of marriages) should require testing for sickle cell anemia and provide basic genetic counseling for those with positive results.
- A similar program was adapted in the Kingdom of Bahrain since 1993, and as a result of this, the annual births of children with sickle cell anemia decreased by 60 % from 2.1 to 0.9 %.

Further Reading

Adams RJ, McKie VC, Hsu L, et al. Prevention of a first stroke by transfusions in children with sickle cell anemia and abnormal results on transcranial Doppler ultrasonography. N Engl J Med. 1998;339:5–11.

Brittenham GW, Cohen AR, McLaren CE, et al. Hepatic iron stores and plasma ferritin concentration in patients with sickle cell anemia and thalassemia major. Am J Hematol. 1993;42:81–5.

Cox JV, Steane E, Cunningham G, Frenkel EP. Risk of alloimmunization and delayed hemolytic transfusion reactions in patients with sickle cell disease. Arch Intern Med. 1988;148:2485–9.

Emre U, Miller ST, Gutierez M, Steiner P, Rao SP, Rao M. Effect of transfusion in acute chest syndrome of sickle cell disease. J Pediatr. 1995;127:901–4.

Hasan MF, Marsh F, Posner G, et al. Chronic hepatitis C in patients with sickle cell disease. Am J Gastroenterol. 1996;91:1204–6.

Kim HC, Dugan NP, Silber JH, Martin MB, Schwartz E, Ohene-Frempong K, Cohen AR. Erythrocytapheresis therapy to reduce iron overload in chronically transfused patients with sickle cell disease. Blood. 1994;83:1136–42.

Rosse WF, Gallagher D, Kinney TR, et al. Transfusion and alloimmunization in sickle cell disease. The Cooperative Study of Sickle Cell Disease. Blood. 1990;76:1431–7.

Silliman CC, Peterson VM, Mellman DL, Dixon DJ, Hambidge KM, Lane PA. Iron chelation by desferrioxamine in sickle cell patients with severe transfusion-induced hemosiderosis: a randomized, double-blind study of the dose-response relationship. J Lab Clin Med. 1993;122:48–54.

Singer ST, Quirolo K, Nishi K, Hackney-Stephens E, Vichinsky E. Erythrocytapheresis for chronically transfused children with sickle cell disease: an effective method for maintaining a low hemoglobin S level and reducing iron overload. J Clin Apher. 1999;14:122–5.

Vichinsky EP, Haberkern CM, Neumayr L, et al. A comparison of conservative and aggressive transfusion regimens in the perioperative management of sickle cell disease. The Preoperative Transfusion in Sickle Cell Disease Study Group. N Engl J Med. 1995;333:206–13.

Wang WC, Kovnar EH, Tonkin IL, et al. High risk of recurrent stroke after discontinuance of five to twelve years of transfusion therapy in patients with sickle cell disease. J Pediatr. 1991;81:1109–23.

20 Blood Transfusion Therapy for Patients with Sickle Cell Anemia

20.1 Introduction

- Sickle cell anemia is an inherited hemoglobinopathy that causes acute and chronic hemolytic anemia.
- Patients with sickle cell anemia have a variable Hb level that may range from 7.0 to 11.0 g/dL in their steady-state condition.
- This however may decrease as a result of several sickle cell anemia-related complications.
- Blood transfusion should be aimed to increase tissue delivery of oxygen.
- Blood transfusion however is not totally safe and short- or long-term complications may occur.
- In patients with SCA, blood transfusion has several advantages:
  - Raises the hemoglobin level for oxygen delivery
  - Lowers the percentage of sickle Hgb (HgbS)
  - Decreases the propensity for vaso-occlusion
  - Suppression of erythropoietin release caused by the rise in Hgb, thereby reducing the production of new HgbS-containing cells
  - Increases in Hgb oxygen saturation levels by approximately 1–6 %, which increases oxygen delivery to the tissues
- The indications of blood transfusion in patients with sickle cell anemia are variable and include acute hemolytic, aplastic, or sequestration crises.
- Chronic blood transfusion is indicated in cases of strokes or high cerebral blood flow on skull Doppler ultrasonic studies, recurrent acute chest syndrome, and recurrent splenic sequestration crisis.
- Exchange blood transfusion is indicated in severe acute chest syndrome (ACS), priapism, or perioperatively.
- Once it is decided to transfuse blood, the transfused blood should be Hb S negative and Rh and Kell antigen matched.

A. Al-Salem, *Medical and Surgical Complications of Sickle Cell Anemia*,
DOI 10.1007/978-3-319-24762-5_20

- Used correctly, blood transfusion can be life-saving and prevent progressive organ damage in patients with sickle cell anemia.
- In patients with sickle cell anemia, blood transfusions are indicated for either episodic events triggered by an acute complication or in the form of chronic blood transfusion therapy.
- Several methods of transfusion are available, including simple blood transfusion, partial exchange transfusion, or erythrocytapheresis.
- The method used depends on the specific indications.
- Fresh blood (less than 3 days old) should be used in exchange transfusions done to improve oxygen delivery because of hypoxia.
- Patients with a history of alloimmunization should be given as few transfusions as possible and phenotypically matched units if practical.
- These patients must carry a record of all documented alloantibodies and show it to any physician contemplating giving them blood transfusion.
- Patients with a history of febrile transfusion reactions should be given leukocyte-depleted units and may be pretreated with acetaminophen and antihistamines if necessary.
- Hyperviscosity from simple transfusion is a dangerous complication in patients with sickle cell anemia and must be avoided. The posttransfusion hematocrit should not exceed 36 %.
- In general, limited phenotypically matched, sickle-negative, leukocyte-depleted packed cells are the blood product of choice to be transfused to patients with sickle cell anemia.
- A comprehensive transfusion protocol should be established for each patient receiving blood transfusion that includes:
  - Accurate medical records
  - The patient's red cell phenotype
  - Alloimmunization history
  - The number of units of blood received
  - Serial hemoglobin S percentages
  - Results of acquired infections
  - Iron overload monitoring results
- There are a number of important complications that may occur with transfusion. These include:
  - Volume overload
  - Alloimmunization
  - Iron overload
  - Exposure to infectious agents
- Identification bracelets should provide information regarding alloantibodies, and the number of blood transfusions is important in sensitized patients.
- Screening for alloantibodies 6–8 weeks after transfusion will document new antibodies that may disappear if there is a prolonged interval without transfusion but still cause delayed transfusion reactions if further transfusions are required.

20.2 Indications for Blood Transfusion

- The two primary goals of blood transfusion are:
  - To correct the low oxygen-carrying capacity caused by severe anemia
  - To improve microvascular perfusion by decreasing the proportion of sickle red cells in the circulation
- The indications for blood transfusion therapy for patients with SCA are divided into two major attacks:
  - Therapeutic
  - Prophylactic/preventive

20.3 Indications for Episodic Blood Transfusion

- Management of severe anemia
  - In severely anemic patients, simple blood transfusions should be used.
  - Packed red blood cell transfusion should be used to avoid volume overload.
  - Patients should be transfused if there is evidence of physiologic derangement, such as heart failure, dyspnea, hypotension, or marked fatigue. Their symptoms may include tachycardia, postural hypotension, dizziness, mental status change, dyspnea, or congestive heart failure.
  - Hemoglobin values of less than 5 g/dL or a 20 % fall below the baseline during an acute illness is indications for blood transfusion.
- Acute splenic sequestration crisis:
  - Major acute splenic sequestration crisis produces hypovolemia and cardiovascular decompensation as a result of pooling of blood into the splenic sinusoids.
  - These patients require immediate blood transfusion to prevent cardiovascular collapse.
  - In general, blood transfusions are indicated when the hemoglobin drops by more than 2 g/dL from the steady state.
  - The rise in hemoglobin following blood transfusion is usually greater than expected as a result of release of sequestered red cells from the spleen.
- Transient red cell aplasia (aplastic crisis):
  - Parvovirus B19 is the primary cause of transient red cell aplasia.
  - Severe anemia develops over a few days secondary to shortened red cell survival without compensatory production of new red cells.
  - While many patients recover spontaneously, red cell transfusions are indicated for those who become symptomatic or whose hemoglobin value falls 2 g/dL below baseline.
- Hyperhemolysis:
  - This is associated with infection, acute chest syndrome, and particularly malaria.

  - Acute chest syndrome, stroke, sepsis, and acute multi-organ failure are leading causes of death in sickle cell disease.
  - A falling hemoglobin value often accompanies these events.
  - Transfusions to improve tissue oxygenation and perfusion are indicated in these seriously ill patients.
  - Acute chest syndrome:
    - When acute chest syndrome is associated with hypoxia and a falling hemoglobin, transfusions are indicated.
    - Early transfusion may prevent the progression of acute chest syndrome.
    - Many patients with acute chest syndrome can be treated with a simple red cell transfusion.
    - In severe cases of acute chest syndrome, exchange blood transfusion/red cell pheresis is recommended.
  - Stroke:
    - Chronic transfusion therapy reduces the rate of recurrent vaso-occlusive stroke.
    - The efficacy of transfusion in the management of acute stroke has not been well studied, but early exchange transfusions may improve perfusion and oxygenation to brain tissue.
  - Management of multi-organ failure:
    - Acute multi-organ failure is a devastating complication of sickle cell anemia.
    - This is usually associated with falling hemoglobin and platelet count, as well as progressive multi-organ failure.
    - Aggressive blood transfusion may improve survival and recovery of organ function.
- Preparation for general anesthesia:
  - Individuals with SCA have a high frequency of serious perioperative complications, some of which may be ameliorated by preoperative RBC transfusion.
  - All sickle cell anemia patients undergoing major surgery should be prepared in advance with simple blood transfusion to correct their anemia to a hemoglobin of approximately 10 g/dL and hemoglobin S percent to approximately 60 %. This simple blood transfusion uses packed RBCs.
  - Indications for preoperative blood transfusion:
    - Preoperative transfusion is the standard of care in children and adults with sickle cell anemia undergoing major surgery.
    - Preoperative transfusion may not be necessary in children and adults undergoing elective, minor, low-risk surgery.
    - Regardless of blood transfusion or type of surgical procedure, attention to the following is necessary to minimize surgical risks:
      - Preoperative hydration
      - Incentive spirometry
      - Optimal management of reactive airway or other underlying chronic lung disease

    - Maintenance of oxygenation during postoperative sedation
    - Avoiding hypoxia, hypothermia, hypercarbia, and acidosis
    - Adequate analgesia
    - Early mobilization
  - Patients undergoing high-risk surgery (cardiovascular, ophthalmic, vascular, or brain surgery) are given preoperative exchange blood transfusion with the aim of lowering HgbS concentration of <30 %.
  - The optimal preoperative transfusion for children and adults with HbSS who are scheduled to undergo major surgery is to give simple blood transfusion to increase the Hgb to 10 g/dL, rather than an aggressive exchange transfusion regimen to reduce the HgbS concentration in the perioperative period.
  - Compared with an aggressive regimen, a conservative approach provides equivalent outcomes, similar rates of major complications, and fewer transfusion-related complications. The aggressive blood transfusion was, however, associated with increased risk of alloimmunization.
  - Minor surgery not requiring prolonged general anesthesia is not an indication for blood transfusion.
- Acute chest syndrome:
  - Transfusion is an important component of the management of acute chest syndrome (ACS), which is one of the most common causes of mortality in patients with SCA.
  - The use of simple versus exchange blood transfusion depends on:
    - The severity and rate of clinical decline in pulmonary function
    - The corresponding increased need for respiratory support
  - In general, exchange blood transfusion rather than simple blood transfusion is required for those with more severe decline in respiratory function (e.g., rapid increase in oxygen requirement or work of breathing over the course of hours, along with abnormalities on chest radiography and declining oxygen saturation).
  - Transfusion can also be used as an adjunct to other measures (e.g., control of asthma, which is the greatest risk factor for ACS) to prevent ACS.
  - Blood transfusions are advocated for patients who continue to have episodes of ACS despite hydroxyurea therapy.
  - For children, prophylactic, regularly scheduled blood transfusions should be given if there are repeated episodes of severe acute chest syndrome despite hydroxyurea therapy and optimal management of asthma.
  - Short-term therapy (e.g., less than 6 months) is often used during high-risk periods, such as winter months, with increased frequency of respiratory illness, or during transition to hydroxyurea therapy.
  - Long-term therapy (greater than 6 months) is used for children with year-round severe ACS episodes.
  - Prophylactic, regularly scheduled blood transfusions are given if there have been two or more episodes of moderate to very severe ACS in the past 24 months despite maximal hydroxyurea therapy.

- Exchange blood transfusions either manually or by automated apheresis is given every 4–6 weeks to maintain a maximum HgbS percentage <30 %.
- Chronic transfusion therapy is continued for 1–2 years. Thereafter, the decision to continue transfusion therapy is based on a reexamination of the risk-to-benefit ratio accounting for factors such as iron overload, alloimmunization, and recent clinical course.

Definite Indications for Blood Transfusion

- Acute neurologic event (stroke)
- Acute splenic sequestration
- Severe pneumonia or pulmonary infarction (acute chest syndrome)
- Severe anemia with cardiac decompensation
- Acute arterial hypoxia
- Aplastic crisis with severe anemia
- Hyperhemolytic crisis
- Preoperative preparation for major surgery including ophthalmological surgery, cardiac surgery, and neurosurgery
- Multi-organ failure

20.4 Chronic Blood Transfusion Therapy

- Chronic blood transfusion therapy programs are indicated for several conditions in patients with sickle cell anemia.
- The goal is to maintain the hemoglobin S at 30–50 %, depending on the specific indication.
- Blood transfusions are usually given every 3–4 weeks.
- Simple blood transfusions can be used.
- Red cell pheresis-exchange transfusions are recommended to decrease iron overload.
- Primary stroke prevention:
  - Chronic blood transfusion therapy reduces the occurrence of first stroke in children with a rate of high blood flow through the circle of Willis cerebral arteries, as measured by Doppler ultrasonography.
- Prevention of recurrence of stroke:
  - Stroke is a leading cause of death in SCA, and stroke prevention is one of the major goals of comprehensive care for individuals with SCA.
  - The approaches to primary stroke prevention include:
    - Screening by transcranial Doppler
    - Prophylactic regularly scheduled transfusion for those with abnormal flow velocity
  - Secondary stroke prevention:
    - Chronic exchange blood transfusion, with a goal of reducing the maximum fraction of HgbS to <30 % of total Hgb and maintaining the total Hgb >9 g/dL

  - Chronic blood transfusion therapy for children who suffer vaso-occlusive stroke decreases the recurrent stroke rate from 90 % to less than 10 %.
  - Initially, the hemoglobin S level is maintained at 30 % or less for approximately 5 years.
- Pulmonary hypertension and chronic lung disease:
  - Chronic blood transfusion therapy has been used to decrease the recurrence of acute chest syndrome.
  - Patients with proven pulmonary hypertension and chronic lung disease should receive long-term chronic blood transfusion therapy.
- Vital organ failure:
  - Transfusion therapy for patients with chronic heart failure, along with interventions to improve cardiac function, enhances quality of life.
  - Severe anemia, secondary to chronic renal failure, often becomes debilitating, necessitating chronic blood transfusion.
- Chronic debilitating pain:
  - A small percentage of patients with sickle cell anemia suffer from unusually protracted and severe pain episodes.
  - These patients have a very poor quality of life and are unable to carry ordinary daily activities.
  - Chronic blood transfusions are beneficial in these patients.
  - Children generally respond better to chronic transfusions than adults do.

20.5 Controversial Indication for Blood Transfusions

- Acute priapism:
  - In priapism, the initial management is conservative, but if this fails, blood transfusions should be considered.
  - Exchange blood transfusions have been advocated for the management of acute priapism not responding to conservative management.
  - It is well known that recurrent priapism often produces impotence.
  - Chronic blood transfusion therapy is advocated for those with recurrent priapism in an effort to prevent impotence.
  - The aim is to maintain hemoglobin S below 30 % for 6–12 months.
- Pregnancy:
  - In the past, blood transfusion therapy was recommended for sickle cell patients because of poor pregnancy outcome.
  - With improved prenatal care, the benefit of blood transfusion therapy is questionable.
  - Currently, blood transfusion therapy is advocated for women who experience frequent complications during pregnancy.
- Management of "silent" cerebral infarct and/or neurocognitive damage:
  - Subclinical infarcts detected by magnetic resonance technology are often associated with neurocognitive defects.
  - These patients appear to be at higher risk of future stroke.

  - Routine chronic transfusion therapy may prove beneficial in these patients by decreasing the risk of subsequent stroke.
- Leg ulcers:
  - These ulcers are difficult to treat in patients with sickle cell anemia.
  - Blood transfusions should be considered in those with recurrent skin ulcers or poorly healing ulcers after failure of conservative therapy.

Relative Indications for Blood Transfusion

- Symptomatic anemia
- Hepatic sequestration
- Leg ulcers refractory to conservative treatment
- Priapism not responding to acute treatment
- Recurrent severe or prolonged pain crisis
- Frequent painful crisis
- Chronic respiratory insufficiency
- High-dose intravenous contrast studies
- High-risk pregnancy

Blood Transfusions Are Not Usually Indicated in the Following Conditions

- Stable chronic anemia
- Painful crisis without absolute or relative indications
- Minor surgery under local or short general anesthesia
- Uncomplicated infections
- Chronic bone disease or organ failure without other indications

20.6 Recommendations for Blood Transfusion

- Standard bank blood is appropriate to be transfused for patients with sickle cell anemia.
- The blood to be used should be not too old and within the set time limit.
- For exchange blood transfusion, the blood should be less than 5 days old.
- All blood to be used should be negative for sickle cell.
- These patients should have red blood cell (ABO, Rh, Kell, Duffy, Kidd, Lewis, Lutheran, P, and MNS groups) antigenic phenotype determined.
- All patients with a history of prior transfusion should be screened for the presence of alloantibodies.
- To limit alloimmunization, all patients should receive blood with limited phenotypic matching for antigens E, C, and Kell. Extensive phenotypic matching is recommended for patients who have already formed alloantibodies.
- The efficacy of a chronic transfusion regimen should be assessed periodically by determining the proportion of hemoglobin S.

20.7 Transfusion Precautions

- Most patients with SCA will receive multiple transfusions over their lifetimes and are thus at risk for transfusion complications.
- To minimize these complications, unnecessary blood transfusions should be avoided.
- Blood to be transfused should be matched for minor RBC antigens (C, E, and Kell) to reduce the risk of alloimmunization.
- Some blood banks also match RBC units for additional minor antigens, such as Duffy, Kidd, and S.
  - Alloimmunization due to minor RBC antigen mismatch is of greater concern in patients with SCA because they may require ongoing transfusions throughout their lifetimes.
  - Alloimmunization to minor RBC antigens can be associated with vaso-occlusive episodes and life-threatening hemolysis.
  - Alloimmunization can result in a greater risk of future transfusion reactions and greater difficulty identifying compatible units of blood for these patients.
- Use a white blood cell filter (leukoreduction) to decrease the rate of febrile nonhemolytic transfusion reactions. Leukoreduction removes most of the white blood cells present in the unit of RBCs, by passing the blood through a filter.
- Use chelation therapy if iron stores reach a high threshold.
- Screen for and use sickle cell trait-negative blood.
- Central venous catheters are frequently required for patients with SCA who receive chronic transfusions. This, however, is associated with risks of infection and thrombosis.

20.8 Types of Blood Transfusions

- Simple blood transfusions:
  - Simple blood transfusions using packed red blood cells can be used to treat acute anemia or hypovolemia.
  - Simple blood transfusion involves transfusion of 1 or more units of blood without removal of the patient's blood.
  - Simple blood transfusions may provide sufficient increase in hemoglobin (Hgb) to increase the oxygen-carrying capacity in the setting of severe anemia.
  - In individuals with severe anemia (i.e., Hgb <5 g/dL), simple blood transfusion may also be effective in lowering the HgbS level without increasing the red cell viscosity.
  - Simple blood transfusion is indicated in the following situations:
    - An uncomplicated drop in Hgb levels resulting in signs or symptoms of decreased oxygen delivery (e.g., tachycardia, hypotension, mild respiratory distress).

    - If the Hgb is <5 g/dL and the patient is critically ill, simple blood transfusion can be used to increase the Hgb level to 10–11 g/dL.
    - Preoperative transfusion to reduce complications of major surgery.
  - Simple blood transfusions can cause hyperviscosity syndrome in children or adults with SCA because they raise the Hgb but only marginally lower the percentage of HgbS. The higher HgbS levels that remain following simple transfusion contribute significantly to higher blood viscosity. This must be kept in mind and overtransfusion should be avoided.
  - Central nervous system hyperviscosity can cause signs of acute neurologic injury and can be associated with central venous thrombosis or cerebral infarcts.
- Chronic simple blood transfusion:
  - Regularly scheduled blood transfusion therapy (also called chronic, prophylactic, or preventive transfusion) involves periodic transfusion of the patient at regularly scheduled intervals, with the frequency guided by the patient's symptoms, Hgb, and HgbS percent.
  - Indications:
    - Regular blood transfusions are effective in reducing morbidity of most complications of SCA.
    - Regular blood transfusions are utilized in the secondary prevention of:
      - Stroke
      - Recurrent acute chest syndrome despite hydroxyurea therapy in severely affected patients
      - Vaso-occlusive pain episodes that are severe, frequent, and not responsive to maximum tolerated doses of hydroxyurea
      - Recurrent priapism
      - Pulmonary hypertension (PH) with progressive clinical symptoms or increasing pulmonary artery pressure documented by right heart catheterization
      - Pregnancy (third trimester for most patients with HbSS and earlier for patients at higher risk of complications)
  - Simple blood transfusions are given at intervals every 2–4 weeks.
  - This is used to maintain HbA level at 60–70 % which is monitored regularly by quantitative hemoglobin electrophoresis.
  - To obviate the risk of hyperviscosity, the posttransfusion hematocrit should not exceed 36 %.
  - Regular blood transfusion is effective in maintaining low levels of Hb S if this is indicated by the clinical situation.
  - Transfusion of 5–10 cc/kg of packed cells every 3–4 weeks is the usual dose.
  - Once the % S is <50, the hematocrit can be increased to 30 vol.% (Hb 10 g%).
  - The patient should then be transfused every 3–4 weeks to keep the minimum hematocrit at 30 vol.%, the reticulocyte count at <4 %, and the percent S approximately 30 %.
  - The goal of regularly scheduled transfusions is to maintain the percent HgbS <30 % of total Hgb and the total Hgb >9 g/dL.

- These patients should have regular monitoring of the Hgb level, the percent HgbS, serum ferritin, and reticulocyte count with every blood transfusion. These should help in deciding the time when the next blood transfusion should be given.
- Regularly scheduled chronic blood transfusion is continued indefinitely when it is used for primary or secondary stroke prevention.
- Patients who have been placed on regular blood transfusion to decrease a high frequency of vaso-occlusive crisis or ACS are given blood transfusion for 6–24 months depending on the actual benefit to the patient.

- Exchange blood transfusion:
  - This type of transfusion reduces the concentration of sickle cells without increasing the hematocrit or whole-blood viscosity.
  - Exchange blood transfusion also reduces iron overload.
  - Chronic automated erythrocytapheresis also reduces iron overload and can be done rapidly and safely. The major concerns include increased red cell utilization, venous access, and increased cost.
  - Hypotension is not a contraindication to exchange blood transfusion.
  - The volumes required for simple and exchange transfusions can be estimated based on patient weight and hematocrit.
    - In children, the general rule is that a transfusion of 10 cc/kg will increase the Hgb 2.5–3.0 g/dL and the hematocrit by 7–9 % points.
    - The general rule for adults is that each unit of RBC infused will increase the Hgb concentration by approximately 1 g/dL and the hematocrit by 3 % points.
    - The following formulas are used for estimation of simple transfusion and partial exchange transfusion volumes:
      - Packed RBC volume for simple transfusion (mL) = ([desired HCT − actual HCT] × total blood volume) ÷ replacement blood HCT.
      - Manual partial exchange volume (mL) = ([desired HCT − actual HCT] × total blood volume) ÷ (replacement blood HCT − [(actual HCT + desired HCT) ÷ 2]).
      - Total blood volume is 60 mL/kg in adult women, 70 mL/kg in adult men, 80 mL/kg in children, and 100 mL/kg in infants.
  - Technique of exchange blood transfusion:
    - Whole blood can be removed from one arm, and at the same time the donor cells are transfused into the other arm.
    - In adults, this procedure can be performed in 500-mL units.
    - In children, the individual exchange volumes are adjusted to a safe and practical level.
    - Exchange transfusions performed with whole blood (or, more commonly, packed cells reconstituted to the volume and hematocrit of whole blood using saline or other diluents) are more efficient than those using packed cells.
    - In children, a practical estimate of the volume required for exchange (whole blood or packed cells reconstituted to a hematocrit of 30–40 %) is 50–60 mL/kg.

- In adults, 500 mL of blood can be removed from the patient, followed by infusion of 500 mL of donor blood; this may be repeated for 6–8 units of transfusion.
- Alternatively, the following technique can be used:
  - Bleed one unit (500 mL) of blood from the patient and infuse 500 mL of saline.
  - Bleed a second unit from the patient and infuse 2 units of blood.
  - Repeat steps 1 and 2; if the patient has a large red blood cell mass, repeat once more.
  - Usually 6–8 units of blood are needed for exchange blood transfusion for an adult.
- Care must be taken to ensure that the final hemoglobin level does not exceed 10–11 g/dL to avoid hyperviscosity.
- The level of hemoglobin and the percentage of hemoglobin A should be monitored.

20.9 Methods of Blood Transfusion

- Simple blood transfusion:
  - Simple blood transfusion is indicated for:
    - Severe anemia
    - Aplastic crisis
    - Hyperhemolytic crisis
    - Chronic transfusion programs
  - For chronic transfusion:
    - Packed red blood cells are given to raise the hematocrit to 30 % (Hb 10 g%) and then every week until the % S is <50 %.
    - When the % HbS is <50, the hematocrit can be increased to 35 % (Hb 11–12 g%).
    - The patient should then be transfused every 3–4 weeks to keep the hematocrit at 30–35 % and the HbS <30 %.
  - To calculate the amount of blood to be transfused, the following formulas can be used:
    - Total blood volume = 70 − 75 cc × weight in kg.
    - Total blood volume to be given: weight in kg × 3 × (Hb desired − actual Hb).
    - Red cell volume of patient = total blood volume × hematocrit.
    - Giving 3 cc/kg of packed red cells will raise the hemoglobin by 1 g/dL.
    - Giving 10 cc/kg of packed red cells will raise the hematocrit by 10 points (vol%) or hemoglobin by about 3 g/dL.
    - Transfusion volume = [total blood volume × (Hcrit desired − Hcrit pre Tx)] / Hcrit of donor unit.

- Exchange blood transfusion:
  - The goal of exchange blood transfusion is to achieve a <30 % Hb S and a hemoglobin of 10 g%.
  - Hemoglobin levels >12 g% during exchange may be associated with increased blood viscosity and complications.
  - The following formulas can be used to estimate exchange transfusion volume:
    - Single volume red cell exchange reduces %Hb S to approximately one-third (33 %) of initial value.
    - Packed red blood cell volume = [total blood volume (75 cc/kg) × desired Hcrit]/Hcrit of donor units.
- Automated red cell exchange:
  - Apheresis can be used to rapidly reduce the Hb S to less than 30 % and give extra packed cells to adjust the final hemoglobin.
  - Two red cell mass exchanges should be performed, and then the patient should be transfused up to a hemoglobin of 10 g%.
  - Hemoglobin electrophoresis with automated red cell exchange quantitation should be obtained to assess the % Hb S.
  - Packed red cells are initially transfused, while whole blood is removed to reduce the percentage of Hb S. Then whole blood or whole blood equivalent is transfused to increase the percentage of Hb S without further increasing the hemoglobin levels.
  - This technique is applicable to adults and children and is based on the initial hematocrit and body weight in kg.
  - The exchange can be done using one or two IV sites by removing and transfusing aliquots adjusted to the total blood volume.
  - Hematocrit up to 19 % (Hb >6.5 g%):
    - Give packed cells equal to 30 cc/kg body weight while removing an equal volume of the patient's whole blood. Then give donor whole blood equivalents cc for cc while removing an additional 40 cc/kg of the patient's whole blood.
  - Hematocrit between 20 and 30 % (Hb 6.6–10 g%):
    - Exchange 10 ml/kg body weight by giving packed cells while removing whole blood and then exchange another 70 ml/kg body weight giving donor whole blood equivalent for the patient's whole blood volume removed.
  - Hematocrit >30 % (Hb >10 g%):
    - Exchange whole blood removed with normal saline to 10 ml/kg body weight and then exchange patient whole blood removed with donor whole blood equivalent.
  - Whole blood equivalent is the whole blood with a hematocrit of 40 % or packed cells and saline or other plasma equivalents reconstituted to a hematocrit of 40 %.
  - Packed cells are assumed to have a hematocrit of 60 % in AdSol.
  - The protocol aim should be an Hb S level of about 30 % and a final hemoglobin being 10 and 12 g%.

20.10 Blood Transfusion Complications

- Specific transfusion complications for sickle cell patients have been reported including:
  - Precipitation of painful crisis
  - Stroke
  - Acute pulmonary compromise
- Hyperviscosity and hypertension
- Volume overload:
  - Volume overload occurs when too much volume is transfused too quickly.
  - Congestive heart failure and pulmonary edema occur in patients who have cardiac dysfunction or minimal cardiac reserve.
  - Intravenous furosemide and partial removal of red cell-preserving fluid before transfusion and a slow transfusion rate can help avoid this serious complication.
- Alloimmunization and delayed hemolytic transfusion reactions:
  - The incidence of alloimmunization to red blood cell antigens in transfused patients with sickle cell anemia is approximately 20–25 %, which is greater than that of the general population.
  - Alloimmunization makes it difficult to obtain subsequent compatible blood and results in a high incidence of delayed hemolytic transfusion reactions.
  - The delayed transfusion reaction occurs 5–20 days after transfusion due to antibodies not detectable at the time of compatibility testing.
  - 30 % or more of antibodies to red blood cell antigens may disappear with time.
  - Alloimmunization also can cause immune-mediated hemolysis, typically as a delayed hemolytic transfusion reaction. This can lead to shortened RBC survival, worsening anemia, and exacerbation of SCA complications.
  - Acute hemolytic transfusion reactions, which are a medical emergency due to rapid intravascular hemolysis of RBCs, can also occur.
  - Delayed hemolytic transfusion reactions can cause severe anemia, precipitate painful crisis, or even lead to death.
- Acute hemolytic transfusion reactions:
  - Acute major hemolytic transfusion reactions in sickle cell patients occur primarily with major blood group (ABO) incompatibilities and must be treated aggressively to maintain blood pressure and glomerular filtration.
  - These occur with errors in crossmatching or transfusion of units from other donors not compatible to the patient.
  - Minor hemolytic reactions occur when the amount of antibody in the serum is limited.
  - These reactions are characterized by:
    - The disappearance of the transfused blood during a period of several days with a consequent decrease in the hemoglobin and hematocrit.
    - The appearance of direct hyperbilirubinemia.

    - No further treatment is necessary except monitoring the hemoglobin and hematocrit level to ensure that it does not fall to a dangerously low level.
- Autoimmune hemolytic anemia following allosensitization:
  - In some highly alloimmunized patients, a syndrome of autoimmune hemolytic anemia can follow allosensitization or a hemolytic transfusion reaction.
  - The patient can become more anemic than before transfusion.
  - The direct antiglobulin (Coombsí) test remains positive even after the incompatible transfused cells have been destroyed.
  - This syndrome occurs because the body produces antibodies against self-antigens.
  - The condition may persist from several weeks to 2–3 months before disappearing.
  - Further transfusion is complicated by the presence of autoimmune antibody, and this makes it difficult to find the "least incompatible" blood for transfusion.
- Alloantibodies to white blood cells, platelets, and serum proteins:
  - Transfused patients can become alloimmunized to antigens specific to leukocytes or platelets.
  - These antibodies can cause febrile reactions.
  - Removal of the leukocytes by filtration or washing reduces the frequency of febrile reactions.
  - Plasma washing to antigenic plasma proteins and administration of antihistamines also help against febrile reactions.
- Infection:
  - There are several infections that are acquired secondary to blood transfusions. These include:
    - Hepatitis B and C
    - AIDS
    - Parvovirus
    - Bacterial infections
    - Malaria
  - Hepatitis and other transfusion-transmitted viral infections occur with the same frequency in sickle cell patients as with other patients receiving transfusions.
    - The increased number of transfusions over the years in these patients contributes to an increased incidence of hepatitis in patients with sickle cell anemia.
  - The consequences of viral infections, however, can be more severe in sickle cell patients because of pre-existing organ damage.
  - Patients who are negative for antibody against hepatitis B should be immunized.
  - Patients receiving multiple transfusions should be serially monitored for hepatitis C, hepatitis B, and other viral infections.
  - Therapy is evolving for hepatitis C and B, and many patients are being successfully treated with interferon in combination with other antiviral agents.

  - Acquired immune deficiency syndrome (AIDS) from transfusion has decreased dramatically in recent years.
  - However, HIV infection has been reported as late as 8 years after transfusion from a donor not known to be infected.
  - Sickle cell patients transfused before blood products should be tested for HIV infection, as well periodic screening for HIV.
  - Parvovirus infections occur in 1 in every 40,000 units of transfused blood and have been associated with acute anemia and multiple sickle cell complications.
  - When available, the parvovirus vaccine should be given for all at-risk patients.
  - Transfusion-induced bacterial infections are uncommon, but these can be acquired through the intravenous lines and improper sterilization.
  - Repeatedly transfused hemoglobinopathy patients are particularly vulnerable to *Yersinia enterocolitica* and bacteremia secondary to ineffective skin cleansing at the time of phlebotomy. *Yersinia enterocolitica* can cause colitis in these patients.
  - All patients developing fever after transfusion must be immediately assessed for potential bacterial and viral infections.
- Iron overload:
  - Excessive accumulation of iron is a serious problem and may be undetected in patients with sickle cell anemia because transfusion therapy may be irregular and episodic.
  - Iron overload in sickle cell patients is often undetected and/or not treated.
  - Most patients with sickle cell anemia are iron overloaded because of intermittent transfusions throughout their life.
  - Therefore, a comprehensive program designed to monitor and treat iron overload is necessary.
  - Many patients with SCA will develop excessive iron stores if chelation therapy is not used.
  - Excess iron is a cause of significant morbidity in patients with SCA. The life expectancy of patients with sickle cell anemia continues to increase with improved management and use of hydroxyurea which makes them liable to develop iron overload-related morbidity and mortality.
  - Hepatic fibrosis and death from hemosiderosis-related cirrhosis of the liver can occur in these patients.
  - For those who receive multiple transfusions, iron chelation therapy is an important part of the transfusion program. Iron chelation prevents the complications associated with iron deposition in the heart and liver.
  - The serum ferritin concentration is a useful test to monitor the status of iron stores.
  - Ferritin levels need to be serially measured at least every 3–4 months in those receiving multiple blood transfusions.
  - Patients receiving chelation therapy measure serum ferritin level prior to every blood transfusion.

- The serum ferritin level, however, is not reliable as it fluctuates. It is important to average three to five serial ferritin measurements as a guide to determine the status of iron stores.
- A serum ferritin value no greater than 1000–1500 ng/mL (1000–1500 mcg/L) is acceptable.
- Other noninvasive ways to measure iron stores is quantitative MRI to assess liver iron.
- Liver biopsy is the most accurate way to assess hepatic iron stores.
- The initiation of chelation therapy in patients with SCA depends upon:
  - The number of transfusions given
  - The degree of iron deposition in the liver and heart
  - The amount of hepatic and cardiac dysfunction present
  - The type of transfusion regimen
- Generally, chelation therapy is started:
  - After 2 years of transfusion in chronically transfused patients
  - After approximately 120 mL of transfused packed RBCs per kilogram
  - When the serum ferritin level exceeds 1000–1500 mcg/L (ng/mL) or the liver iron is >7 mg/g dry weight
- There are three available iron chelators:
  - Deferiprone
  - Deferoxamine
  - Deferasirox
- Deferasirox (DFX; Exjade) is an orally available iron chelator that appears to have efficacy similar to deferoxamine in decreasing liver iron concentration. Deferasirox is orally active and has a good therapeutic index.
- The side effect of deferasirox includes:
  - Diarrhea
  - Nausea
  - Vomiting
  - Abdominal pain
  - Dose-dependent rise in serum creatinine, which is reversible
  - Liver dysfunction
  - Rare reports of renal failure and Fanconi syndrome
- The starting dosage for oral deferasirox is 20 mg/kg/day once daily.
  - The dose is increased by 5–10 mg every 3–6 months based on iron stores.
  - Toxicities such as skin rash, nausea, and diarrhea are dose related.
  - These adverse effects may be decreased by giving the same total dose twice a day, rather than once a day, and accompanied with food.
- Deferiprone (DFP; Ferriprox) is also orally active.
- Its major side effect is the risk of agranulocytosis.
- Other side effects of deferiprone include:
  - Arthralgia
  - Gastrointestinal symptoms
  - Hepatotoxicity

- The standard dosage of deferiprone is 75 mg/kg three times a day.
  - After 6 months, it may be increased up to 100 mg/kg/day in nonresponding or high-risk patients.
- Deferoxamine (DFO; Desferal) is effective and available but requires daily subcutaneous infusions.
- It can also be given intravenously for more rapid iron chelation.
- Desferrioxamine is known to be associated with side effects but these are rare. These include:
  - Ototoxicity
  - Ophthalmologic toxicity
  - Allergic reactions
  - Growth failure
  - Unusual infections
  - Pulmonary hypersensitivity
- In general, in stable patients without iron-induced cardiac dysfunction, the starting dosage of deferoxamine is 30 mg/kg given daily over 8–12 h, 5 days per week.
  - This dose can be modified by 5–10 mg every 3–6 months depending on the individual patient's transfusion burden and iron status.
- A formal audiology exam should be given prior to initiation of iron chelation therapy.
  - A screening hearing exam should be performed in clinic every 6 months and a formal audiogram every 12 months.
  - Hearing loss is most frequently seen in those receiving deferoxamine, especially when given at higher doses.
- Visual loss is also reported in those receiving deferoxamine, especially at high doses. An annual evaluation by an ophthalmologist should be performed.
- Creatinine, BUN, serum electrolytes, and urine protein and creatinine should be monitored monthly in individuals on deferasirox and every 3 months in those on deferoxamine.
  - Treatment should be discontinued immediately if the serum creatinine is greater than two times the upper limit of normal.
  - Any patient with a serum creatinine increase >50 % above baseline level should stop the drug temporarily.
  - If there is an increase in serum creatinine of 33–50 %, the dose should be reduced.
  - The chelator should be stopped temporarily if the urine protein/creatinine ratio is >0.6 mg/mg.
- Those on deferiprone require weekly complete blood count to detect serious neutropenia/agranulocytosis.
  - A neutrophil count below 1000 cells/μL requires stopping the drug and reassessing future use.
  - All individuals with fever who are on deferiprone require an immediate reevaluation of their white blood cell count.

- Deferasirox has been associated with neutropenia, agranulocytosis, worsening anemia, and thrombocytopenia, including fatal events.
    - Deferasirox should be stopped in patients who develop cytopenias until the cause of the cytopenias has been determined.
    - Deferasirox is contraindicated in patients with platelet counts below 50,000/μL.
- Growth can sometimes be affected by chelation therapy.
- Hepatic enzymes should be monitored monthly for those receiving deferasirox and every 3 months for those receiving other chelators.
    - Chelation therapy should be stopped if the serum alanine aminotransferase (ALT) is greater than five times the upper limit of normal.
- Other complications that require immediate temporary withdrawal of chelation therapy include:
    - Acute respiratory distress
    - Stevens-Johnson syndrome
    - Acute gastrointestinal bleeding
- It was also found that chelating agents may affect the growth of some microorganisms (e.g., *Yersinia enterocolitica*) and they should be held temporarily in patients with fever or active infection until the patient becomes afebrile.

Complications of Blood Transfusions

- Specific transfusion complications including:
    - Precipitation of painful crisis
    - Stroke
    - Acute pulmonary compromise
- Hyperviscosity and hypertension
- Volume overload
- Alloimmunization
- Iron overload
- Coombs-negative hemolysis
- Infections
    - Hepatitis B and C
    - AIDS
    - Parvovirus
    - Bacterial infections
    - Malaria
- Acute hemolytic transfusion reactions
- Autoimmune hemolytic anemia following allosensitization
- Autoantibody-mediated hemolysis
- Alloantibodies to white blood cells, platelets, and serum proteins

- Autoantibody-mediated hemolysis
  - Autoantibodies (antibodies that recognize the patient's own RBCs) have been reported in 7–47 % of patients receiving blood transfusions.
  - An autoantibody is more likely to develop in patients who have already been alloimmunized.
  - The development of new autoantibody can cause marked hemolysis.
- Coombs-negative hemolysis
  - Patients with SCA are prone to develop direct antiglobulin-negative (i.e., Coombs negative) hyperhemolysis that acts as an autoimmune hemolytic transfusion reaction.
  - Patients with severe autoimmune transfusion reactions may respond to immunosuppressive therapy with intravenous gamma globulin, steroids, or rituximab.

Further Reading

Alvarez O, Yovetich NA, Scott JP, et al. Pain and other non-neurological adverse events in children with sickle cell anemia and previous stroke who received hydroxyurea and phlebotomy or chronic transfusions and chelation: results from the SWiTCH clinical trial. Am J Hematol. 2013;88:932.

Beverung LM, Strouse JJ, Hulbert ML, et al. Health-related quality of life in children with sickle cell anemia: impact of blood transfusion therapy. Am J Hematol. 2015;90:139.

Brittenham GM. Iron-chelating therapy for transfusional iron overload. N Engl J Med. 2011;364:146.

Davies SC, Roberts-Harewood M. Blood transfusion in sickle cell disease. Blood Rev. 1997;11:57.

Goldstein AR, Anderson MJ, Serjeant GR. Parvovirus associated aplastic crisis in homozygous sickle cell disease. Arch Dis Child. 1987;62:585.

Howard J, Malfroy M, Llewelyn C, et al. The Transfusion Alternatives Preoperatively in Sickle Cell Disease (TAPS) study: a randomised, controlled, multicentre clinical trial. Lancet. 2013;381:930.

Josephson CD, Su LL, Hillyer KL, Hillyer CD. Transfusion in the patient with sickle cell disease: a critical review of the literature and transfusion guidelines. Transfus Med Rev. 2007;21:118.

Miller ST, Wright E, Abboud M, et al. Impact of chronic transfusion on incidence of pain and acute chest syndrome during the Stroke Prevention Trial (STOP) in sickle-cell anemia. J Pediatr. 2001;139:785.

Quirolo K. How do I transfuse patients with sickle cell disease? Transfusion. 2010;50:1881.

Vichinsky EP, Earles A, Johnson RA, et al. Alloimmunization in sickle cell anemia and transfusion of racially unmatched blood. N Engl J Med. 1990;322:1617.

Vichinsky E, Bernaudin F, Forni GL, et al. Long-term safety and efficacy of deferasirox (Exjade) for up to 5 years in transfusional iron-overloaded patients with sickle cell disease. Br J Haematol. 2011;154:387.

Wayne AS, Kevy SV, Nathan DG. Transfusion management of sickle cell disease. Blood. 1993;81:1109.

Hydroxyurea Treatment for Sickle Cell Anemia

21

21.1 Introduction

- Sickle cell anemia is one of the common hemoglobinopathies worldwide.
- Till now, there is no widely available cure.
- The current management is directed toward relieving their symptoms and treating complications.
- The goals of treating patients with sickle cell anemia include:
  - To relieve pain
  - To prevent infections
  - To prevent organ damage
  - To prevent stroke
  - To control and treat complications
- The modern management of sickle cell anemia is based on these therapeutic approaches:
  - Symptomatic treatment of painful crisis
  - Blood transfusion
  - Immunization and penicillin therapy
  - Treatment of complications
  - Hydroxyurea
  - Bone marrow transplant
- It was found that patients with sickle cell anemia and high levels of HbF have a relatively milder disease than those with low HbF. Fetal hemoglobin helps prevent red blood cells from sickling and improves anemia.
- Increased fetal hemoglobin (HbF) production has long been recognized as one of the key factors which can ameliorate SCA, and in the 1970s, 5-azacytidine was investigated as an HbF promoting agent because of its potential ability to reactivate silenced γ-globin genes by inhibiting the methylation of deoxycytidine.
- Although 5-azacytidine successfully increased HbF levels in patients with SCA and thalassemia, it was found to be relatively toxic.

A. Al-Salem, *Medical and Surgical Complications of Sickle Cell Anemia*,
DOI 10.1007/978-3-319-24762-5_21

- Hydroxyurea was used to treat leukemia and showed particular activity in myeloproliferative disorders.
- Hydroxyurea was also found to promote HbF synthesis.
- Hydroxyurea was developed as a safer alternative to 5-azacytidine and showed significant increase in both HbF and total hemoglobin.
- In 1995, a multicenter study evaluated the value of hydroxyurea for patients with sickle cell anemia. In this, the hydroxyurea group showed reductions in the rate of acute pain (median 2.5 vs. 4.5 episodes per year, $P<0.001$), acute chest syndrome (25 vs. 51, $P<0.001$), and blood transfusion (48 vs. 73, $P<0.001$) when compared to the placebo group.
- Hydroxyurea also reduced the number of hospitalizations ($P=0.0016$) and total days in hospital ($P=0.0027$) in patients with sickle cell anemia.
- There was also an increased survival associated with long-term hydroxyurea use. A 40 % reduction in mortality was reported in those who continued using hydroxyurea after 9 years ($P=0.04$).
- Blood and bone marrow stem cell transplants:
  - This may offer a cure for a small number of patients with sickle cell anemia.
  - Blood and bone marrow stem cell transplants usually are used for young patients who have severe sickle cell anemia.
  - The transplant must come from a closely matched donor. This limits the number of people who may have a donor.
  - The transplant is expensive and not readily available.
  - The transplant is risky and can lead to serious side effects or even death.
- Research on blood and bone marrow stem cell transplants, gene therapy, and new medications for sickle cell anemia is ongoing.
- Gene therapy is being studied as a possible treatment for sickle cell anemia.
- Researchers are also studying several medications for the treatment of sickle cell anemia. They include:
  - Decitabine
  - Adenosine A2a receptor agonists
  - 5-HMF
  - Butyric acid
  - Clotrimazole
  - Nitric oxide

21.2 Hydroxyurea

- Hydroxyurea was first synthesized in 1869 in Germany by Dressler and Stein.
- A century later, phase I and II trials began testing the safety of this drug in humans with solid tumors.
- It was first approved by the FDA in 1967 for the treatment of neoplastic diseases.
- In subsequent years, clinical trials demonstrated the efficacy of this drug for the treatment of chronic myeloid leukemia, psoriasis, and polycythemia vera.
- In February 1998, hydroxyurea was used for the treatment of sickle cell anemia.

- It is approved for use in reducing the frequency of painful crises and the need for blood transfusions in adult patients with recurrent moderate-to-severe painful crises (generally at least three during the preceding 12 months).
- Hydroxyurea is also approved for use in the treatment of melanoma, resistant CML, and recurrent, metastatic, or inoperable carcinoma of the ovary.

21.3 Mechanism of Action

- The precise mechanism by which hydroxyurea produces its varied effects is unknown.
- Assays conducted in cell-free bacterial systems have demonstrated that its target is the enzyme ribonucleotide reductase, with hydroxyurea acting as a free radical that is specific for the tyrosyl groups of this enzyme.
- Ribonucleotide reductase is essential for deoxyribonucleic acid (DNA) synthesis, and its inhibition by hydroxyurea results in S-phase cell cycle arrest.
- Hydroxyurea is an S-phase cytotoxic agent which does not demethylate DNA; it is thought to directly reduce DNA synthesis by inhibiting ribonucleotide reductase activity.
- This nonspecific interruption of the cell cycle probably accounts for most of the HbF promoting activity.
- Hydroxyurea acts on both early and late erythroid progenitors to increase the total intracellular hemoglobin, γ-globin mRNA, and HbF levels.
- Other mechanisms may be responsible for the fact that this drug acts as a radiation sensitizer, inhibiting the repair of damaged DNA.
- The efficacy of hydroxyurea in the treatment of sickle cell anemia is generally attributed to its ability to increase the levels of fetal hemoglobin (HbF, $\alpha 2\gamma 2$).
- This lowers the concentration of Hb S resulting in less polymerization of the abnormal hemoglobin.
- However, the mechanisms by which it increases HbF are unclear.
- Early studies suggested that hydroxyurea is cytotoxic to the more rapidly dividing late erythroid precursors, an effect that leads to the recruitment of early erythroid precursors with an increased capacity to produce HbF.
- Others have suggested that it acts directly on late precursors to reprogram them to produce HbF.
- Alternatively, it may interrupt the transcription factors that selectively bind to promoter or enhancer regions around the globin genes, thereby altering the ratio of Hb A to HbF.
- There is also evidence that hydroxyurea can act as a nitric oxide donor and increase cGMP levels which accelerates translation of the γ-globin gene.
- A recent study has provided evidence for a nitric oxide-derived mechanism for HbF induction by hydroxyurea.
- Another study has suggested that it increases HbF production by inhibiting ribonucleotide.
- Hydroxyurea may be of benefit in sickle cell anemia for reasons unrelated to HbF production, including:
  - Its ability to increase the water content of red blood cells

  - Decrease the neutrophil count
  - Alter the adhesion of red blood cells to the endothelium
- The effects of hydroxyurea on the blood in SCA are dose dependent and include:
  - Increases HbF levels
  - Increases erythrocyte volume
  - Increases hemoglobin content
  - Decreases reticulocyte count
  - Decreases white cell count
  - Increases segmentation of the neutrophil nucleus
  - Reduces RBC dehydration by increasing their water content
  - Reduces phosphatidylserine exposure
  - Reduces expression of adhesion molecules and alters the adhesion of red blood cells to the endothelium
- The clinical benefit of hydroxyurea is directly related to the increased HbF levels and reduced hemoglobin polymerization within the red cell, resulting in reduced red cell damage.
- Hydroxyurea acts directly on vascular endothelium to decrease the expression of some adhesion molecules, which is clearly independent of any effects on the β-globin gene family.
- Hydroxyurea may be more effective in preventing acute pain caused by microvascular complications than cerebrovascular disease in large blood vessels.
- Hydroxyurea may improve hypoxemia, prevent cerebrovascular disease, and reduce proteinuria.

21.4 Indications for Hydroxyurea Treatment

- The two main indications for hydroxyurea treatment are:
  - More than three episodes of acute pain each year, which are causing significant disruption to education, or family life
  - Recurrent or severe acute chest syndrome
- Other less established indications include:
  - Conditional velocities on transcranial Doppler scans.
  - Significant cerebral vasculopathy when blood transfusions are unacceptable.
  - Progressive cerebral vasculopathy despite adequate blood transfusions.
  - Persistent low hemoglobin (<6 g/dL).
  - Hypoxemia.
  - Significant proteinuria.
  - Patients keen to avoid blood transfusions if at all possible.
  - Preoperative preparation when blood transfusions are not acceptable.
  - There are those who believe that hydroxyurea should be recommended for all children with sickle cell anemia regardless of symptomatology in order to prevent organ damage.

21.5 Evaluation and Investigations

- Each patient must be evaluated carefully before starting hydroxyurea.
- Baseline investigations include:
  - Complete blood count and reticulocytes
  - HbF%
  - Renal function
  - Hepatic function including ALT

21.6 Monitoring of Patients

- Complete blood count, reticulocytes, and renal and hepatic functions should be checked 2 weeks following the start of hydroxyurea.
- Complete blood count, reticulocytes, HbF%, and renal and hepatic functions should be checked every 1–3 months.
- If the dose is increased, blood tests should be performed after 2 weeks on the higher dose, before resuming the 1–3 monthly monitoring.
- Patients on hydroxyurea should still have annual review blood tests and investigations performed, including transcranial Doppler scanning.
- Stop hydroxyurea if toxicity occurs.
- Markers of toxicity include:
  - Hematological:
    - Neutrophils <1.0 × 109/L
    - Platelets <80 × 109/L
    - Reticulocytes <80 × 109/L
  - Renal:
    - 50 % or more increase in serum creatinine
  - Hepatic:
    - 100 % increase in ALT
- The patients should be assessed and investigated if they develop symptoms suggestive of sepsis or unusual bruising or bleeding, because of the possible risk of bone marrow suppression.

21.7 Withdrawal of Hydroxyurea

- Patients usually are treated for at least 6 months before deciding to stop hydroxyurea because of the lack of benefit.
- When hydroxyurea is associated with clinical improvement, it is typically continued for at least 2–3 years; consideration is then given to stopping it, depending on the initial indication.
- In general, it is better to stop hydroxyurea during school holidays and not just before important events such as school examinations.

21.8 Treatment and Dosage

- When used to treat sickle cell anemia, hydroxyurea is administered orally and is readily absorbed.
- The peak plasma levels are reached in 1–4 h after an oral dose.
- The drug is distributed rapidly and widely in the body and concentrates in leukocytes and erythrocytes.
- The therapeutic dose of hydroxyurea ranges from 15 to 35 mg/kg daily.

Indications for Hydroxyurea

Definite Indications

1. More than three episodes of severe acute pain per year
2. Two or more episodes of acute chest syndrome

Probable Indications

1. Frequent episodes of acute pain requiring analgesia
2. Persistent albuminuria or other evidence of renal disease
3. Hypoxemia or other evidence of lung disease
4. Sickle hepatopathy
5. Tricuspid jet velocity >2.5 m/s on echocardiography or pulmonary hypertension
6. Primary or secondary stroke prevention when blood transfusions are unacceptable
7. Hemoglobin <7 g/dL

Possible Indications

1. Poor growth
2. Conditional transcranial Doppler velocities
3. Patient or family request
4. Elevated steady-state white cell count
5. Preoperative management
6. Significant coexisting disease likely to exacerbate SCA like bronchial asthma and systemic lupus erythromatosis
7. Strong wish to avoid blood transfusion, including Jehovah's Witnesses
8. Living in low-income country with greatly increased early mortality

- Most children should be started on a dose of 15–20 mg/kg daily, unless there is particular concern about the risk of myelosuppression, when lower doses should be used.
- For most patients, the lowest effective dose as assessed by clinical improvement is used.

- However, for some indications, such as those involving cerebrovascular disease, the dose should be increased until limited by myelosuppression.
- The patient's blood count is monitored every 2 weeks.
- If the blood counts are in an acceptable range, the dose may be increased by 5 mg/kg/day every 2–3 months until the maximum dose of 35 mg/kg/day is reached.
- If blood counts are between the acceptable range and the toxic range, the dose is not increased.
- If blood counts are found to be in the toxic range, treatment is discontinued until blood counts return to normal.
- It may then be resumed after the dose is reduced by 2.5 mg/kg/day from the last dose that was associated with hematologic toxicity.
- The drug may then be titrated up or down every 2–3 months in increments of 2.5 mg/kg/day until the patient reaches a stable dose that does not result in hematologic toxicity.
- Blood counts considered to be acceptable are:
  - Neutrophils greater than or equal to 2500 cells/mm^3
  - Platelets greater than or equal to 95,000/mm^3
  - Hemoglobin greater than 5.3 g/dL
  - Reticulocytes greater than or equal to 95,000/mm^3 if the hemoglobin concentration is less than 9 g/dL
- Blood counts considered to be toxic are:
  - Neutrophils less than 2000 cells/mm^3
  - Platelets less than 80,000/mm^3
  - Hemoglobin less than 4.5 g/dL
  - Reticulocytes less than 80,000/mm^3 if the hemoglobin concentration is less than 9 g/dL

21.9 Benefits of Hydroxyurea for Patients with Sickle Cell Anemia

- Hydroxyurea is the only approved drug for treatment of sickle cell anemia.
  - Hydroxyurea can be given safely, and it improves anemia and hemoglobin F levels while reducing complications of sickle cell anemia.
  - The hemoglobin level was found to be higher in hydroxyurea recipients than placebo recipients after 2 years (difference, 6 g/L).
  - There was a relative increase in fetal hemoglobin of 4–20 % in hydroxyurea recipients.
  - Hydroxyurea reduces the frequency of painful sickle cell crises.
  - The median number of painful crises was 44 % lower than in the placebo group and a relative reduction in crisis rates by 68–84 %.
  - Hydroxyurea reduces the frequency of acute chest syndrome.
  - It also reduces the need for blood transfusions.
  - Hydroxyurea reduces the overall hospital visits.
  - It also reduces the overall hospital admissions.
  - There was a reduction in hospital admissions by 18–32 % in hydroxyurea recipients.

21.10 Side Effects of Hydroxyurea

- Short-term side effects are few, but the theoretical possibilities of an increased risk of malignancy and reduced fertility continue to cause concern, particularly when hydroxyurea is given for young children who may take it for many years.
- Hydroxyurea may impair spermatogenesis.
- The limited evidence indicates that hydroxyurea treatment in adults with sickle cell anemia is not associated with leukemia.
- The limited evidence suggests that hydroxyurea and leg ulcers are not associated in patients with sickle cell anemia.
- The evidence is insufficient to estimate the risk for skin neoplasms and hydroxyurea.
- Hydroxyurea can cause bone marrow suppression
- The following are known side effects of hydroxyurea:
  - Nausea, vomiting, loss of appetite, mouth sores, diarrhea, and constipation
  - Painful or difficult urination
  - Confusion, hallucinations, seizure
  - Fever, chills, body aches, flu symptoms, sores in the mouth and throat, pale skin, feeling light-headed or short of breath, rapid heart rate, and trouble concentrating
  - Severe upper abdominal pain spreading to the back, nausea and vomiting, tachycardia
  - Nausea, upper abdominal pain, itching, feeling of tiredness, loss of appetite, dark urine, clay-colored stools, jaundice

Side Effects of Hydroxyurea

Common Side Effects

1. Cough or hoarseness
2. Fever or chills
3. Lower back or side pain
4. Painful or difficult urination

Less Common Side Effects

1. Black, tarry stools
2. Blackening of the fingernails and toenails
3. Blood in the urine or stools
4. Pinpoint red spots on the skin
5. Sores in the mouth and on the lips
6. Unusual bleeding or bruising

Rare Side Effects

1. Confusion
2. Convulsions (seizures)
3. Difficulty with urination
4. Dizziness
5. Headache
6. Joint pain
7. Seeing, hearing, or feeling things that are not there
8. Swelling of the feet or lower legs

Further Reading

Berthaut I, Guignedoux G, Kirsch-Noir F, et al. Influence of sickle cell disease and treatment with hydroxyurea on sperm parameters and fertility of human males. Haematologica. 2008;93: 988–93.

Charache S, Terrin ML, Moore RD, et al. Effect of hydroxyurea on frequency of painful crises in sickle cell anemia. N Engl J Med. 1995;332:1317–22.

Fitzhugh CD, Wigfall DR, Ware RE. Enalapril and hydroxyurea therapy for children with sickle nephropathy. Pediatr Blood Cancer. 2005;45:982–5.

Singh SA, Koumbourlis AC, Aygun B. Resolution of chronic hypoxemia in pediatric sickle cell patients after treatment with hydroxyurea. Pediatr Blood Cancer. 2008;50:1258–60.

Strouse JJ, Lanzkron S, Beach MC, et al. Hydroxyurea for sickle cell disease: a systematic review for efficacy and toxicity in children. Pediatrics. 2008;122:1332–42.

Zimmerman SA, Schultz WH, Burgett S, Mortier NA, Ware RE. Hydroxyurea therapy lowers transcranial Doppler flow velocities in children with sickle cell anemia. Blood. 2007;110: 1043–7.

Hematopoietic Stem Cell Transplantation for Patients with Sickle Cell Anemia

22

22.1 Introduction

- Sickle cell anemia is an inherited hemoglobinopathy that is known to be associated with long-term complications and reduced life expectancy.
- The treatment of patients with sickle cell anemia generally aims to relieve their pain and manage or prevent sickle cell-related complications.
- In the recent years, the management of patients with sickle cell anemia has improved markedly. This is reflected in prolonged survival of these patients, and it is attributed to several factors including:
  - Improvement in conservative management policies of these patients
  - The use of hydroxyurea
  - The availability of extended phenotyping of transfused donor red cells to reduce alloimmunization risks
  - Erythrocytapheresis to reduce iron overload in chronically transfused patients
  - The availability of oral chelating agents
- In spite of this, patients with sickle cell anemia continue to suffer from sickle cell-related complications including the ongoing sickle cell vasculopathy.
- Sickle cell anemia progression, organ damage, and sudden death can occur in these patients despite adequate supportive care measures.
- Add to this the cost and availability of medical resources for lifelong medical care of these patients.
- Hydroxyurea does ameliorate the disease and has been shown to reduce painful crises, acute chest syndrome, and the need for blood transfusions, but it does not provide cure.
- In 1982, at St. Jude hospital, there was a patient who had leukemia and sickle cell disease. This patient had transplant using bone marrow donated from the patient's brother. The patient was cured of both leukemia and sickle cell disease.
- Hematopoietic stem cell transplantation (HSCT) is currently the only established curative treatment modality for SCA.

A. Al-Salem, *Medical and Surgical Complications of Sickle Cell Anemia*,
DOI 10.1007/978-3-319-24762-5_22

- The benefits of HSCT are now well established, but it is associated with complications including:
  - HSCT-related organ toxicities
  - Graft-versus-host disease (GVHD)
  - Graft rejection (GR)
  - Donor availability
- HSCT can establish donor-derived erythropoiesis and, more importantly, can stabilize or restore function in affected organs such as the central nervous system (CNS) and lung and prevent further deterioration of their functions.
- For over two decades, hematopoietic stem cell transplantation was offered only to patients with severe SCA and only if a matched sibling donor was available.
- Though human leukocyte antigen (HLA)-matched sibling donor (MSD) transplants offer the best outcomes for SCA, less than 14 % of patients with SCA have such available donors.
- Currently, there are three main types of stem cell donors:
  - Matched related:
    - A brother or sister who has the same bone marrow type and the same mother and father.
    - Brothers and sisters are matched through special blood tests called HLA typing.
  - Matched Unrelated:
    - Volunteers who have the same bone marrow type as the patient.
    - Usually these types of donations are matched through national organizations that match donors and patients who have the same type of bone marrow.
  - Haploidentical:
    - Half-matched family members (usually a mother or father).
    - This type of donation is still considered experimental.
    - Stem cells can be obtained from the donor's bone marrow or peripheral blood.
    - Or in some cases, stem cells are collected from the umbilical cord at the time of birth.
- There are however several factors that makes bone marrow transplant not readily available option. These include:
  - Bone marrow transplant is not available in every country and in specialized centers within the same country. This limits accessibility.
  - It is a very expensive method of treatment.
  - Patients with sickle cell anemia are less likely to find a matching donor. This is because of the genetic complications associated with sickle cell anemia.
  - Regular blood transfusions which are common in patients with sickle cell anemia lead to the production of antibodies which could potentially affect the success of a future transplant.
  - Bone marrow transplantation is a risky procedure with a high morbidity and mortality, including the chance that about one child in ten will die from the procedure itself. The risks of bone marrow transplantation are higher in older children and adults.

- One option for many patients who cannot find a suitable bone marrow match is umbilical cord blood transplant, which involves the use of blood taken from the umbilical cord and placenta minutes after the birth of a baby.
- A good match is less important with cord blood transplants and known to be associated with lower risk of graft-versus-host disease or rejection.
- Although bone marrow transplant is the only known cure for sickle cell anemia, the complications from a traditional bone marrow transplant can be life threatening.
- Traditionally, bone marrow transplantation requires heavy doses of chemotherapy prior to transplant in order to destroy the recipient's bone marrow so it will not reject the donated marrow. As a result of this, transplant recipients become vulnerable to life-threatening complications.

22.2 History of Bone Marrow Transplantation

- Georges Mathé, a French oncologist, performed the first European bone marrow transplant in 1959 on five Yugoslavian nuclear workers whose own bone marrow had been damaged by irradiation caused by an accident at the Vinča Nuclear Institute, but all of these transplants were rejected.
- Mathé later pioneered the use of bone marrow transplants in the treatment of leukemia.
- Stem cell transplantation was pioneered using bone-marrow-derived stem cells by a team at the Fred Hutchinson Cancer Research Center from the 1950s through the 1970s led by E. Donnall Thomas, whose work was later recognized with a Nobel Prize in physiology or medicine.
- Thomas' work showed that bone marrow cells infused intravenously could repopulate the bone marrow and produce new blood cells. His work also reduced the likelihood of developing a life-threatening complication called graft-versus-host disease.
- The first physician to perform a successful human bone marrow transplant on a disease other than cancer was Robert A. Good at the University of Minnesota in 1968.
- In 1975, John Kersey, M.D., of the University of Minnesota, performed the first successful bone marrow transplant to cure lymphoma. His patient, a 16-year-old boy, is today the longest-living lymphoma transplant survivor.
- The first successful hematopoietic cell transplantations (HCT) in beta-thalassemia major were reported in 1982. Since that time, more than 3000 of such transplants have been performed worldwide.
- Prof. Guido Lucarelli in the 1980s was the one who popularized bone marrow transplantation (BMT) from compatible donor as the main cure for thalassemia.
- Dr. Pietro Sodani used bone marrow transplantation (BMT) from haploidentical mother to child using protocol 30 to cure thalassemia.
- The first patient with SCA to be treated with HCT was an 8-year-old girl who had both acute myeloid leukemia (AML) and recurrent vaso-occlusive crises. After HCT, in addition to having a normal bone marrow with no evidence of

AML, her hemoglobin S level decreased to the level of the donor, who had sickle cell trait, and she had no further vaso-occlusive crises. This was published in the New England Journal of Medicine in 1984 by Johnson et al.

- Additional studies with larger numbers of patients were reported in 1994 by Vermylen C and Cornu G from Belgium, with an overall and disease-free survival of 96 and 89 %, respectively.
- Similar results were reported in a French study involving 14 patients by Bernaudin et al. in 1993.
- Dr. Lakshmanan Krishnamurti:
  - Dr. Lakshmanan Krishnamurti is clinical director of hematology in the Division of Hematology/Oncology at Children's Hospital of Pittsburgh of UPMC.
  - His research has focused on sickle cell disease.
  - Dr. Krishnamurti and his colleagues reported that six of seven sickle cell patients who received RIC bone marrow transplants in the last decade now have donor marrow and are free from symptoms of their sickle cell disease.
  - Dr. Lakshmanan Krishnamurti in 1999 performed the first successful bone marrow transplant on a patient with sickle cell disease at Children's Hospital, using a rare approach known as reduced-intensity transplant.
  - "Bone marrow transplant is the only known cure for sickle cell disease. But doctors have avoided performing them in these patients because complications from a traditional bone marrow transplant can be life-threatening," said Dr. Krishnamurti, director of the Sickle Cell Program at Children's Hospital. "Through the reduced-intensity approach we developed the potential for complications is dramatically lessened".
- The first multicenter trial from the United States, published in 1996, reported results in 22 patients younger than 16 years of age who received a HLA-matched sibling HCT.
  - Patient selection was based on strict criteria, including patients with severe debilitating clinical events such as stroke, recurrent acute chest syndrome, and recurrent painful vaso-occlusive crises.
  - The conditioning regimen avoided total body irradiation and included cyclophosphamide, busulfan, and T cell depletion using either antithymocyte globulin or Campath antibodies.
  - A combination of methotrexate and cyclosporin or cyclosporin and prednisone was used for prophylaxis against graft-versus-host disease (GVHD).
  - An increased incidence of neurologic complications, with seizures in some patients, occurred; these complications were mostly resolved after prophylaxis with anticonvulsant medication.
  - Of the 22 patients reported, 20 survived; 16 had stable engraftment of donor hematopoietic cells, and 1 had stable mixed chimerism.
  - Four patients (18 %) had graft rejection, similar to the 13 % rejection rate reported among children with beta-thalassemia major who received HLA-matched sibling HCT.
  - Two patients died of central nervous system hemorrhage or GVHD.
  - The overall survival and event-free survival at 4 years were 91 and 73 %, respectively.

22.3 Selection Criteria and Indications for Hematopoietic Stem Cell Transplantation

- Sickle cell anemia is a disease with an unpredictable clinical course.
- This makes it difficult to choose candidates who are at significant risk for disease-related complications before they exhibit them and will benefit from bone marrow transplantation.
- Taking in consideration the significant morbidity and mortality associated with bone marrow transplantation, it should be offered only to those who suffered significant sickle cell-related complications but without an end organ damage.
- Hematopoietic stem cell transplantation was initially offered only to patients with severe SCA and only if a matched sibling donor was available. This is to insure better success of transplant and taking in consideration the morbidity and mortality associated with bone marrow transplant.
- In the absence of a matched sibling donor, donor options include:
  - A matched (MUD) or mismatched unrelated donor (mMUD)
  - An umbilical cord blood (UCB) product
  - A haploidentical donor from the family
- Each of these transplant approaches is associated with complications and includes graft rejection, GVHD, and delayed immune reconstitution, each of which can result in unacceptable outcomes.
- HSCT should be considered only in the presence of predetermined disease criteria and minimal risks of transplant that outweigh the perceived benefits.
- The indications for HSCT must take in consideration:
  - The risk/benefit ratios for each of these indications
  - The donor availability
  - The patient age
  - The severity of the disease
- Increasing age of the patient at the time of transplant as well as suboptimal HLA matching increases the risks of organ toxicity, GVHD, morbidity, and transplant-related mortality exponentially. This is attributable to the already established organ dysfunction and comorbidities expected with increasing age.
- HSCT has the best outcome prior to already established irreversible organ damage. This calls for early recognition of these patients prior to the disease declaring its severity.
- The dilemma faced with SCA patients is the absence of a good marker that predicts disease severity prior to its development. Add to this the clinical variability from the time of onset and the eventual degree of morbidity. This poses a unique problem in defining which patients are eligible and ideal timing for HSCT.
- The disease-free survival following HSCT is currently more than 80 % and graft rejection rates are less than 10 %.
- More importantly, on long-term follow-ups (2 or more years after transplant), it was found that most patients:
  - Were relieved of pain
  - Had no further strokes or acute chest syndrome

  - Had stabilized pulmonary function
  - Had stable neurologic and cognitive evaluations
- It is important to:
  - Minimize transplant-related toxicities to be able to offer bone marrow transplant to larger numbers of patients
  - Utilize alternative donor sources in the absence of a sibling donor
  - Improve safety and efficacy of HSCT
  - Minimize areas of risk
- It was also found that patients with SCA are more prone to develop CNS toxicity early posttransplant.
- These are seen in 23–50 % and include:
  - Seizures
  - Cognitive impairment
  - Intracranial hemorrhage
- These are seen especially in those with previous pretransplant CNS involvement such as stroke.
- Other posttransplant effects include:
  - Growth failure
  - Sterility
  - Ovarian failure
  - Poor spermatogenesis
  - Poor performance
  - Organ dysfunction
  - Second cancers
- The following criteria were suggested as guidelines for selecting sickle cell anemia patients for bone marrow transplantation:
  - They must be children or very young adults.
  - They already experienced at least one stroke or recurrent episodes of acute chest syndrome or painful crises.
  - None of them had yet developed end-stage organ failure.
  - They have a matched sibling.
- Patients who have not undergone long-term transfusion therapy and who do not have severe complications related to sickle cell anemia are optimal candidates for bone marrow stem cell transplantation.
- Graft rejection after transplantation of hematopoietic stem cells occurs in patients with hemoglobinopathy more frequently than in patients with other hematologic disorders, such as:
  - Aplastic anemia
  - Severe combined immune deficiency
  - Malignant conditions
- In these conditions, the rate of rejection after the transplantation of bone marrow from HLA-identical siblings is less than 3 %.
- The cause of this difference is not known, but transfusion-induced sensitization in these patients could be a contributing factor.

- Patients candidate for bone marrow transplantation:
  - Patients <16 years of age with sickle cell anemia
  - The patient suffered one or more of the following complications:
    - Stroke or CNS event lasting longer than 24 h
    - Recurrent acute chest syndrome
    - Recurrent vaso-occlusive crisis
    - Impaired neuropsychologic function and abnormal cerebral MRI scan
    - Stage I–II sickle lung disease
    - Sickle nephropathy (GFR 30–50 % of predicted normal values)
    - Osteonecrosis of multiple joints
- Patients not candidate for bone marrow transplantation:
  - Patients >16 years of age (currently, this is not a strict criteria)
  - HLA-non-identical donor
  - One or more of the following conditions:
    - Lansky performance score <70 %
    - Acute hepatitis or biopsy evidence of liver cirrhosis
    - Renal impairment (GFR <30 % of predicted normal values)
    - Stage III–IV sickle lung disease
- The results of bone marrow transplantation are best when performed in children with a sibling donor who is HLA identical.
- While there appears to be a considerable benefit to those who survive with stable engraftment of donor cells, there are also significant health risks to those who undergo bone marrow transplant.
- A careful discussion with families by healthcare professionals experienced in the care of patients with sickle cell anemia and with bone marrow transplantation should be conducted to ensure that they understand the risks and benefits and sign an informed consent for this procedure.
- Presently, bone marrow transplantation is reserved for patients who have experienced significant complications of sickle cell anemia, such as:
  - Stroke
  - Recurrent episodes of acute chest syndrome
  - Intractable vaso-occlusive crisis
- Currently, children with sickle cell anemia who experience significant, noninfectious complications caused by vaso-occlusion should be considered for bone marrow transplantation.
- Families should also receive counseling about the collection of umbilical cord blood from future pregnancies. This is in case a suitable bone marrow match is not available.
- For severely affected children who have HLA-identical sibling donors, families should be informed of the risks, benefits, and alternatives to interventions such as bone marrow transplantation. These selected patients should be offered the option of bone marrow transplantation.

Indications for Hematopoietic Stem Cell Transplantation

Matched sibling donor	Matched unrelated donor or minimally mismatched good-quality cord product	Mismatched marrow donor, haploidentical donor
Stroke	Stroke	Recurrent stroke despite adequate chronic transfusion
Elevated transcranial Doppler velocity	Elevated transcranial Doppler velocity	Inability to tolerate supportive care, e.g., alloimmunization, severe veno-occlusive episode, and inability to tolerate hydroxyurea
Acute chest syndrome	Recurrent acute chest syndrome despite supportive care	
Veno-occlusive episode	Recurrent severe veno-occlusive episode despite supportive care	
Pulmonary hypertension/tricuspid regurgitation jet velocity >2.5 m/s	Alloimmunization plus established indication for chronic transfusion therapy	
Osteonecrosis/avascular necrosis	Pulmonary hypertension	
Alloimmunization		
Silent stroke with cognitive impairment		
Recurrent priapism		
Sickle nephropathy		

22.4 Outcome of Bone Marrow Transplantation

- The experience and success of hematopoietic cell transplantation for patients with beta-thalassemia major have been successfully extended to sickle cell anemia.
- Hematopoietic cell transplantation is a treatment with curative potential for sickle cell anemia.
- The goal of this treatment is to eliminate the sickle erythrocyte and its cellular progenitors and replace them with donor hematopoietic pluripotent stem cells that produce erythrocytes expressing at best no sickle hemoglobin or at worse quantities similar to the sickle trait condition.
- The risk of severe adverse events after transplantation is weighed against the possibility of preventing serious complications from sickle cell anemia. These complications can produce extensive morbidity and, in some cases, early death.

- Children were felt to be better candidates for bone marrow transplantation than adult patients because of their lower risk of transplant-related complications such as graft-versus-host disease (GVHD) and because of a presumed lower burden of sickle-related organ damage.
- Currently, more than 90 % of patients survive following bone marrow transplant.
- Approximately 85 % survive free from sickle cell anemia.
- Sickle cell anemia reoccurs in approximately 10 % of patients after transplantation.
- Neurologic complications such as seizures occurred frequently after transplantation, requiring development of preventative measures.
- Among patients who had stable engraftment of donor cells, no subsequent sickle cell-related clinical events occurred and their pre-existing sickle cell-related organ damage stabilized.
- Splenic function also recovered.
- Some patients developed mixed donor-host hematopoietic chimerism after transplantation that was stable. Interestingly, these patients also had no symptoms from sickle cell anemia.
- Primary and secondary amenorrhea were common among females after transplantation, and most patients likely will be infertile.
- The risk of secondary cancers after bone marrow transplantation remains uncertain, but it is estimated to be less than 5 %.
- Linear growth was normal or accelerated after transplantation in most patients.

22.5 Transplantation from Alternative Sources of Stem Cells

- Umbilical cord blood (UCB) and hematopoietic cells from volunteer donors are alternative sources of hematopoietic stem cells that could increase the number of donors for sickle cell anemia patients.
- UCB transplantation for sickle cell anemia has been successful. It possibly produces less graft-versus-host disease than does standard bone marrow transplantation.
- UCB transplantation, however, is known to be associated with slower hematopoietic engraftment and perhaps a higher rate of graft rejection.
- The relatively low number of hematopoietic stem cells recovered from UCB effectively limits the procedure to children.
- Non-myeloablative preparation before hematopoietic cell transplantation could clinically correct sickle cell anemia with lower risk of severe complications. The aim of this is to establish stable donor-host hematopoietic chimerism after transplantation, which might provide a significant clinical benefit to patients. If successful, this approach might improve the safety profile of hematopoietic cell transplantation for older patients with advanced organ damage from sickle cell anemia.

Further Reading

Abboud M, Jackson S, Barredo J, Beatty J, Laver J. Bone marrow transplantation for sickle cell anemia. Am J Pediatr Hematol Oncol. 1994;16:86–9.

Abboud MR, Jackson SM, Barredo J, Holden KR, Cure J, Laver J. Neurologic complications following bone marrow transplantation for sickle cell disease. Bone Marrow Transplant. 1996;17:405–7.

Bernaudin F, Souillet G, Vannier JP, et al. Bone marrow transplantation (BMT) in 14 children with severe sickle cell disease (SCD): the French experience. GEGMO. Bone Marrow Transplant. 1993;12 Suppl 1:118.

Brichard B, Vermylen C, Ninane J, Cornu G. Persistence of fetal hemoglobin production after successful transplantation of cord blood stem cells in a patient with sickle cell anemia. J Pediatr. 1996;128:241–3.

Davies SC. Bone marrow transplantation for sickle cell disease. Arch Dis Child. 1993;69:176–7.

Ferster A, Bujan W, Corazza F, et al. Bone marrow transplantation corrects the splenic reticuloendothelial dysfunction in sickle cell anemia. Blood. 1993;81:1102–5.

Ferster A, Christophe C, Dan B, Devalck C, Sariban E. Neurologic complications after bone marrow transplantation for sickle cell anemia. Blood. 1995;86:408–9.

Gluckman E, Rocha V, Boyer-Chammard A, et al. Outcome of cord-blood transplantation from related and unrelated donors. Eurocord Transplant Group and the European Blood and Marrow Transplantation Group. N Engl J Med. 1997;337:373–81.

Johnson FL, Look AT, Gockerman J, et al. Bone-marrow transplantation in a patient with sickle-cell anemia. N Engl J Med. 1984;311:780.

Lubin BH, Eraklis M, Apicelli G. Umbilical cord blood banking. Adv Pediatr. 1999;46:383–408.

Lucarelli G, Polchi P, Izzi T, et al. Allogeneic marrow transplantation for thalassemia. Exp Hematol. 1984;12:676–81.

Lucarelli G, Polchi P, Galimberti M, et al. Marrow transplantation for thalassaemia following busulphan and cyclophosphamide. Lancet. 1985;1:1355–7.

Lucarelli G, Galimberti M, Polchi P, et al. Marrow transplantation in patients with advanced thalassemia. N Engl J Med. 1987;316:1050–5.

Mentzer W, Heller S, Pearle P, Hackney E, Vichinsky E. Availability of related donors for bone marrow transplantation in sickle cell anemia. Am J Pediatr Hematol Oncol. 1994;16:27–9.

Milpied NHJ, Garand R, David A. Bone-marrow transplantation for sickle-cell anaemia. Lancet. 1988;ii:328–9.

Nagel RL. The dilemma of marrow transplantation in sickle cell anemia. Semin Hematol. 1991; 28:233–4.

Rocha V, Chastang C, Souillet G, et al. Related cord blood transplants: the Eurocord experience from 78 transplants. Eurocord Transplant group. Bone Marrow Transplant. 1998;21 Suppl 3:S59–62.

Sullivan K, Walters MC, Patience M, Leisenring W, Buchanan GR, et al. Collaborative study of marrow transplantation for sickle cell disease: aspects specific for transplantation of hemoglobin disorders. Bone Marrow Transplant. 1997;19 Suppl 2:102–5.

Thomas ED. The pros and cons of bone marrow transplantation for sickle cell anemia. Semin Hematol. 1991;28:260–2.

Thomas ED, Buckner CD, Sanders JE, et al. Marrow transplantation for thalassaemia. Lancet. 1982;2:227.

Vermylen C, Cornu G. Bone marrow transplantation for sickle cell disease. The European experience. Am J Pediatr Hematol Oncol. 1994;16:18–21.

Vermylen C, Cornu G, Philippe M, et al. Bone marrow transplantation in sickle cell anaemia. Arch Dis Child. 1991;66:1195–8.

Vermylen C, Cornu G, Ferster A, et al. Haematopoietic stem cell transplantation for sickle cell anaemia: the first 50 patients transplanted in Belgium. Bone Marrow Transplant. 1998;22: 1–6.

Walters MC, Sullivan KM, Bernaudin F, et al. Neurologic complications after allogeneic marrow transplantation for sickle cell anemia. Blood. 1995;85:879–84.

Walters MC, Patience M, Leisenring W, Eckman JR, Scott JP, Mentzer WC, Davies SC, Ohene-Frempong K, Bernaudin F, Matthews DC, Storb R, Sullivan KM. Bone marrow transplantation for sickle cell disease. N Engl J Med. 1996;335:369–76.

Walters MC, Storb R, Patience M, et al. Impact of bone marrow transplantation for symptomatic sickle cell disease: an interim report. Blood. 2000;95:1918–24.

MIX
Papier aus verantwortungsvollen Quellen
Paper from responsible sources
FSC® C105338

If you have any concerns about our products, you can contact us on
ProductSafety@springernature.com

In case Publisher is established outside the EU, the EU authorized representative is:
Springer Nature Customer Service Center GmbH
Europaplatz 3, 69115 Heidelberg, Germany

Printed by Libri Plureos GmbH
in Hamburg, Germany